MODULES FOR

BASIC NURSING SKILLS

Fourth Edition

Volume I

MODULES FOR
Basic Nursing Skills

Fourth Edition

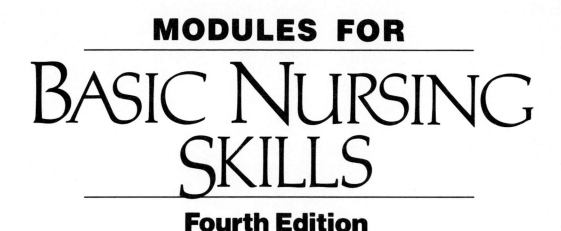

Janice Rider Ellis, R.N., M.N.
Elizabeth Ann Nowlis, R.N., M.N., Ed.D.
Patricia M. Bentz, R.N., M.S.N.

Shoreline Community College
Seattle, Washington

Volume I

Houghton Mifflin Company   Boston
Dallas   Geneva, Illinois   Palo Alto   Princeton, New Jersey

Illustrations by Brooke Dickson, Educational Media Center, Tufts New England Medical Center, and E. Penny Pounder, Medical Illustrator

ISBN: 0–395–35656–3
ABCDEFGHIJ-AP-9543210-8987

CONTENTS

Contents

LIST OF SKILLS

The following skills are included in this volume. For easy reference, a module number and a page number are provided for each skill.

Skill	Module	Page

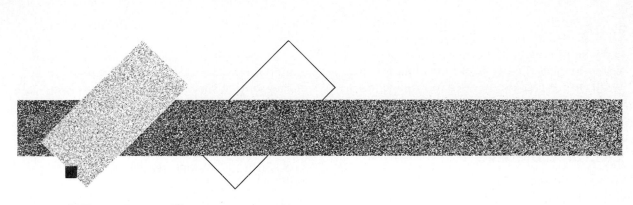

To the Instructor

Modules for Basic Nursing Skills, Fourth Edition, is a two-volume text designed to teach beginning nursing students how to perform basic skills and procedures. It can be used in the clinical practice laboratory of an introductory nursing course or in any other suitable setting.

COMPREHENSIVE SKILLS COVERAGE

There are now 57 modules in two volumes. Volume 1 contains the most basic skills and is appropriate by itself for some courses enrolling LPN/LVN students, as well as for courses for nursing aides and nursing assistants. Volumes 1 and 2 together are most useful in programs for RN students. Because programs vary considerably from state to state and from institution to institution, we have tried to make the two volumes as adaptable as possible to many different programs by offering comprehensive coverage of nursing skills.

ORGANIZATION

The modules are organized into units that reflect broad concepts of nursing care. This structured presentation will help the student understand how individual skills relate to particular human needs and to the nursing pro-

cess. The first unit focuses on skills that students must master in order to deal safely and effectively with patients. As in the previous edition, throughout the two volumes skills are arranged in a progression from simple to complex, but each module is self-contained so that skills can be omitted or reordered according to the needs of particular programs.

SELF-INSTRUCTIONAL FORMAT

By consistently emphasizing the nursing process and appropriately highlighting rationale, the format of the modules focuses on the student's practice and mastery of skills and procedures. The elaborate program of features is designed to encourage understanding, independent learning, and self-instruction.

Module Contents

An outline of the module contents helps the student identify the information and specific skills that are included in the module.

Prerequisites

The list of prerequisites lets the student know what other modules and significant material are essential to successful completion of the particular module. This information is especially helpful when the order of modules is adjusted to meet the needs of individual nursing programs. It can also be used advantageously by the student who wishes to prepare for a particular patient-care situation.

Overall Objective

A general statement of the overall objective concisely describes what the student can expect to learn in the module.

Specific Learning Objectives

Arranged in tabular form, the outline of learning objectives previews the important steps in the skill and indicates what basic knowledge and application of knowledge are required in addition to psychomotor skills.

Learning Activities

The learning activities provide additional guidance to the student about what steps to take in order to accomplish the desired objectives.

Vocabulary

A list of key terms for each skill is provided. These terms are defined in the Glossary at the back of each volume.

Module Core

The discussion of each procedure includes necessary background information and step-by-step instructions, with carefully chosen photographs and technically precise illustrations. Instructions are presented in a nursing process format when the skill is one that is used with patients and when the nursing process is appropriate to the skill. The steps in the process—Assessment, Planning, Implementation, Evaluation and Documentation—are clearly delineated by headings. This emphasis reinforces for students the fact that nursing process is relevant to practice. Rationale for the use of each skill is explained at the beginning of every module, and rationale for the specific actions that are part of the procedure are highlighted

throughout the discussion by the use of italic type.

Because the approach to many skills is the same, whenever possible a general procedure for a group of specific procedures has been identified. The purpose of this is to facilitate the student's ability to transfer basic principles from one situation to another. We have tried to do this in a way that does not create confusion and which can be followed when practicing the skill.

References

In the fourth edition, we have included a list of references at the end of the module core. These references include articles from other sources that are quoted in the module. The instructor may desire to read a specific article in its entirety, or may use the list collectively as a bibliography for those wishing to expand their knowledge of the subject being discussed.

Performance Checklist

The performance checklist follows the nursing process approach and can be used for quick review and for evaluation of the student's performance in terms of psychomotor skills. To facilitate review and evaluation, all steps of each procedure, including those which are first presented as part of a general procedure, are outlined in the performance checklist.

Quiz

A self-test is provided at the end of each module to allow students to test their mastery of the material in the module. The quizzes may also be used by instructors for evaluation purposes.

Glossary

The terms in the vocabulary lists are defined in the glossary at the back of each volume. The glossaries are a convenient reference source for students.

Answers to Quizzes

Answers to the quizzes are given at the end of each volume.

Index

An index is provided at the back of each volume.

CONVENIENT PACKAGING

The pages of both volumes are three-hole punched and perforated, so students can either tear them out and hand them in or keep them in notebooks.

TESTING SUPPLEMENT

A test bank accompanying Volumes 1 and 2 includes multiple-choice questions for all the skills that are covered.

Modules for Basic Nursing Skills, Volumes 1 and 2, Fourth Edition, can be used in conjunction with the text by Ellis and Nowlis, *Nursing: A Human Needs Approach*, Third Edition, which treats the theory behind nursing practice. However, the two volumes of modules are designed to stand alone and can be used by themselves in a course addressing nursing skills. *Modules for Basic Nursing Skills* can also be used in con-junction with any other text covering nursing theory or fundamentals.

We would like to thank the following individuals for their reviews of the manuscript at various stages and for their many useful suggestions:

Diane Craine, Macon Junior College
Barbara Engelhardt, Youngstown State University
Brenda McMillan, California State University at Fresno
Catherine Libert Peterson, San Diego City College
Carolyn Wyss, Walters State Community College

We are especially grateful to our students and colleagues who used the modules as they were originally written, worked through the changes made for the first three editions, and assisted in the planning of this revision. Their constant feedback has been essential to us.

J.R.E.
E.A.N.
P.M.B.

To the Student

The modules in these two volumes are designed to enable you to learn the procedures that are basic to your role as a health care provider. Each module contains the following parts, unless they are not applicable to a particular skill:

Module Contents

The outline of the module contents provides you with an overview of all the information and specific skills contained in the module. Often a module contains several skills, and these will all be listed in the contents.

Prerequisites

The list of prerequisites describes the specific skills or abilities needed to master the new skill and indicates other modules that contain information necessary to an understanding of the skill.

Overall Objective

A general statement of the overall objective describes the basic skill that is taught in the module.

Specific Learning Objectives

A table of specific learning objectives breaks down the basic skill you are studying into specific subskills that you can test yourself on after completing the module.

Learning Activities

The learning activities are designed to help you progress safely and gradually into performing the new skill. Practice, in whatever setting is available, is essential to skillful performance. The amount of practice needed by each student will differ, depending on manual dexterity and previous experience. If your school provides audiovisual aids to use with the module, view them after reading the module but before actually practicing the skill. Do not hesitate to contact your instructor if you encounter difficulties.

Vocabulary

The vocabulary list gives special terms used in the module. A glossary at the back of each volume gives the definitions of these terms, though some are best understood in the context of the module itself.

Module Core

A statement of rationale for the use of the module skill appears in italic type at the beginning of the module core. Rationale for specific actions is incorporated throughout the description of the procedure and is emphasized by the use of italic type. Background information and a step-by-step guide to performing the skill, including photographs and illustrations where necessary, are contained in this section. Note that a nursing process approach is used when it is appropriate for the skill being presented. The steps in the process—Assessment, Planning, Implementation, Evaluation, and Documentation—are keyed into the discussion to make you aware of the importance of the nursing process in the performance of skills. Because the approach to many skills is the same, whenever possible a general procedure for a group of specific procedures has been identified. The purpose of this is to facilitate your ability to transfer basic principles from one skill to another. We have tried to do this in a way that does not create confusion and which can be followed when practicing the skill.

References

A list of references is provided at the end of each module core for those who wish to obtain more material on a particular subject.

Performance Checklist

The performance checklist is used as a guide for practicing the skill and judging your performance of it.

Quiz

The quiz is a brief review for self-testing.

Glossary

The glossary at the back of each volume provides definitions for the key vocabulary terms.

Answers to Quizzes

The answer key at the end of each volume allows you to score yourself on the quizzes.

Index

An index is provided at the back of each volume.

We hope you will find gaining these essential skills to be a satisfying endeavor, and we wish you our best as you begin your studies.

J.R.E.
E.A.N.
P.M.B.

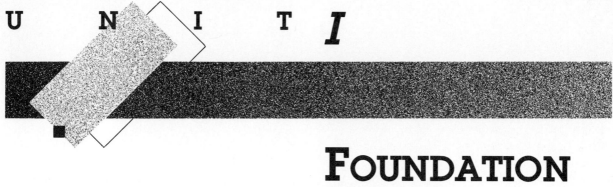

U N I T *I*

FOUNDATION SKILLS

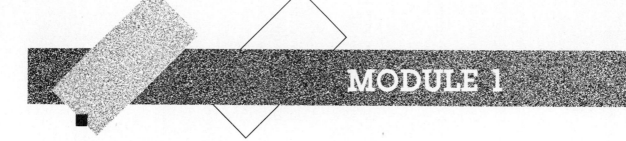

MODULE 1

An Approach to Nursing Skills

MODULE CONTENTS

OVERALL OBJECTIVE

To understand how patients' rights and the nursing process relate to performing nursing skills with technical proficiency and safety.

SPECIFIC LEARNING OBJECTIVES

	Know Facts and Principles	Apply Facts and Principles	Demonstrate Ability	Evaluate Performance
1. *Patient rights*	List patient rights in eight major areas that are of special concern to nurses	Give an example of a nursing behavior that supports each right listed	Consistently strive, in contacts with patients, to maintain patient rights	Evaluate with instructor
2. *Nursing process*	List the major steps of the nursing process Define each step of the nursing process	Give an example of a nursing behavior that demonstrates each step of the nursing process	Write an outline of the nursing process you used in relation to a simple patient problem	Evaluate your process with your instructor
3. *Technical proficiency*	List four components of technical proficiency Identify which component is most critical	Give an example of behavior you can use to enhance your ability in each component of technical proficiency Identify a way to increase your technical proficiency in each skill approached	Demonstrate increased technical proficiency in each skill practiced	Evaluate your technical proficiency with your instructor

LEARNING ACTIVITIES

1. Review the Specific Learning Objectives.
2. Look up the module vocabulary terms in the Glossary.
3. Read the material on patient rights, the nursing process, and direct care skills in Ellis and Nowlis, *Nursing: A Human Needs Approach*, or comparable material in another text.
4. Read through the module.
5. Check the policy manual of the facility where you will practice for information on:
   Confidentiality/privacy
   Patient rights
   Consent
   Patient complaints
6. Arrange to go to a nursing unit as an observer. Make observations in the following three categories:
   a. Patient rights
      (1) Identify and record staff actions that support any of the patient rights listed in the module.
      (2) Identify and record any behaviors that appear to interfere with patients' rights.
   b. Nursing process
      (1) Record examples of nurses performing each step of the nursing process.
   c. Technical proficiency
      (1) Arrange to observe a simple procedure (such as bedmaking) done by two different staff members. Be sure that you have their consent for observing.
      (2) Time each person doing the task.
      (3) Identify the factors that contributed to finishing rapidly and those that interfered with finishing rapidly.
      (4) Compare the dexterity of the two staff persons.
      (5) Compare the organization of the two staff persons.
7. In a discussion group with other students, discuss your observations.

VOCABULARY

advocate
assessment
confidentiality
consent
data
dexterity
dignity
ethical
evaluation
health care system
health status
implementation
nursing diagnosis
nursing process
objective
ombudsman
organization
planning
privacy
sanction
self-care
self-determination
subjective
technical proficiency

AN APPROACH TO NURSING SKILLS

Rationale for the Use of This Information

*T*he patient in the health care system has both ethical and legal rights. Failure to recognize those rights in care can result in ethical sanctions and even in legal action against the care provider and the institution. The nursing student, therefore, must approach every patient with these rights in mind. Nursing is more than just performing skills. The nursing process provides a framework for the total role of the nurse and must be the underlying framework in all activities. A concern for patient rights and the nursing process must always be part of your approach to any nursing skill. Technical proficiency is important, but it must be situated within the broad context of the nursing role.

Although each nursing skill is presented separately for learning purposes, no single nursing skill exists in a vacuum, as an entity by itself. Nursing skills will be most valuable when the rights of the patient as an individual, the importance of the nursing process, and the value of technical proficiency are kept in view.

You will note that rationale for action is emphasized throughout the module by the use of italics.

Patient Rights

Patient rights include both rights that are supported by law and would be upheld in court and ethical rights that the health care community recognizes as important to the patient's well-being. Various groups, such as the American Hospital Association, individual health care agencies, and state nurses' associations, have adopted lists of what they see as patient rights. These lists differ slightly, since each focuses on the health care services provided by a particular agency or group. Here we will present some general concepts that are usually included in any discussion of patient rights and focus on how you can support these in your nursing practice.

Rights Supported by Law

These rights either are specifically stated in the laws of a particular state or jurisdiction or have consistently been supported in court.

Right to Self-Determination/Consent   The patient has a right to make personal decisions regarding health care. This is often called the right to consent. *All adults over the age of eighteen—twenty-one in some states—have the right to make their own decisions about health care. Only those who have been declared incompetent by a court and who therefore have a court-appointed guardian and those who are unconscious do not have this personal right.* Old age alone is never a valid reason for ignoring the right to self-determination. *For children, parents exercise these rights.* After the age of seven or eight, however, *children are often included in the decision-making process. This enhances their ability to participate in care, even though final authority rests with the parents.*

Some minors do have the right to self-determination. Examples include those who are considered to be emancipated because they are married and those who are living independently of parents as prescribed by law. In most states, minors can give consent for care related to reproduction, such as birth control, abortion, and treatment for sexually transmitted disease. The facility where you practice should have specific policies that are based on applicable state law and court decisions to guide you in knowing who can legally give consent for care. One of your responsibilities is to review these policies.

Self-determination means that the patient has the right to accept or refuse any aspect of care—the right to decide whether to use the health care system at all, to use any part of the system, to ask for adaptations of the system, or to totally refuse the care available. It is the responsibility of the care provider to provide enough information to enable the patient to make the decision with an adequate understanding of all its consequences. For example, if you ask the patient to consent to having a procedure such as an enema done, it is your responsibility to make sure the patient understands the purpose of the enema as well as the possible consequences of not having it at this time. Then the patient's choice is truly informed.

Sometimes consent is implied by the previous actions or statements of the patient. When a patient consents to have surgery, there is implied consent to those procedures and routines that are necessary for successful preparation for and recovery from the surgery. *Although the patient is free at any time to change his or her mind with regard to the original procedure or to refuse any aspect of care,*

care proceeds on the basis of the implied consent. Another factor to be considered in such a situation is the patient's current health status. *The individual who has just had surgery and is weakened and in pain is not in a position to make the best decisions about care.* Thus, immediately after surgery, you do not ask a patient if he or she is willing to turn. You say, "It is time to turn now." When you believe that pain medication is needed, you say, "It is time for your pain medication. This will help you to rest more comfortably and move as you need to." The patient does have the right to refuse the pain medication, but this seldom happens; he or she is interested in recovery and willing to accept the judgment of the care provider as to the best action.

Consent is also implied by the actions the patient performs in response to your statements. If you say, "It is time for your injection," and the patient rolls over to receive the injection, this is considered implied consent. If you hand the patient an oral medication and he or she reaches for it, implied consent is present.

Decision making is shared between the care provider and the patient in some situations. Nurses instruct new diabetics in how to give an insulin injection. At some point, the patient will need to perform the procedure independently. Together, nurse and patient will consider the progress the patient has made in learning, and together they will agree on when the patient is ready to take on this responsibility. The nurse must agree that the patient has the necessary knowledge and skill, and the patient must agree that he or she is ready to undertake the task. There are many situations in nursing in which joint decision making is the most appropriate course of action.

Nurses and other care providers do make all the decisions for some patients in some situations. The elderly person who is disoriented as to time and place is sometimes not able to make decisions about safety and care. In such cases the nurse will decide that, for example, raised side rails or restraints are necessary to prevent falls. For the newborn infant, nurses must decide on the amount of covering needed to maintain proper body temperature, position for safety, and other details of the infant's daily routine. If the patient is unconscious, all aspects of his or her daily life must be controlled by those responsible for care. Decisions such as the amount of a feeding and the length of time to lie in one position, as well as more technical aspects of care, must all be made by care givers.

Correctly assessing the patient's ability to make decisions is a very important responsibility for the nurse. Consult with your instructor and with more experienced staff nurses to make sure that you are providing maximum self-determination consistent with the patient's health status.

Right to Information upon Which to Base Decisions *The patient has a right to information upon which to base decisions.* This means that the nurse has an obligation to provide information related to the care that he or she is personally giving. When you take blood pressure, you have an obligation to tell the patient what the reading is, if he or she asks. You do not, however, speak for others. Thus, when the patient asks what the medical diagnosis is, explain that this question should be directed to the physician who has made the diagnosis. It is then the physician's responsibility to discuss the diagnosis with the patient.

There is often a reluctance to give information to patients for fear that it will upset them and increase their anxiety. This fear is usually groundless. *Not knowing what is happening usually produces much more anxiety than knowing the truth. Fear of the unknown can be paralyzing to the patient. Some people prefer not to have information about their health status because it would make them anxious. These people will simply avoid asking for information with which they are not ready to cope.* Therefore, the patient should be your guide in deciding how much information to share.

There are some instances in which it is essential that a patient have information regarding his or her current health status. A patient who is on a special diet, for example, must have information in order to manage self-care. In these instances, the nurse does not wait for the patient to ask questions but initiates discussion and specifically plans for health teaching.

Right to Privacy/Confidentiality *The patient has a right to have information of a confidential nature carefully protected.* In today's complex society, it is all too easy for confidential information to spread to those who have no need for it. Keep in mind that *people can be harmed when information is spread unnecessarily.* The information might cause a change in someone's attitude toward the

7

patient, adversely affect the patient's employment opportunities, or result in financial loss, to name only a few possibilities. *Even when no objective harm is demonstrated, the individual may feel exposed and vulnerable.*

To maintain patient privacy, you should discuss information about a patient only with those who have a need for that information, such as nurses or the health care team. Discussions should take place only where you will not be overheard by others. An appropriate place might be a conference room, a patient room, or the nurses' station. Even these places, however, may be inappropriate. For example, a nurses' station with several visitors at the desk might be too public.

Written communication must also be safeguarded. Watch your notes carefully, and do not leave them in patient rooms or in the cafeteria. When you no longer need informal notes, they should be discarded in the waste basket, not left around on desks. Charts should be read only by those involved in care, those who have the permission of the patient, and those involved in health care education. This means that you should not read a patient's chart or access a computer record if you do not have a valid need to know about that patient.

The use of patient information for learning experience is valid but requires you to take special care. Do not identify patients by name when you are using them as subjects for a paper. *This would be a breach of confidentiality.* When using a patient as an example in a class discussion, share only information that is pertinent to the topic. *Recognize that some information of a very personal or private nature should perhaps not be shared.*

When gathering information from a patient, explain that you will be sharing information you receive with the nurse assigned to the patient's care or with your instructor. Since you are a beginner, you should not accept the responsibility of receiving confidences that cannot be shared in this manner. Doing so might put you in a situation that would be difficult to handle. If the patient asks you to promise to tell no one what is said, explain that you cannot make that promise. State that to plan appropriate care, you need to be free to discuss concerns with your instructor or the staff nurse, and if the patient does not want the information shared in this way, then perhaps it should not be told to you. This does not indicate rejection of the patient but clearly outlines your responsibilities. *The patient is then free to choose what to share, and you are free to consult with others as necessary.*

Right to Safe Care *The patient has a right to expect that those who are providing care are knowledgeable and competent and will provide safe care.* This means that the patient will receive safe care no matter who is providing it. Therefore, as a student nurse you are held to the same standard of safety in care as a registered nurse. The patient cannot be expected to accept poor-quality care because you are learning. It is your responsibility to learn skills before you perform them, to know the safety precautions that must be taken, and to seek supervision. *These actions safeguard the patient and protect you from legal action.* To function safely at all times requires a constant attitude of self-evaluation and a willingness to accept help and strive toward excellence.

Rights Supported by Ethics

These rights are based on ethical beliefs as to what constitutes high-quality care. *They are concerned with supporting optimum health in the patient, not merely with ensuring the absence of harm.* In most cases, these rights would not be upheld by a court. If they were violated, recourse would come only from appeal within the health care system or from pressure from the community.

Right to Personal Dignity *The patient has a right to care that respects the dignity and worth of the person, unrestricted by considerations of nationality, race, creed, color, status, age, or sex.* Respecting the individual dignity of the person does not mean that everyone is treated in the same way. It does mean that people are treated as if each has intrinsic value at all times, regardless of nationality, race, creed, color, status, age, or sex. Although the attitude is an internal characteristic, you give it meaning through your behavior.

One behavior that reflects this attitude is calling the person by the name that he or she chooses to use. Therefore, the older person who prefers to be addressed as Mr. or Mrs. ——— is so addressed, and the person who asks to be called by a nickname is addressed in that way. *You can also show respect for the dignity of the patient by showing concern for his or her privacy and modesty by knocking on closed doors, pulling curtains, and providing appropriate garments and draping. You show respect for individual dignity when you help a person to have the best possible appearance through careful attention to hygiene and personal care. By doing so you reflect your view of the patient as a human being who is valuable to you and to others.*

The attitude you convey to patients by the manner in which you communicate with them is very important. *Listening to the thoughts and concerns of the patient conveys respect. An attentive, concerned listener says, by his or her attitude, "What you have to say is important." Explaining expectations and new situations so that the patient is more able to cope reflects your recognition that he or she is capable of coping when given the opportunity and the necessary information.*

Accepting the individual's feelings as real without judging them as right or wrong is still another way of exhibiting respect. Everyone has feelings. They are personal and arise from things within as well as from external circumstances. Even though you do not understand the feelings expressed, you can accept them.

Right to Individualized Care

The patient has a right to individualized care related to his or her unique needs and life style. Each of us is unique, with a different combination of physical attributes, thoughts, feelings, and beliefs. *Care that is precisely uniform will fit no one precisely. Adaptations in plans of care are made to provide for each patient's special needs and attributes.* You might adapt a method of bathing to respect a patient's attitude about modesty. You might alter visiting hours to help maintain an important family bond. You might request a special dietary consultation to plan diet modifications to fit the patient's cultural background. The patient has the right to expect this kind of individualized approach to planning care.

Right to Assistance Toward Independence

Being able to care for oneself is important in building one's self-esteem and is critical in being able to function as an independent person. The patient has a right to expect that care will have the goal of returning him or her to maximum independence. Nurses can support this right in a wide variety of ways. In a simple way, this means that you will allow the patient to perform self-care whenever possible. In bathing a patient, you might encourage the patient to wash his or her own face. When you are helping the patient to move in bed, take the extra time to give directions carefully *so that the patient can move independently without strain. In order to function independently at home, the person with a health problem may need consider-*

able knowledge and skill. The nurse is frequently the person who must plan and carry out the teaching program.

Right to Complain and Obtain Changes in Care

The patient has a right to complain when care has not been of high quality and to obtain changes that improve the quality of care. To do this, the patient needs some knowledge of what constitutes good care. *Providing health care consumers with this knowledge provides them with more power.* In the past, some health care providers have been reluctant to share this information with consumers for fear of being harshly evaluated. The reality is that health care consumers will always evaluate the providers, but if they have no objective standards, they will do so on the basis of physical attractiveness, pleasantness of demeanor, or other superficial criteria. Some hospitals now provide patients with a form that lists evaluation criteria and asks the patient to respond. In a less formal way, patients may be given information on admission as to what they can expect with regard to care. Some facilities provide patients with a list of their rights as patients so that they can knowledgeably exercise them. *Although legal recourse is always available when care has been so poor as to cause harm, this is a very complex process that is not suited to lesser issues that are nevertheless important to the patient.* Some facilities now have someone in the position of "patient advocate" or "ombudsman." It is this person's responsibility to discuss problems with the patient and then work with the health care system to bring about improved care for the patient. In many facilities, however, no one is officially designated to do this job, and the role of patient advocate falls to the nurse. It is logical for the nurse to fulfill this role, since nurses are the only care providers who are in contact with the patient 24 hours a day, 7 days a week. Nurses are also in a position to understand the institutional structure and to interface with that structure on behalf of the patient. This role is not an easy one. It demands a great deal of understanding of human behavior, understanding of the institution, and great skill in communication.

You can support this right by listening carefully to patients' concerns and complaints and then discussing them with your instructor or a knowledgeable nurse on the unit. There may be simple remedies that you can implement, or you may begin the process by which others will resolve the patient's concerns.

9

When you are criticized, do not become defensive, but carefully consider how this information might help you to provide better care not only to this patient but to others.

Research Base for Nursing Practice

Although nursing is moving toward a research base for its practice, this does not yet exist for many of the procedures and skills that we use. References to the research that is available to support certain methods or approaches to a skill are given in the modules. Remember that research is an ongoing process and that future research may further refine what we do or significantly alter how we proceed. For a great many nursing skills, there is little or no research base. In these instances, recommended practices are based on past practice and sound deductive reasoning from known facts. In the future, when these practices are the subjects of research, we may find that the research supports them, or we may learn that even though our reasoning seemed correct from a logical point of view, the actual research did not support it.

Because nursing is an applied science, we must care for patients in the present even though our knowledge is incomplete. Given this reality, it is the responsibility of all nurses to be aware of the reasoning or rationale underlying what they do, to evaluate this rationale, and to be willing to alter their practice when research brings more specific information.

The Nursing Process

The nursing process is a thoughtful, deliberate use of a problem-solving approach to nursing. This process will form the structure by which you function. You will need to consult a text on nursing theory for a complete understanding of the nursing process. Here we will simply define each step and then discuss how that step is used in the performance of technical skills.

Assessment

Assessment is the process of gathering information, analyzing information, and identifying problems. The basic purpose of some skills is to gather information. These skills are grouped together in

Unit III. For every skill that you utilize, however, you must gather appropriate information in order to implement the skill correctly and safely. In each module, directions for carrying out the skill begin by indicating the assessment data you must gather before you proceed.

In addition to carrying out the specific assessment listed, you should always be observant while performing the procedure. It is an excellent time to gain further information about the patient. You may extend your knowledge of existing problems or gain insight that will lead you to identify new ones.

Nursing Diagnosis

Nursing diagnosis may be considered either an entirely separate step in the nursing process or the second phase of assessment. *Nursing diagnosis includes the intellectual processes of sorting and classifying the data collected, recognizing patterns and discrepancies, comparing these with norms, and identifying patient responses to health problems that are amenable to nursing intervention.* The problem-solving process embodied in assessment, planning, implementation, and evaluation is always appropriate, but in the context of specific skills, nursing diagnosis may not be appropriate. The purpose of the assessment is to enable you to gather data, individualize the procedure to the patient, and assure safety. Although you may identify concerns, these may not fall into the classifications currently accepted by the North American Nursing Diagnosis Association (NANDA). Of course, during the process you may uncover data that contribute significantly to the development of nursing diagnoses for the patient. In many instances a skill is used to help resolve a patient problem or nursing diagnosis that has already been made.

Planning

Planning is the phase during which you identify specific desired outcomes for the individual patient and determine what actions will be needed to reach those outcomes. Planning will often include a group of nursing measures needed to combat a particular problem. Many of the actions planned will require specific technical skills. Within each skill there is also a planning phase. The general guidelines given for evaluation must be examined and translated into specific desired outcomes for this specific patient. Equipment must be identified and obtained. Timing must be determined. Careful planning is the main factor in organization.

Implementation

This is the phase of the nursing process during which the actions planned are actually carried out. The specific nursing skills you use are only part of the implementation for a given problem. Nursing implementation includes your attitude toward and communication with the patient as well as the task you carry out. Since implementation is the most visible part of nursing, there are those who make the mistake of thinking that it is the most important. It certainly is important, but it can never be more important than the careful data gathering and planning that went before.

For each technical skill presented, step-by-step instructions are given to guide you in your implementation of the skill. The implementation phase is the "hands on," "doing" segment of any procedure.

Evaluation

Evaluation is the process by which the outcomes of your nursing action are identified. The central aspect of evaluation is the evaluation of the patient. However, you will also want to evaluate your own nursing ability and whether you functioned well.

For each skill, specific factors that can help you to identify outcomes are listed. You will need to adapt those factors to the specifics of individual cases. For example, if one of the steps of evaluation states that you should recheck the patient's vital signs to determine response, it is essential to identify what the specific desired vital signs are for this particular patient.

Documentation

Documentation is establishing a written record of the assessment, the care provided, and the patient's responses. It is usually considered not as an independent step in the nursing process, but rather as an extension of each of the other steps. That is, you assess and then you record your assessment, you plan and then you record your plan, and so forth. For the beginner, it is often much

easier to consider all documentation at the same time. Therefore, we have grouped all information about documentation as a fifth section in each skill. You will find more complete information about documentation in Module 6.

Technical Proficiency

Technical proficiency has four components: the technique, the organization, the dexterity, and the speed with which you implement nursing skills.

Correct Technique

Correct technique is always the most important component of technical proficiency because it maintains safety and is most likely to achieve the appropriate outcome for the patient. In each module, the correct technique is outlined and discussed in detail in the implementation phase. Some elements of each procedure may be done differently depending upon the circumstances and the policy in your facility. These elements are carefully pointed out. In practicing a skill, the most important element is to make sure that you always practice the correct technique, regardless of how slow or awkward it may be at first.

Organization

Having an organized approach to technical skills has many advantages. First of all, *if you are well organized, you do not waste your time or the time of others.* Second, *being well organized makes you appear competent and enhances the patient's trust in your skill.* Third, *you are less likely to make errors in technique when you are well organized, and therefore you will give safe care.*

During the planning of any procedure, you will be organizing your work. One part of this is carefully identifying all the equipment you will need so that you can obtain it all at once. Nothing makes a person look more disorganized than repeated trips to get items that are needed and were forgotten. Trips of this kind also take time and energy that can be better spent in other ways. The equipment needed for each skill is listed in the planning phase of the directions.

Another part of organization is determining when in your schedule it would be most appropriate to carry out a task. For example, an irrigation that is likely to result in a wet bed should be done before the bed linen is changed so that you do not end up changing the bed twice. *The patient's schedule and needs must also be considered in deciding when to perform a procedure.* The patient may wish to have a bath after a procedure in order to feel fresher. In other instances, the patient should have the bath before the procedure so that after the procedure he or she can rest without interruptions. Since planning for the timing of any procedure is a highly individual matter, it is not included in the directions for each skill. You will need to keep it in mind, however, in the clinical setting.

Dexterity

Dexterity refers to your skill or adroitness in the use of your hands. When you are dexterous, your movements are deliberate, coordinated, and purposeful. You do not use awkard or inappropriate movements. Dexterity requires practice. *To increase your dexterity, you must work with the equipment enough to develop the neural pathways that coordinate your movements.* You develop your sense of touch to provide accurate feedback about the position of your hands and the equipment. Although some people are naturally more dexterous than others, everyone needs practice to develop dexterity with a new skill. Going slowly and thinking carefully about your movements at first will help you to develop dexterity.

Speed

The speed with which you carry out a nursing skill is important. *When you perform a procedure quickly, you help yourself in terms of overall time management, and, more importantly, you also help the patient.* If a procedure is uncomfortable and you perform it in five minutes instead of fifteen, the patient is only uncomfortable for five minutes. If a procedure creates anxiety, the anxiety is lessened if you are quick and dexterous. The value to yourself in terms of time management is a serious consideration. Nurses often find that the many demands on their time can lessen the quality of patient care. *When you perform an individual skill more quickly, you are more free to plan for all the needs of the patients.* Be very cautious, however, in your quest for speed. Never sacrifice correct technique or neglect patient rights. Developing your organizational ability and your dexterity are the first steps in gaining speed in performance. After you have mastered the correct technique, developed your organizational ability, and achieved some dexterity, you can work on speed alone.

12

QUIZ

Short-Answer Questions

1. List patients' rights in eight major areas that are of special concern to nurses.

    a. _____

    b. _____

    c. _____

    d. _____

    e. _____

    f. _____

    g. _____

    h. _____

2. Give an example of a behavior that demonstrates respect for the individual.

    _____

3. List the steps of the nursing process.

    a. _____

    b. _____

    c. _____

    d. _____

4. Define assessment _____

5. List four components of technical proficiency.

    a. _____

    b. _____

    c. _____

    d. _____

6. If research is not available, how is the decision made as to what nursing action is correct?

    _____

    _____

7. What is the purpose of evaluation in nursing practice?

    _____

    _____

MODULE 2

Medical Asepsis

PREREQUISITES

Successful completion of the following modules:

VOLUME 1

Module 1 / An Approach to Nursing Skills

OVERALL OBJECTIVE

To apply principles of medical asepsis when practicing all aspects of nursing, with particular emphasis on handwashing.

SPECIFIC LEARNING OBJECTIVES

	Know Facts and Principles	Apply Facts and Principles	Demonstrate Ability	Evaluate Performance
1. *Movement of microorganisms*	State five ways in which microorganisms move from one area to another	Given a situation, state methods to prevent microorganisms from moving from dirty to clean items or areas		
2. *Medical asepsis related to general nursing* *a. Handling linens* *b. Disposition of soiled articles*	State medical asepsis guidelines related to handling linens and disposition of soiled articles	State rationale for holding linen away from uniform, not shaking or tossing linen, and keeping clean items separate from dirty items	Hold linen away from uniform. Do not shake or toss linen. Keep clean items separate from dirty items.	Evaluate own performance with instructor using Performance Checklist
3. *Handwashing*	State when handwashing is indicated	State rationale for washing hands before and after each patient contact, before handling food, after using toilet, after blowing nose or sneezing, and after touching hair	Wash hands at appropriate times	Evaluate own performance with instructor using Performance Checklist
4. *Procedure* *a. Friction* *b. Running water* *c. Cleansing agents*	State effect of friction, running water, and cleansing agents on handwashing. Describe correct handwashing techniques.	State rationale for use of friction, running water, and cleansing agents during handwashing	Employ friction, running water, and cleansing agents when washing hands, using correct handwashing techniques	Evaluate own performance with instructor using Performance Checklist
5. *Personal hygiene* *a. Hair* *b. Fingernails* *c. Jewelry*	State personal hygiene guidelines related to hair, fingernails, and jewelry	Describe manner of fixing own hair that conforms to guidelines given	Wear hair short or restrained. Keep fingernails clean and trimmed. Do not wear jewelry in clinical facility.	Evaluate own performance with instructor using Performance Checklist

LEARNING ACTIVITIES

1. Review the Specific Learning Objectives.
2. Read the section on asepsis (in the chapter on infection) in Ellis and Nowlis, *Nursing: A Human Needs Approach,* or comparable material in another textbook.
3. Look up the module vocabulary terms in the Glossary.
4. Read through the module.
5. Arrange for time to practice handwashing techniques.
6. In the practice setting, practice safe handwashing techniques, using the procedure as a guide and the Performance Checklist as an evaluation tool. When you are satisfied with your ability, have your instructor evaluate you.
7. In the clinical setting, demonstrate handwashing to your clinical instructor.

VOCABULARY

bacteria
barrier
body substances
contaminate
droplet nuclei
friction
immunosuppression
interdigital
invasive
medical asepsis
microorganism
nosocomial
pathogenic organism
subungual

MEDICAL ASEPSIS

Rationale for the Use of This Skill

Medical asepsis may be defined as the practice of techniques and procedures designed to reduce the number of microorganisms in an area or on an object and to decrease the likelihood of their transfer. The practice of medical asepsis takes on added importance in the presence of individuals who have been made more susceptible to infection by illness, surgery, or immunosuppression.

Because the nurse may be in contact with a number of patients during any given day, it is especially important to be aware of the principles of medical asepsis in order to avoid transferring microorganisms from a patient to the nurse, from the nurse to a patient, from the nurse to a coworker, or from one patient to another. Microorganisms can also be transferred by way of equipment.[1]

Principles of Medical Asepsis

How Microorganisms Spread

Microorganisms move through space on air currents. Because of this movement, avoid shaking or tossing linens, motions that create air currents on which microorganisms can be transported. To reduce the spread of microorganisms, most hospitals are built in such a way that the ventilation system does not circulate air from one section to another. Be sure that all doors leading to isolation rooms are kept closed to stop air currents.

Microorganisms are transferred from one surface to another whenever objects touch. There are both clean and dirty items in a hospital. Even among ostensibly clean items, some are more clean than others. When a clean item touches a less clean item, it becomes "dirty," because microorganisms (which are not visible) are transferred to it. Therefore, keep your hands away from your own hair and face, keep linens away from your uniform, and always keep clean items separate from dirty ones. If you drop anything on the floor, consider it dirty.

Microorganisms are transferred by gravity when one item is held above another. Avoid passing dirty items over clean items or areas because it is possible for

microorganisms to drop off onto a clean item or area. When storing items in a bedside stand, place clean items on upper shelves and potentially dirty items, such as bedpans, on lower shelves.

Microorganisms are released into the air on droplet nuclei whenever a person breathes or speaks. Coughing or sneezing dramatically increases the number of microorganisms released from the mouth and nose. Avoid having a patient breathe directly into your face, and avoid breathing directly into a patient's face. Whenever you have coughed, sneezed, or blown your nose, wash your hands before you touch anything else. If you handle tissues that a patient has used when coughing or sneezing, always wash your hands thoroughly.

Microorganisms move slowly on dry surfaces but very quickly through moisture. For this reason, use a dry paper towel when you turn off faucets, and dry a bath basin before you return it to a bedside stand for storage.

Proper handwashing removes many of the microorganisms that would be transferred by the hands from one item to another. Wash your hands, therefore, not only when they are obviously soiled, but whenever you move from one patient to another, or from patient contact to contact with the general environment or vice versa.

Handwashing

The single most important procedure for preventing the transfer of microorganisms, and, therefore, nosocomial infection, is correct and frequent handwashing. Properly done, handwashing protects the patient, your coworkers, you, and your family.

For medical aseptic purposes, the CDC recommends at least a vigorous ten-second handwashing procedure that includes "a rubbing together of all surfaces of lathered hands followed by rinsing under a stream of water." Further, they comment that in situations in which hands are visibly soiled, "more time" may be required (Garner & Favero, 1985, p. 7).

Handwashing should be done at the beginning of every work shift, before and after prolonged direct contact with a patient, before invasive procedures, before contact with especially susceptible patients, and before and after touching wounds, as well as at the end of every shift before leaving the health care facility. In addition, it is recommended that clean gloves be worn whenever direct or indirect contact with an individual's body substances is anticipated. How-

---

[1]You will note that rationale for action is emphasized throughout the module by the use of italics.

ever, hands should be washed after contact with body substances even when gloves are worn. The CDC goes on to recommend that hands should also be washed any time you are in doubt about the necessity for doing so. While these recommendations may not be supported or practiced by everyone with whom you work, it is your responsibility to carry out proper technique based on your knowledge.

Friction, running water, and a cleansing agent are necessary to remove microorganisms or other material that may be present on the hands. The cleansing agent may be plain soap in all situations except those involving the care of newborns, between patients in high-risk units, and before the care of immunosuppressed patients. In these situations, antimicrobial products should be used. A deep sink with controls that can be operated by foot, leg, or elbow is ideal for handwashing. Where faucets are operated by hand, it is common practice to use a dry paper towel as a barrier when turning the water off *because a dirty hand was used to turn it on. Because the handwashing procedure causes microorganisms to accumulate in the sink,* it is important that you avoid touching the sink as you wash and also that you avoid splashing dirty water on your uniform.

Procedure for Handwashing

1. Roll your sleeves above your elbows and remove your watch. If your watch has an expansion band, you may simply move it up above your elbow *to allow you to wash well up your arms.* After the initial handwash of the shift, simply wash your hands and well above the wrists, unless you have been in a situation that you feel necessitates more thorough washing.
2. Turn on the water and adjust the temperature. *Warm water removes fewer oils from the skin than hot water, and removes microorganisms more effectively than cold water.*
3. Dispense liquid or powdered soap, preferably with a foot control. Bar soap is not recommended *because it may harbor microorganisms.* If only bar soap is available, lather and rinse the bar thoroughly *to remove the outside layer of soap before you use it.*
4. Lather your hands and arms well.
5. Clean your fingernails as needed with a nail file or orange stick. (If these utensils

are not provided, do this before you leave home.) *The subungual area has been shown to be especially important, as it is an area where bacteria multiply that is thought to be frequently missed in handwashing* (Larson, 1986). It is not necessary to clean your nails each time you wash your hands.

6. Wash your hands and arms up to your elbows, adding soap as needed *to maintain a lather. Microorganisms are suspended in the lather and later rinsed off.* Keep your hands lower than your elbows at all times.
   a. Rub briskly, using friction and a rotary motion (as opposed to a back-and-forth motion) *to contact all surfaces more effectively.*
   b. Pay particular attention to the areas between your fingers (the interdigital spaces), your knuckles, and the outside surfaces of the fifth or "little" fingers, *because these areas are often missed.*
7. Holding your hands and forearms lower than your elbows, rinse thoroughly, starting at one elbow and moving down the arm (see Figure 2.1). Then repeat this

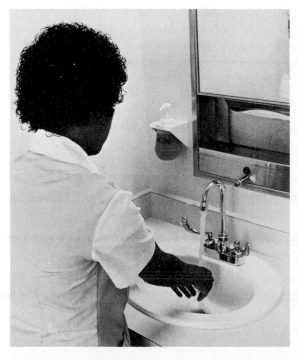

FIGURE 2.1 *HANDWASHING WITH HANDS LOWER THAN ELBOWS*
Courtesy Ivan Ellis

step for the other arm. *This position prevents microorganisms from being rinsed up your arms from your hands, which are frequently the most contaminated.*

8. Dry your hands thoroughly. Most facilities provide paper towels for this purpose. Blotting with a paper towel *is easier on the skin* than rubbing.

9. Use a dry paper towel to turn off the faucet if it is hand operated.

10. Use lotion if needed *to maintain your skin condition. Since frequent handwashing can lead to dry, cracked skin in some individuals,* lotion may be encouraged *to help keep skin intact, thus preventing possible invasion by microorganisms.* In some settings, however, you may be asked not to use lotion *because it can be an excellent medium for bacterial growth.*

Personal Hygiene

Obviously, *in order to enhance medical asepsis,* you must practice good personal hygiene. *Also, it is much more pleasant for patients to be near someone who smells fresh and who is wearing a clean uniform.* Use the following important guidelines for personal hygiene:

1. Arrange hair in such a way that it does not fall forward when you lean forward (as, for example, when you examine a patient). *When hair falls over an area, microorganisms can drop from the hair (by gravity) onto the patient, or the hair itself may fall onto trays or wounds.* Keep your hair short or restrain it in some way *so that it does not fall forward.*

Also avoid any style in which you are constantly brushing your hair out of your eyes. Your hair is usually less clean than your hands *because it is not washed as frequently.* In addition, if your hands have been contaminated by contact with a patient, *you will transfer microorganisms from them to your hair and near your face.*

2. Keep your fingernails clean and trimmed or filed short, *so as not to endanger patients by scratching them or by harboring bacteria.* If you use polish, it must be intact; *chipped polish is also a place for bacteria to lodge.*

3. *Jewelry, too, is a place for microorganisms to lodge;* therefore, wear only a minimum. Plain studs or posts for pierced ears and plain wedding bands are the most jewelry you should wear in a clinical setting. *Necklaces and large hoop or dangling earrings are a hazard not only in terms of medical asepsis: a patient can grab them and hurt both you and the jewelry. These guidelines often are not enforced by the employing agency;* therefore, your knowledge of the rationale for such guidelines and your conscience must guide your actions.

REFERENCES

Garner, Julia S., and Martin S. Favero. *Guideline for Handwashing and Hospital Environmental Control, 1985.* Atlanta: Centers for Disease Control, 1985.

Larson, Elaine, et al. "Physiologic, Microbiologic, and Seasonal Effects of Handwashing on the Skin of Health Care Personnel." *American Journal of Infection Control,* 14, No. 51 (April 1986), 51–59.

PERFORMANCE CHECKLIST

Medical asepsis related to general nursing

	Unsatisfactory	Needs More Practice	Satisfactory	Comments
1. Hold linen away from uniform.				
2. Do not shake or toss linen.				
3. Keep clean items separate from dirty ones.				

Handwashing

	Unsatisfactory	Needs More Practice	Satisfactory	Comments
1. Roll sleeves above elbows and remove watch.				
2. Do not touch outside or inside of sink.				
3. Turn on water and adjust temperature.				
4. Lather hands and arms well, using rotary motion.				
5. Clean fingernails.				
6. Hold hands and forearms lower than elbows. Wash with running water, using rotary motion and giving special attention to areas between fingers. Leave water running during entire procedure.				
7. Wash hands and arms to elbows.				
8. Rinse thoroughly, keeping hands lower than elbows.				
9. Dry hands thoroughly.				
10. Turn off water with paper towel if faucet is hand operated.				

Personal hygiene

	Unsatisfactory	Needs More Practice	Satisfactory	Comments
1. Keep hair restrained.				
2. Keep fingernails clean and short.				
3. Do not wear jewelry, or wear only a minimum.				

QUIZ

Multiple-Choice Questions

_____ 1. In which of the following situations should the nurse wash his or her hands?

   a. At the beginning of the shift
   b. Before going to lunch
   c. After removing gloves used while handling body substances
   d. All of these

_____ 2. Which of the following are essential components of the handwashing procedure? (1) friction; (2) running water; (3) foot-operated water controls; (4) cleansing agent

   a. 1 only
   b. 1 and 4
   c. 2, 3, and 4
   d. 1, 2, and 4

_____ 3. Which of the following areas should the nurse *not* touch during the handwashing procedure? (1) the inside of the sink; (2) the outside of the sink; (3) a hand-controlled faucet; (4) his or her own hair

   a. 1 only
   b. 2 only
   c. 1, 2, and 3
   d. All of these

_____ 4. Which of the following should receive attention during the handwashing procedure? (1) palms; (2) elbows; (3) spaces between the fingers; (4) fingernails

   a. 1 and 4
   b. 1, 3, and 4
   c. 2, 3, and 4
   d. All of these

Short-Answer Questions

5. State the rationale for the following actions.

   a. Avoid shaking or tossing linens. _____

   _____

b. Keep your hands away from your hair and face. _____

_____

c. Avoid passing dirty items over clean items or areas. _____

_____

d. Use a dry paper towel when you turn off faucets. _____

_____

MODULE 3

Safety

PREREQUISITES[1]

Successful completion of the following modules:

VOLUME 1

Module 1 / An Approach to Nursing Skills
Module 2 / Medical Asepsis
Module 21 / Applying Restraints

[1]The need for safety is implicit in the skills outlined in all the modules. Keep safety in mind at every step.

OVERALL OBJECTIVE

To provide a safe environment for patients, staff, and visitors within the hospital community by constantly being vigilant for unsafe conditions that may be a threat to the safety of others.

SPECIFIC LEARNING OBJECTIVES

	Know Facts and Principles	Apply Facts and Principles	Demonstrate Ability	Evaluate Performance
1. *Safe behavior*	State seven behaviors that are important to safety	State rationale for each behavior and explain the consequences if safety measures are not carried out	In the clinical setting, document own behavior and that of others	Discuss documentation with instructor
2. *Safety in working spaces, halls, and corridors*	List five physical aspects of safety in working spaces, halls, and corridors	State rationale for each aspect	In the clinical setting, document safety by describing: a. a working space b. a hallway c. a corridor	Discuss documentation with instructor
3. *Safety in the patient's room*	Name seven safety precautions specific to patients' rooms	State rationale behind each precaution as it relates to the patient	In the clinical setting, identify and document safe and unsafe conditions in a patient's room	Discuss documentation with instructor

4. Protecting the dependent patient	Discuss additional safety precautions to protect dependent patients	Identify reason for each precaution or action	If the opportunity to care for a dependent patient is available, add any appropriate safety measures to the care plan	Evaluate with instructor
5. Smoking policy in the health care facility	State policies that health care facilities use to contain or monitor smoking behavior	Give rationale underlying policies regarding smoking behavior	In the clinical setting, observe which policies regarding smoking are in effect	Identify whether changes in policies regarding smoking in your facility are needed. Share with instructor.
6. Fire plans	List the eleven steps of most fire plans	Read the plan currently in use in your facility, and compare steps with module list	In the clinical setting, identify specific fire procedures for assigned unit	Evaluate with instructor using Performance Checklist
7. Disaster plans	Briefly discuss disaster plans, both internal and external	Explain how each type of disaster plan applies to the staff nurse	In the clinical setting, identify specific disaster plan for your department	Evaluate with instructor
8. Incident reports	Give the three main purposes of incident reports	State rationale regarding legal importance of reporting	In the clinical setting, fill out an incident report, using the facility's form and a hypothetical situation	Discuss the completed report with the instructor

LEARNING ACTIVITIES	VOCABULARY

LEARNING ACTIVITIES

1. Review the Specific Learning Objectives.
2. Read the sections on safety in Ellis and Nowlis, *Nursing: A Human Needs Approach,* or comparable material in another textbook.
3. Read through the module.
4. In the practice setting, form groups of three to five students. Taking turns, discuss what steps in the following modules could lead to unsafe conditions for the patient, visitors, or staff. You may refer to the modules.
   7 / Bedmaking
   8 / Moving the Patient in Bed and Positioning
   9 / Feeding Adult Patients
   11 / Hygiene
   21 / Applying Restraints
   22 / Transfer
   27 / Applying Heat and Cold
5. In the clinical setting:
   a. Read the sections of the policy or procedure manual dealing with general safety.
   b. Read the fire plan.
   c. Examine the incident report forms used by the facility.
   d. Find out whether your facility has a printed disaster plan, internal or external; if so, read it.
   e. Visit a patient in a room. Observe potential safety hazards. After the visit, list these on a piece of paper and share with your instructor.
   f. Note on paper any risks to safety you see in the hallways, work spaces, or nursing station. Share these observations with your instructor.

VOCABULARY

acute care
AIDS
antineoplastic
caustic
critical care
external disaster
fetal
internal disaster
isotope
pavilion
scalpel
triage
vesicant

28

SAFETY

Rationale for the Use of This Information

Because of its complexity, the hospital setting is a potentially dangerous one. The physical plant itself is usually spacious in design, with heavily traveled hallways, steps, and elevators. For reasons of economy, most hospitals are constructed on a high-rise or pavilion plan. Monitoring areas for unsafe conditions and needed maintenance constantly poses problems and requires the vigilance and assistance of staff.

Patient rooms, on the other hand, usually are not spacious but confining—even more so if special equipment is needed for care. The space provided for nurses' stations has also been encroached upon by the records and monitoring equipment that have been added as nursing and medical practice have grown more sophisticated.

The variety of equipment used within the hospital adds to the difficulty of maintaining safety. Equipment as diverse as a simple thermometer and a complicated ventilator is included in the repertory of practicing nurses today. The nurse must be skillful both in operating equipment and in detecting and correcting any problems that arise.

The unfamiliarity of hospital surroundings to most who are cared for or visit adds to the potential for accident or injury. The nursing staff must not only protect itself but also act as a guardian or stabilizing group for others.

More serious dangers are fire and natural disasters. These are a constant worry and threat in any facility containing a large number of people, especially when many of these people are ill or dependent. An important goal for every practicing nurse is to be knowledgeable and prepared in all aspects of safety.[2]

Safety In Institutions

The patient has a right to a safe environment during hospitalization. Whether you are in a patient's room, traveling the hallways, working in utility rooms, or at the nurses' station, similar safety precautions apply. These precautions include safe behavior at all times, constant vigilance for unsafe conditions, and the protection of dependent patients. When a breach in safety occurs and an incident results, it is also important to know how to report such a happening *to protect the patient, the staff, and the hospital.*

Safe Behavior

Many of the habits of safe behavior may seem to be nothing more than common sense, but they are of great importance to safety.

Use Good Body Mechanics Although you will learn good body mechanics in connection with moving patients, using proper body mechanics in daily practice is just as important. As you carry out your duties, which require much standing and walking, an erect posture in good body alignment *protects you from strain.* Stretching and reaching, as well as carrying or moving heavy objects, can take their toll on poorly aligned muscles. Using good body mechanics and reminding others of their importance is a basic part of safe behavior.

Walk; Avoid Running It is sometimes imperative that you run—in a patient emergency, for example. Even at these times, however, remember that *running is risky and leads to falls.* Often the same task can be accomplished just as rapidly by brisk walking, which is much safer. *For safe movement,* well-fitting shoes are essential. Clogs and other ill-fitting shoes can prove hazardous, particularly if running becomes necessary, *because they may slip off and trip the wearer.*

Keep to the Right in Hallways *It is easy to run into someone else* whose attention is diverted. Therefore, as a general practice, always walk to the right. This provides for a smoother flow of traffic.

Turn Corners Carefully *Most collisions take place when two people are rounding a corner.* Always keep to the right, slow your pace, and turn corners carefully. This is of particular importance when you are pushing a stretcher or cart. In some hallways, mirrors are placed high on the intersecting walls *to allow you to see around the corner and avoid such collisions.*

---

[2]You will note that rationale for action is emphasized throughout the module by the use of italics.

Open Doors Slowly *An opening door may easily strike someone on the other side. If it is opened slowly, it is less likely to cause injury.* With swinging doors that have a glass insert, it is possible to see whether anyone is on the other side of the door. Even with this safety precaution, however, *distractions can interfere with full vision,* and a door can strike another person.

Use Stretchers Properly When pushing a patient on a stretcher, keep the patient's head toward your body and the feet in front. This is done *so that the head, which is highly vulnerable to impact injury, is protected and the feet, which are less vulnerable, are outward.*

When pushing a stretcher, occupied or unoccupied, or a cart or conveyance of any kind, keep your eyes to the front at all times. *Looking away for even a second can result in a collision and possible injury to another.*

Use Brakes on Beds, Wheelchairs, and Stretchers When beds, wheelchairs, and stretchers are stationary, apply the brake or brakes. On beds and stretchers, the brake is usually a flat metal "rocking" bar near the wheels. Pushing down on one side of the bar with your foot applies the brake, and pushing on the opposite side releases it. On wheelchairs, the brake is usually a small handle near the wheel. Moving the handle toward the occupant causes a bar to compress the rubber wheel and prevent it from moving. When a patient is being transferred to one of these pieces of equipment or when it is standing still, *the braking action prevents accidental movement that may lead to injury.*

Place Elevators on "Hold" when Loading or Unloading When you are pushing a patient in a wheelchair or stretcher, place elevator operating buttons on "hold." *This will keep the doors open until you and the patient are safely in or out of the elevator.* Back into the elevator with an occupied wheelchair *so that if the door does not hold with the hold request button, you, rather than the patient, will receive the impact.*

Safety in Working Spaces, Halls, and Corridors

Lighting These spaces should always be lighted well enough *to allow objects and people to be seen clearly.* (See Figures 3.1 and 3.2.) During

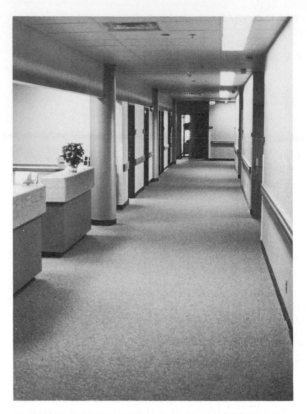

FIGURE 3.1 UNCLUTTERED HOSPITAL CORRIDOR
Courtesy Ivan Ellis

the late evening hours, hallways are sometimes dimmed *so that patients can rest more comfortably,* but lighting should always be at a level *that will ensure clear visibility.*

Floor Surfaces Whether the flooring is of tiling, linoleum, or carpeting, surfaces should be smooth. Cracked tiles, raised linoleum, or torn carpeting *can easily lead to falls.* Highly polished floors *can also cause skidding, falls, and injury.* Dropped materials such as tissues or food substances should be retrieved immediately, *since they also can cause a staff member, a visitor, or a patient to skid.* It is very important to wipe up spills of liquids immediately. Calling a custodian or maintenance person *could cause a delay long enough to expose someone to the danger of a fall.* If mopping is in progress, "Danger, Wet Floor" signs should always be posted.

Cords When an appliance such as an electric polishing machine is being used in a hallway or

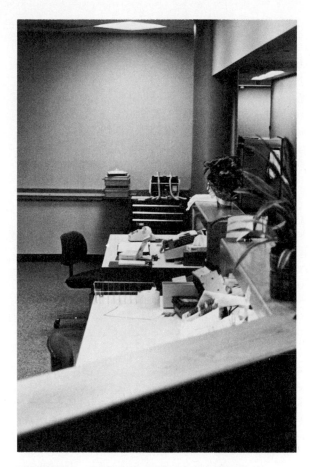

FIGURE 3.2 SPACIOUS NURSES' STATION
Courtesy Ivan Ellis

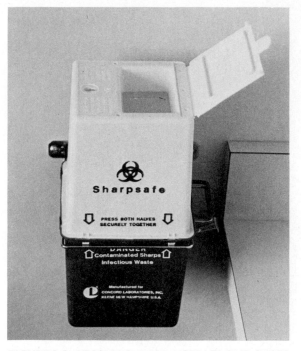

FIGURE 3.3 RECEPTACLE FOR NEEDLES AND SHARP OBJECTS
Courtesy Ivan Ellis

work area, the cord should not lie in such a way that people can trip over it. A cord or plug that is frayed or damaged should never be used *because it may cause sparks or fire, endangering the surrounding area or injuring the operator.*

Needles and Other Sharp Objects   Studies have shown that most "needle sticks" are sustained when the nurse is attempting to recap a needle. *To prevent transmission of blood-carried infections (such as hepatitis and AIDS) through needle sticks,* the Centers for Disease Control (CDC) recommend that needles never be recapped but be placed in a special receptacle with the syringe still attached (CDC, 1983, p. 7). Razor blades and scalpels (surgical knife blades) may also be put in these receptacles. Many hospitals are installing such receptacles in all patients' rooms *to ensure maximum protection.* (See Figure 3.3.)

Dangerous or Caustic Substances or Materials All such products should be clearly labeled to warn of any risks or dangers. They should never be left within easy reach of others in hallways or work spaces, including nurses' stations. *They could be ingested by children or by persons who are confused or incompetent.* A liquid substance could be spilled, *causing burns or injury.*

Equipment   Government codes usually prohibit the presence of equipment in hallways. *In a fire or emergency, such equipment could block the access of emergency personnel and equipment and the evacuation of patients and staff.*

Some hospitals, however, have hallways with "nurse servers" attached to the corridor walls for each patient or for several patients in adjacent rooms. These contain charts, medications, and supplies, and provide a charting area. *Making such items more accessible greatly saves staff time,* and this placement is in compliance with fire codes.

Safety in the Patient's Room

Many of the precautions taken in other areas of the hospital also pertain to safety in the patient's

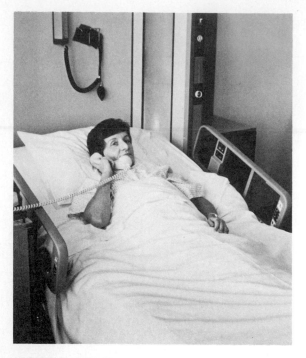

FIGURE 3.4 PATIENT IN A SAFE ENVIRONMENT
Courtesy Ivan Ellis

room. It is well to mention these important considerations again briefly in order to provide a complete inventory of safety precautions involving the patient in our care. Most patients experience some mild difficulty in accommodating to a new, unfamiliar environment. We should do everything possible to decrease the risk of injury (see Figure 3.4).

Lighting   Patient rooms need enough light *to allow the patient who is ambulatory to easily see objects that may be in the way and to allow staff to work without difficulty.* At night most patients who have slept in complete darkness at home are not disturbed by the use of a nightlight (a very small light extending from an electric socket near the floor). *This light helps to orient both the bedfast patient and the patient who is able to get out of bed to use the bathroom.*

Floor Surfaces   Again, floor surfaces should be smooth, whether they are of tile, linoleum, or carpeting. Liquids should be mopped or wiped up immediately, and foreign items picked up and disposed of. *The unsteady patient can slip even more easily than an able-bodied visitor or staff member.*

Remember, too, to provide nonslip mats or

a bath towel for use on the floor of a shower or on the bottom of a bathtub *to prevent slipping.* It is also a good idea to have hand rails and a call cord within reach *to ensure the safety of the patient.*

Oxygen   If oxygen is in use, special precautions have to be taken *to ensure that sparks and flames never occur in the vicinity.* While oxygen, as a gas, does not itself explode, *it supports very rapid combustion, and materials will burn at an explosive rate in its presence.* These precautions, therefore, are of the utmost importance for safety.

Cords   Examine cords and plugs used on equipment in the patient's room. This is especially important when the patient is receiving oxygen. As a general rule, any electrical appliance brought into the institution by the family should be checked by the engineer of the hospital *to ensure that it is working correctly.* All appliances must be grounded with a three-prong adapter if they are not already grounded.

Furniture   All furniture in the patient's room should be arranged to allow easy access to the wash basin, bathroom, closet area, and door. *This protects both ambulatory patients and staff members from bumps or falls.* Newer hospital beds may have a bedside stand that contains a console used for summoning the nurse and operating the television. This stand is attached in such a way that it swings out away from the bed. Although *consoles are more convenient for the patient,* remember that stretching toward a stand that is just out of reach has caused serious falls for many patients.

Medications and Dangerous Substances   Medications and dangerous substances should be removed from the patient's bedside. If a liquid used in treatment, such as a saline or hydrogen peroxide solution, is to be kept at the bedside, the container should be clearly marked. Medications should be removed from the bedside *to prevent a visitor or someone for whom they were not intended from ingesting them.* At times there is an order for a patient to keep at the bedside one or more medications taken regularly at home. If this is the case, they should be out of sight of others.

Doors   Entrance doors and bathroom, closet, and cabinet doors should be either fully open or fully closed at all times *to eliminate the possibility of people running into them.* If latches are not in repair, have them fixed or replaced.

Protecting the Dependent Patient

The Dependent Adult

It is part of the nursing role to protect those in our care who are partially or completely unable to protect themselves. It is useful to know which patients are at special risk for falls and injury. A study by Janken (1984, p. 215) has identified such patients. These high-risk patients include those who are elderly or confused; those who have sensory deficits, impaired mobility, a history of falls, or a history of substance abuse; and those who are receiving medications that interfere with normal functioning. A few important considerations are discussed below.

Position of the Bed   All occupied beds should remain in the low position unless bed height is needed for care procedures. In this way, *if the patient should fall, the distance is lessened.*

Side Rails   *Side rails ensure that the patient does not fall out of bed.* They should be used thoughtfully. If there is any doubt about the patient's safety, however, a nursing judgment can be made to use them. In some facilities, side rails are raised to protect every patient over the age of sixty-five. Those who do not wish them are required to sign a "Release from Liability" form. However, this policy varies from institution to institution.

Many falls occur when patients attempt to climb over raised rails. *To prevent this,* a device (usually known by the brand name Bed Check) can be obtained that will alert the nurse when a patient attempts to climb over a rail or abruptly get out of bed. The device consists of a slim, plastic-covered rod placed widthwise under the mattress. An electric alarm box fits underneath the bed. If the patient suddenly lifts up and reduces the pressure on the mattress, the alarm sounds. Casual movements such as position changes and turning will not activate the alarm. These devices are usually obtained from departments such as housekeeping or central supply.

Restraints   Restraints are designed *to protect patients or staff from injury.* They should be used only when careful assessment of the patient indicates that they are needed. Studies have shown that some patients who are restrained are at greater risk of injury *because in resisting the restraint, they apply undue pressure upon dependent extremities.* Resisting the restraint can also lead to sudden release of the device and a fall. Any patient who is restrained should be checked frequently, at least every two hours, *to make sure the restraint is still properly in place.* In addition, all restrained patients should have the devices removed every two hours *for exercise and position change* and to assess the circulatory status of the restrained extremity. (Refer to Module 21, Applying Restraints.)

Positioning   The unconscious or immobile patient must be positioned *so that extremities are not caught beneath the heavier portions of the body or on the side rails. Failure to do this could lead to nerve impingement and permanent damage.*

Protection from Sharp Objects   Dropped instruments, utensils, pieces of debris, fingernail clippings, and even minute loose hairs between the patient's body and the bed *can cause irritation and eventual skin breakdown.* Ensuring that such items are not dropped into the bed and inspecting and rearranging linens frequently *can safeguard the dependent patient.*

Nurses should be discouraged from wearing nail polish, but if they do, it must be kept in good repair *so that it does not chip and fall into the bed.*

Eyes   The eyes of the comatose patient should be routinely examined not only for irritation but for the *presence of foreign bodies that may cause harm.* All sharp objects must be kept away from eyes. If the eyes of the patient in coma are open and do not blink enough *to lubricate the cornea,* it is sometimes necessary to pad and tape the lids closed *to protect the eyes from ulceration.*

In caring for contact lenses, follow the guidelines for the specific lens worn. Removal and care of contacts for patients who are unable to care for their own lenses is discussed in Module 11, under Eyes, Ears, Hair and Nails. *Failure to properly remove and clean contact lenses can lead to damage to and/or infection of the eyes.*

Air Passages   *To eliminate the risk of aspiration,* lint from cloth or loose cotton balls and caustic substances should never be used around the air passages of the dependent patient. The patient's airway must be protected at all costs.

The Dependent Child

All the precautions just discussed for the dependent adult patient are applicable to the dependent child. There are also some additional responsibilities. Each situation requires careful assessment and the use of discretion.

To prevent falls, infants and small children should never be left unattended when they are lying on a high surface, such as an examining table. They should never be left unattended in tubs, *where they might slip and drown.* All medications and products used on the unit must be locked or made inaccessible *so that nothing can be taken unintentionally* and cause harm. A glass oral thermometer is used with children only when they can safely hold it in the mouth without biting it. The airway must be protected at all costs *to maintain adequate ventilation.* Foods should be of a consistency that allows it to be chewed and swallowed without choking. Mints, nuts, and popcorn are not appropriate for a small child *because of the high risk of choking.* Toys should be inspected for evidence of loose small parts *that could be detached and swallowed.* Protectors should be placed over electrical outlets *to prevent a child from inserting fingers or small objects, which could lead to electric shock.* Nurses caring for infants or children must intensify their vigilance for possible dangers to safety.

Other Safety Considerations

Several environmental considerations are important for those working and being cared for in the hospital environment. Unstable temperature control, inadequate ventilation, and improper food preparation or waste disposal are just a few examples of conditions *that could endanger patients, staff, and visitors.* Any of these conditions should be reported immediately to the supervisor of that area, such as the engineer or custodian responsible for temperature control, ventilation, or waste disposal. Notify the nutritionist or kitchen manager of any concerns you may have about food preparation.

Many patients are treated with radioactive substances called isotopes. Most of these are of low-grade activity and are not dangerous to those who are in close contact with them for short periods. *The potential risk depends on the substance used.* Because of this, special guidelines for the safe limits of exposure for staff and visitors are available. Very often, these guidelines include instructions about handwashing or the wearing of gowns and gloves. In many cases, limiting the time of exposure is sufficient. In some facilities, badges that monitor excessive exposure are worn or can be requested by health care personnel. Pregnant women should avoid any exposure, however, *since the potential danger to the fetus is as yet unknown.*

Also of potential danger to the patient or nurse is the improper use of vesicants. Vesicants are antineoplastic agents that can cause blistering, necrosis, or the sloughing of tissues. When handling these drugs, precautions should be taken. If clean gloves do not arrive on the unit with the drug, you must secure a pair for handling the equipment and/or the drug. When you put the medication into a syringe, cover the tip of the needle with sterile gauze or cotton when you rid the syringe of air *so that the agent is not dispersed into the air, where it might come in contact with the respiratory system.* Any spills should be wiped up immediately with paper towels, which should then be placed in a marked plastic bag. Although it does not seem likely at this time that these drugs produce prolonged injurious effects upon nurses who routinely administer them, data are still being compiled.

To protect the patient who is receiving vesicants intravenously, frequent assessment is essential *to detect any sign of infiltration.* If infiltration into the tissue occurs, stop the flow immediately, elevate the extremity, apply ice *so that the vesicant does not spread,* and notify the physician. (Refer to Module 54, Administering Intravenous Medications.) Specific nursing interventions for individual vesicant infiltrations are usually outlined in the procedure manual of each health care facility.

Protection against harmful microorganisms is a constant concern and responsibility for the nurse. This subject is covered in Volume 1, Module 2, Medical Asepsis, and in Volume 2, Module 34, Isolation Technique. As discussed under medical asepsis, the Centers for Disease Control (CDC) strongly recommend wearing clean gloves when any care or procedure is undertaken that places the nurse in contact with body fluids or discharges of any kind.

There are many things nurses can do to become more resistant to the many disease-causing organisms that are always present to some extent in the hospital environment. General good health habits such as proper nutrition, adequate rest, and lessened stress *enhance the body's immune system and decrease the chances of infection.*

Smoking as a Hazard in the Health Care Facility

Smoking has become a major health hazard in our society, and it can pose unique problems in a health care facility. Not only can fires be started accidentally, but smoking is known to have harmful effects on both those who smoke and those around them. (The American Lung Association and the American Cancer Society have clearly documented harmful physical effects upon nonsmokers who inhale smoke produced by others.) For some time, cigarettes have not been sold in health care facilities *in order to discourage what is recognized as a major health risk.*

Many hospitals have established a complete "no smoking" policy on their premises. There are, of course, exceptions. Smoking may be allowed in designated areas, such as a section of the cafeteria. Certain patients are allowed to smoke with a doctor's order. This is permitted because *the stress to a long-term smoker of not being able to smoke, when added to the many stresses of being ill, can compound the patient's problems.* A patient who smokes cannot be placed in the same room with a nonsmoker without the nonsmoker's permission, *to protect the nonsmoker's right to a smoke-free environment.* Any patient who is confused or medicated and has an order to permit smoking should do so only under the supervision of a staff person, *to prevent accidental fires.* If the staff does not have time to closely monitor smoking, ask the patient to refrain from smoking until a staff member is available. Only nonflammable containers should be used as ashtrays.

Patients on oxygen should not be allowed to smoke under any circumstances. *Oxygen supports combustion, and a spark or flame can rapidly become a life-threatening fire.*

Fire Plans

Medical facilities are being renovated and built in accordance with fire code standards. As a result, disastrous fires that encompass entire struc-

tures are becoming rare. As nurses with patients in our care, however, it still behooves us to be knowledgeable about what to do in the event of a fire of any size. Fire plans vary somewhat in different facilities, but all have similar basic principles. The plan is written into the procedure or policy manual of the facility. Basically, most plans follow the fire code procedure given below.

Fire Code Procedure

1. *In order to avoid alarming patients and visitors,* a code is used both to report the fire and to notify others in the building. There may be a special number on the telephone that signals the telephone operator in the building to call the Fire Department and notify those in the facility. The overhead paging system is commonly used to voice-page a code, frequently in the form of a number or code name. Some facilities have a fire bell that sounds softly but insistently. Whatever the system, become familiar with it.
2. If you are actually at the location of the fire, first and foremost remove any patient to a safe distance before taking the time to "call" the fire code. *This prevents harm to the patient.*
3. Then initiate the fire code according to the policy at your facility.
4. If you do not "call" the fire code yourself, but hear the code paged or the fire bell, return immediately to your nursing unit. The intention of this procedure is to mobilize all personnel who might be useful in the emergency.
5. Never use elevators to return to your unit or for any other purpose. They must remain free *so that firefighters and emergency equipment can be transported. Also, elevators may cease to work if the fire involves electrical wiring and can act like chimneys in a fire, rapidly filling with smoke.*
6. On the unit, return patients who are in the hallways to their rooms. Close all doors to rooms. *This is done to contain the fire and keep smoke from spreading through the environment.*
7. Be available to calm patients.

8. Follow any additional directions of the person in charge.

   If the danger is immediate, take action. This may include the use of fire extinguishers. Although all fire extinguishers now are red rather than color-coded, each has its classification clearly designated on the container along with both words and pictures of the items against which it is effective. Class A is a water or solution type, designed to be used on paper and linens; Class B is a foam extinguisher, designed to be used on grease and other chemicals; and Class C is a carbon dioxide or a dry chemical type, designed to be used on electrical fires. Currently, on the patient units most facilities have a variation of the Class C extinguisher that is multipurpose and can be used for paper or linens or on electrical fires. Some facilities hold in-service classes on using fire extinguishers. If your facility does not, this equipment is usually described for you in the unit manual. Read this section closely and locate and examine any fire extinguishers that are on your unit *so that you are prepared if the need arises.*

9. If there are no specific directions, stand quietly in the hallway, where you will be visible in case an evacuation of patients is ordered.

10. *Because smoke as well as fire is a real danger to the health of patients,* those in charge may order an evacuation. *The goal is to move the most patients in the shortest period of time.* To accomplish this, those who are ambulatory are directed to exits first *because they can move more rapidly.* Then those in wheelchairs or using assistive devices are helped out, and finally those who are bedridden and who need transfer are moved. Remaining calm is essential. Lifting patients is sometimes more hazardous to both the patient and the nurse than simply lowering patients to blankets on the floor and pulling them to safety. Remember to assure any person who is restrained or in a confining device such as a cast to be calm, they will also be promptly evacuated. Your actions during this time will depend on those in charge and on your own decision-making ability.

Being prepared ahead of time can be both comforting and useful should the need arise.

11. Remain calm.

12. Wait for further directions or the sound of the all-clear signal.

Disaster Plans

Disaster plans usually cover hazardous occurrences other than fire. Disaster plans are of two types: internal and external. Internal disasters include explosions, collapse of a part of the building, earthquakes, flooding, or toxic fumes. External disasters may affect the facility but have more to do with disaster in the community. In this category are such happenings as aircraft, train, and transit crashes; earthquakes; collapses of buildings; uncontained fires involving sections of a city; extensive flooding; landslides; and widespread toxic fumes.

   To differentiate between external and internal disaster codes, facilities use one of several methods. Some call them by color—a "Red" or "Green" disaster code; others may call the internal code "A" and the external one "B."

Internal Disaster Codes

Just like fire plans, disaster plans assign a specific role to each staff person in the event of a disaster. Usually, this again involves a return to the unit, where further assignments may be given. A special part of the facility is designated as a "triage" area. Triage means prioritization of patients according to their injuries *so that the most expedient and appropriate treatment can be given to a large number of people.*

   Personnel with special skills, such as starting intravenous therapy or suturing wounds, for example, may have specific assignments. Others may transport or maintain patients who are injured or emotionally upset. *Because internal disaster plans vary,* you should carefully read and become knowledgeable about the plans of the facility in which you practice.

External Disaster Codes

These plans are regional so that several facilities within the community can respond. In large urban areas, one hospital takes responsibility for continually monitoring the availability of critical

COPIES PROVIDED
TO:_____
_____
_____
_____

GROUP HEALTH COOPERATIVE OF PUGET SOUND

INCIDENT / HAZARD REPORT

(For use in all cases <u>except</u> personal injury)

DATE OF INCIDENT
_____

TIME OF INCIDENT
_____

TYPE OF INCIDENT / HAZARD: _____
(i.e. theft, safety hazard, flood, loss,fire, Property damage, etc.)
G.H.C. LOCATION_____ FACILITY _____
EXACT LOCATION OF INCIDENT_____

```
I    WHAT HAPPENED (GIVE DETAILS OF INCIDENT) _____
N    _____
C    _____
I    _____
D    _____
E    PROPERTY INVOLVED(MAKE,MODEL, SERIAL NO.,G.H.C. ID. NO.,PURCHASE DATE & COST)
N    _____
T
```

```
H    DESCRIBE FAULTY EQUIPMENT OR OTHER HAZARD IN DETAIL _____
A    _____
Z    _____
A    _____
R    RECOMMENDATION _____
D
```

```
LIST ALL PERSONS INVOLVED IN INCIDENT INCLUDING WITNESSES
_____ PHONE _____
_____ PHONE _____
_____ PHONE _____
NOTIFIED:*SAFETY & SECURITY yes( ) no( )*POLICE yes( ) no ( )*FIRE DEPT. yes( ) no( )
ACTION TAKEN BY ABOVE _____
```

REPORT PREPARED BY _____ TITLE _____ PHONE _____
DATE
```
ACTION TAKEN ( )TO BE TAKEN( ) _____
BY WHOM _____
SUPERVISOR_____ DEPT_____ DATE_____
```
ACTION _____
REFERRED TO SAFETY COMMITTEE YES( ) NO( )
LOSS CONTROL _____ DATE _____
DA-455 (3-80)
Send Original to Loss Control Department via Regional Safety and Security Office.

FIGURE 3.5 PATIENT/VISITOR ACCIDENT REPORT
Courtesy Group Health Cooperative of Puget Sound

care beds for those who need immediate life-saving medical intervention and acute care beds for those who need close monitoring and more intensive nursing care than is provided in general wards. The hospital supervisor or coordinator, after notifying the administrator, usually has the responsibility of activating the plan within the facility. All personnel are categorized according to their skills, and travel times from home are catalogued so that additional personnel can be summoned quickly. Different facilities may take on responsibility for different types of care—a hospital with a burn unit, for example, may receive patients with burns while other facilities receive patients with other types of injuries. Again, become acquainted with the policy in your facility and community.

Incident Reports

The incident report is used to document any unusual occurrence, accident, or error, not just errors in administering care or medications. Some facilities use different forms for different kinds of events—for example, medication errors and falls—whereas others use one standard form for all incidents. Figure 3.5 is an example of a patient/visitor accident report.

Incident reports serve several purposes. First, they *objectively document the event.* Second, because of this, *they serve as a record for insurance and legal reference.* Last, *they help identify the need to modify or correct procedures, policies, or situations within the health care facility.*

The incident report is completed by the staff person who discovers or is involved in the incident. *Because it may become a legal document,* it should contain good usage of language, pertinent facts, and the exact times and proper sequence of events. Only facts—not opinions or conclusions—are documented. If a report concerns a patient, the report itself is not incorporated into the patient's chart but is sent to the immediate supervisor and finally to administration. A notation about the incident itself is made in the chart. The report, in itself, does not constitute an admission of liability, and the fact that one was filed is not documented in the chart. It is important to complete and file an incident report in timely fashion, *for recall is more difficult if time has elapsed.*

REFERENCES

CDC Guidelines for Infection Control in Hospital Personnel. U.S. Dept. of Health and Human Services, 1983, p. 7.

Doll, Ann. "What to Do After an Incident." *Nursing '80,* 10, No. 1 (January 1980), 73–79.

Janken, Janice K., Betty Ann Reynolds, and Kristy Swiech. "Patient Falls in the Acute Care Setting: Identifying Risk Factors." *Nursing Research,* 35, No. 4 (July/August 1986), 215–217.

Jones, Marilee K. "Fire!" *American Journal of Nursing,* 18, No. 11 (November 1984), 1368–1371.

Wyatt, Delia M. "Are You Prepared for a Hospital Fire?" *Nursing '85,* 15, No. 2 (February 1985), 51.

PERFORMANCE CHECKLIST

	Unsatisfactory	Needs More Practice	Satisfactory	Comments
Safe behavior				
1. Use good body mechanics.				
2. Walk; avoid running.				
3. Keep to the right in hallways.				
4. Turn corners carefully.				
5. Open doors slowly.				
6. Use stretchers properly.				
7. Use brakes on beds, wheelchairs, and stretchers.				
8. Place elevators on "hold" when loading or unloading.				
Safety in working spaces, halls, and corridors				
1. Obtain adequate lighting.				
2. Floor surfaces should be in good repair, smooth, and free of spills and foreign material.				
3. Inspect electrical cords and do not use those that are frayed or damaged.				
4. Never recap needles. Dispose of needles and other sharp objects in designated receptacles.				
5. Never leave dangerous or caustic substances unattended.				
6. Equipment should never block hallways.				
Safety in the patient's room				
1. Obtain adequate lighting. Encourage the use of a nightlight.				
2. Ensure that floor surfaces are in good repair, smooth, and free of spills and foreign material.				
3. Keep oxygen away from sparks or flames. Check electrical equipment. Make sure that no one is smoking.				
4. Examine all electrical cords and plugs for damage or fraying.				

	Unsatisfactory	Needs More Practice	Satisfactory	Comments
5. Be sure furniture allows free access to wash basin, bathroom, and closet area.				
6. Never leave medications and caustic substances in full view at the patient's bedside.				
7. Fully open or close entrance, bathroom, closet, and cabinet doors to prevent collisions with them.				

Protecting the dependent patient

1. Ensure that beds remain in low position unless height is needed for a care procedure.				
2. Use side rails only to protect the patient from possible fall and injury.				
3. Use restraints cautiously and only after accurate assessment.				
4. Position the patient so that extremities are not caught beneath body or on side rails.				
5. Prevent sharp objects and foreign materials from falling into the bed.				
6. Protect the eyes from foreign materials and fumes.				
7. Protect air passages from aspirating foreign substances, materials, and fumes at all costs.				

Fire plans

1. Know the fire code and initiating procedure in your facility.				
2. If you are at location of fire, remove any patient in the vicinity.				
3. Call the fire code.				
4. If you are not near the fire or if you did not call, return immediately to your unit.				
5. Do not use elevators.				
6. Return patients to their rooms, closing doors.				
7. Be available to calm patients.				
8. Follow directions of person in charge.				

	Unsatisfactory	Needs More Practice	Satisfactory	Comments
9. Stand quietly in hallway, available for any duties.				
10. If there is an evacuation, move patients according to procedure.				
11. Remain calm.				
12. Wait for further directions or sound of all clear.				

QUIZ

Short-Answer Questions

1. Give three reasons why providing a safe environment in the health care facility is important.

   a. _____

   b. _____

   c. _____

2. List five of the seven behaviors that demonstrate a concern for safety on the part of the nurse.

   a. _____

   b. _____

   c. _____

   d. _____

   e. _____

3. Describe a safe floor surface. _____

   _____

4. Discuss electrical safety precautions. _____

   _____

5. State why attempting to recap the needle on a syringe is unsafe and how needles and syringes are disposed of properly. _____

   _____

6. Describe a safe environment for the patient who is bedfast. _____

   _____

7. What is the most important safety precaution for the dependent patient in your care?_____

8. What rules or policies do health care facilities have about smoking?

   _____

9. Briefly, give the steps of responding to a fire code. _____

   _____

10. What might be the role of the staff nurse in a disaster plan? _____

   _____

11. What are the three purposes of incident reports?

   a. _____

   b. _____

   c. _____

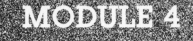

MODULE 4

Basic Body Mechanics

PREREQUISITES

Successful completion of the following modules:

VOLUME 1

OVERALL OBJECTIVE

To apply the principles of body mechanics so as to conserve energy; to decrease the potential for strain, injury, and fatigue; and to promote safety.

SPECIFIC LEARNING OBJECTIVES

	Know Facts and Principles	Apply Facts and Principles	Demonstrate Ability	Evaluate Performance
1. *Principles of body mechanics*	State principles of body mechanics	Given a situation, correctly identify which principles could apply, and state why	In the clinical setting, use body mechanics correctly	Evaluate own performance with instructor using Performance Checklist

LEARNING ACTIVITIES

1. Review the Specific Learning Objectives.
2. Read the section on posture and body mechanics for the nurse (in the chapter on activity and rest) in Ellis and Nowlis, *Nursing: A Human Needs Approach,* or comparable material in another textbook.
3. Look up the module vocabulary terms in the Glossary.
4. Read through the module.
5. In the practice setting, with a partner observing:
   a. Stand with your weight balanced over your base of support.
   b. Stand 3 feet from a table or counter. Try to place a book on the table without enlarging your base of support. Begin again and place the book on the table using an enlarged base of support. Compare your stability in the two situations.
   c. Stand in a normal position. Have your partner take your arms and pull until you begin to tip forward. Using the same base of support, squat low and have your partner pull again. Compare the force needed to disrupt your stability in the two positions.
   d. Stand with your feet 8 inches apart, but side by side, and try to push a bed. Now enlarge your base of support in the direction in which you are pushing and note the difference.
   e. Practice tightening your abdominal muscles upward and your gluteal muscles downward. Relax. Tighten the muscles again. Do this before you attempt any task.
   f. Face the bed. Turn your upper body 90 degrees to the right as if reaching for something while keeping your feet in the same position. Note the feeling of strain and pull on your back muscles. Try bending from this position. Note the lack of stability.

   Face the bed. Turn 90 degrees to the right by moving your right foot and turning your whole body. Note that your back is straight. Now try

   bending and reaching. Note the increased stability in this position.
   g. Pick an object up from the floor or other low surface, bending your knees and keeping your back straight.
   h. With your partner as an assistant, try to move another person up in bed with the head of the bed at a 30-degree angle. Now place the bed in a flat position and repeat the activity. Compare the amount of energy required. Have your "patient" evaluate his or her experience.
   i. Again with your partner as your assistant and with the bed in a flat position, move your "patient" up in bed without a turn sheet and against a wrinkled bottom sheet. Now tighten the bottom sheet and use a turn sheet for the same activity. Compare the experiences. Ask your "patient" to comment.
   j. Hold a 10-pound object (brick, book) with both hands directly in front of and close to your body for three minutes. Now do the same thing holding the object at arm's length from your body. Compare the amount of energy required for each task.
   k. With a turn sheet, turn your "patient" from a supine position to a lateral position, using your weight as a counterbalance. Note the ease with which you can do this.
   l. Have one person lie in the bed. Try to move the patient's shoulders closer to the far edge of the bed by pushing. Then push the hips and feet toward the far side of the bed. Next, move the patient's shoulders toward you by slipping your arms under the shoulders and pulling. Do the same for the hips and feet. Note the difference in ease of movement when pushing and pulling.

   Trade places with the person in the bed and repeat the exercise of pushing and pulling. Compare how it felt to be pulled and how it felt to be pushed.
   m. When you feel you have practiced enough, perform all the above tasks

correctly for your instructor, using your
partner as a "patient" when necessary.

6. In the clinical setting, apply basic body
mechanics whenever possible. If you are
unsure or need help, consult your
instructor.

VOCABULARY

base of support
body mechanics
center of gravity
internal girdle
torsion

BASIC BODY MECHANICS

Rationale for the Use of This Skill

A nurse engaged in clinical practice daily performs a variety of physical tasks, including reaching, stooping, lifting, carrying, pushing, and pulling. Practiced incorrectly, any of these has the potential to cause strain, fatigue, or injury to the nurse and to threaten the safety of patients. With practice, using the principles of body mechanics, the nurse will move smoothly and surely, minimizing personal strain and enhancing the safety, comfort, and confidence of patients.[1]

Principles of Basic Body Mechanics

The following principles of body mechanics have been selected because of their applicability to commonly encountered nursing situations. Examples of how they can be applied are included as illustrations.

1. *Weight is balanced best when the center of gravity is directly above the base provided by the feet. In this position, you can maintain balance and stability with the least amount of effort.* When this posture is *not* maintained, the potential for strain, fatigue, and poor stability is increased (see Figure 4.1).
2. *Enlarging the base of support increases the stability of the body.* Changes in position should not cause the center of gravity to fall beyond the edge of the base. Therefore, when you assist a patient to move, you will be more stable if your feet are apart than if they are close together.
3. *A person or an object is more stable if the center of gravity is close to the base of support.* Apply this principle when picking an object up from the floor by bending at the knees and keeping your back straight (thus keeping the center of gravity directly above and close to the base of support), rather than by bending forward at the waist.
4. *Enlarging the base of support in the direction of the force to be applied increases the amount of force that can be applied.* Place one foot forward when you push a heavy object (such as a bed with a patient in it), or place one foot back when you move a patient toward the side of the bed.

[1]You will note that rationale for action is emphasized throughout the module by the use of italics.

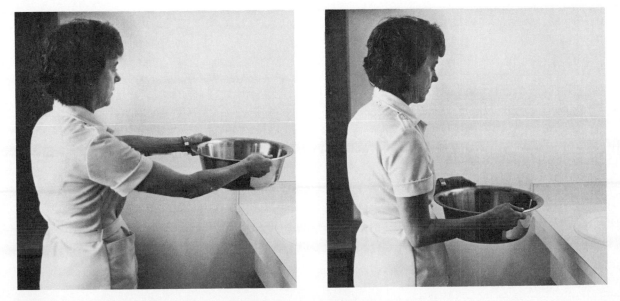

FIGURE 4.1 CONSERVING ENERGY *Left:* Holding basin at a distance from body (incorrect). *Right:* Holding basin close to body (correct).
Courtesy Ivan Ellis

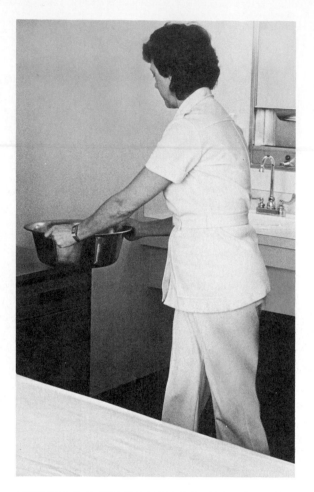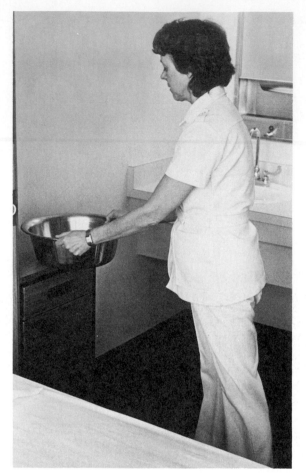

FIGURE 4.2 AVOID TORSION OF THE SPINE   *Left:* Nurse twisting to lift basin from bed to table (incorrect). *Right:* Nurse turning whole body to lift basin from bed to table (correct).
Courtesy Ivan Ellis

5. *Tightening the abdominal muscles upward and the gluteal muscles downward before undertaking any activity decreases the chance of strain or injury to ligaments and muscles.* (We call this putting on the "internal girdle.") If you practice this continually, you will eventually do it automatically when you prepare for any activity.

6. *Facing in the direction of the task to be performed and turning the entire body in one plane (rather than twisting) lessens the susceptibility of the back to injury. Also, the spine functions less effectively when it is twisted* (see Figure 4.2).

7. *Lifting is better undertaken by bending the legs and using the leg muscles than by using the*

back muscles. *Because large muscles tire less quickly than small muscles, you should use the large gluteal and femoral muscles rather than the smaller muscles of the back* (see Figure 4.3).

In addition, if the back muscles are strained, they may be injured, and injury to ligaments, tendons, and even the intervertebral discs may occur. Back injuries are one of the major health problems in adult workers, resulting in pain, disability, and economic loss to the individual, the employer, and society as a whole.

8. *It is easier to move an object on a level surface than to move it up a slanted surface against the force of gravity.* Therefore, you will

50

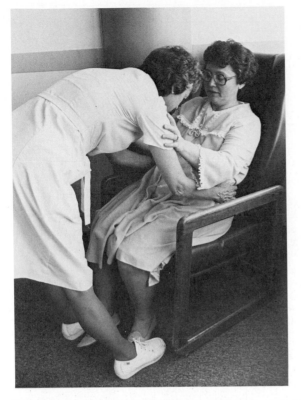 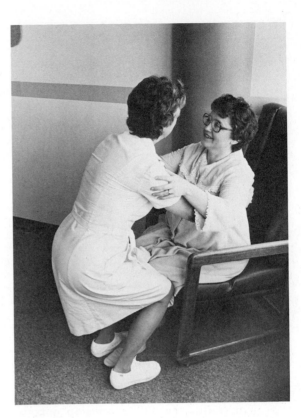

FIGURE 4.3 LIFTING WITH THE LEG MUSCLES   *Left:* Nurse assisting patient to stand, hands under patient's arms, body bent over from waist (incorrect). *Right:* Nurse assisting patient to stand, hands under patient's arms, back straight, knees flexed (correct).

Courtesy Ivan Ellis

need less effort to move a patient up in bed if you first lower the head of the bed.

9. *Less energy is required to move an object when friction between the object and the surface on which it rests is minimized. Because friction opposes motion,* you can make the task of moving a patient in bed easier by working on a smooth surface.

10. *It takes less energy to hold an object close to the body than at a distance from the body; it is also easier to move an object that is close. Muscles are strongest when contracted and weakest when stretched.* Therefore, hold heavy objects close to your body, and move the patient near to your side of the bed (for bathing, for example) to conserve energy.

11. *The weight of the body can be used to assist in lifting or moving.* When you help a patient to stand, you can use the weight of your body by rocking back, counterbalancing the patient's weight, as illustrated in Figure 4.3. You can use the patient's weight by placing his or her legs in a knees-up position before moving the patient from side to side or up in bed.

12. *Smooth, rhythmical movements at moderate speed require less energy than rapid, jerky ones. Smooth, continuous motions also are more accurate, safer, and better controlled than sudden, jerky movements.*

13. *When a soft object is pushed, it absorbs part of the force being exerted, leaving only part of the force available to do the moving. When a soft object is pulled, all of the force exerted is available for the task of moving.* Think of patients to be moved as soft objects, and try to use a pulling motion whenever possible.

PERFORMANCE CHECKLIST				

Basic body mechanics	Unsatisfactory	Needs More Practice	Satisfactory	Comments
1. Keep weight balanced above base of support.				
2. Enlarge base of support as necessary to increase body's stability.				
3. Lower center of gravity toward base of support as necessary to increase body's stability.				
4. Enlarge base of support in direction in which force is to be applied.				
5. Tighten abdominal and gluteal muscles in preparation for all activities.				
6. Face in direction of task and turn body in one plane.				
7. Bend hips and knees (rather than back) when lifting.				
8. Move objects on level surface when possible.				
9. Slide (rather than lift) objects on smooth surface when possible.				
10. Hold objects close to body and stand close to objects to be moved.				
11. Use body's weight to assist in lifting or moving when possible.				
12. Use smooth motions and reasonable speed when carrying out tasks.				
13. When moving patients, use a pulling motion whenever possible.				

QUIZ

True-False Questions

_____ 1. The body is less stable when the center of gravity falls beyond the edge of the base of support.

_____ 2. Stability is increased when the center of gravity is close to the base of support.

_____ 3. Facing in the direction of the task to be performed is not recommended.

_____ 4. Friction cnhances movement.

_____ 5. It takes less energy to hold an object close to the body than at a distance from the body.

_____ 6. When carrying out a task, the faster one moves, the better.

Short-Answer Questions

7. Why is lifting or pulling using the back muscles contraindicated?

_____

_____

8. Which principle of body mechanics is the basis for a decision to put the head of the bed down before moving the patient?

_____

_____

9. Which principle of body mechanics is the basis for a decision to spread your feet farther apart before trying to lift a patient?

_____

_____

10. Which principle of body mechanics is the basis for a decision to move closer to the patient's bed before attempting to move the patient?

_____

_____

MODULE 5

Assessment

PREREQUISITES[1]

Successful completion of the following
modules:

VOLUME 1

Module 1 / An Approach to Nursing Skills
Module 2 / Medical Asepsis
Module 3 / Safety

[1]The other modules in Unit III should be consulted for
specific skills relating to assessment.

OVERALL OBJECTIVES

To perform a beginning-level assessment of individual patients, systematically collecting data for all pertinent areas and using all senses, and to correctly state nursing diagnoses from the data collected.

SPECIFIC LEARNING OBJECTIVES

	Know Facts and Principles	Apply Facts and Principles	Demonstrate Ability	Evaluate Performance
1. Methods of gathering data	State five methods of gathering assessment data	Given a list of information needed, identify appropriate assessment method for that information	Gather assessment data using all five methods	
2. Areas of assessment	Using the human needs approach, list and define eleven areas to be assessed. Using the body systems approach, list and define nine areas to be assessed.	Given patient data, determine to what areas data are pertinent	Gather assessment data in all areas	Evaluate own performance using Assessment Guide
3. Analysis of data a. Objective data (signs or objective symptoms) b. Subjective data (symptoms or subjective symptoms)	Differentiate between objective and subjective data	Given data and their source, identify them as subjective or objective	Include and appropriately identify both subjective and objective information	Evaluate differentiation of data with instructor
4. Statement of nursing diagnoses	State components of nursing diagnosis	Given a list of assessment data, identify problem area and state nursing diagnosis correctly	In clinical setting, correctly identify nursing diagnosis and state on patient's record	Verify accuracy of nursing diagnosis with instructor

LEARNING ACTIVITIES

1. Review the Specific Learning Objectives.
2. Read the chapter on the nursing process and the section on interviewing in Ellis and Nowlis, *Nursing: A Human Needs Approach,* or comparable material in another textbook.
3. Read through the module.
4. Review the format of the Basic Data Gathering Guides, pages 70–75.
5. Arrange to practice the following activities with a partner:
   a. Select an assessment approach and write its assessment categories on one side of a blank piece of paper.
   b. Observe each other without speaking or touching. Write all the data you can gather for each area. You may use the module as a reference while observing each other.
   c. Compare your lists. Discuss the differences and similarities in the data collected. Go through your lists together and star each item that is truly objective.
   d. Show your lists to your instructor for suggestions or corrections.
   e. Next, gather additional data without speaking but using touch and contact. Compare your lists again, discuss the data collected, and star objective data. Show your lists to your instructor again for suggestions or corrections.
   f. As a final step, interview each other to gather further data in each area.
   g. Discuss these data. What data gathered by interview would cue you to make further observations? Also, what data gathered by observation over a longer period of time might be needed? What data are unique and obtainable only by interview? Underline the subjective data.
   h. Show these lists of data to your instructor.
6. In the clinical setting:
   a. Again, select an assessment approach and write its assessment categories on one side of a blank piece of paper.
   b. Consult with your clinical instructor before choosing a patient to observe. Choose a patient who will not be upset or disturbed by your visit.
   c. When you are with the patient, explain your task in a way that will make him or her feel comfortable. You can simply say that you are trying to improve your observational skills. Observe the patient for five or ten minutes. Write all data gathered by observation. You may socialize with the patient during this time, but do not do an interview. At the end of the time period, excuse yourself and look over your list. If it will not upset the patient, two students may work together. In that instance, you could compare lists.
   d. Consult with your instructor regarding the data collected. If you or your instructor feel it would be beneficial to you, repeat the activity with another patient.
7. Look at an available clinical record. From the record, gather only what you feel to be pertinent assessment data. List the data under appropriate assessment areas. Mark each item *O* for objective or *S* for subjective. From these assessment data, identify and write down what you consider the patient's problems to be and formulate nursing diagnoses. Consult with your instructor regarding your determinations.
8. For a patient assigned in the clinical area, use the Basic Data Gathering Guides to gather data from all five sources. Have your instructor review this assessment.
9. Continue to use the guide to assess all patients assigned in the clinical area.

VOCABULARY

asymmetry
bruit
caries
cerumen
cranium
dorsiflexion
gravida
Homan's sign
lesion
nares
nasal speculum
ophthalmoscope
otoscope
para
patellar tendon
pectoralis muscles
periphery
pinwheel
ptosis
reflex hammer (percussion hammer)
Snellen chart
stethoscope
tuning fork
turgor
uvula
vaginal speculum

ASSESSMENT

Rationale for the Use of This Skill

*A*ssessing patients is a major responsibility of the registered nurse. In every nursing care setting, the nurse is called on to gather data in order to determine patients' problems, formulate nursing diagnoses, establish treatment priorities, and plan care. A systematic method of assessment provides a framework for doing this in an orderly, comprehensive way. Without some kind of system, significant areas may be omitted accidentally. This module provides only an initial framework; experience and further education will allow you to expand it.[2]

Methods of Gathering Data

Assessment involves the gathering of all possible data regarding patients in order to identify problems. Methods of gathering data include (1) interview, (2) observation, (3) physical examination, (4) consultation with other members of the health care team through records and reports related to the patient and through verbal interaction, and (5) review of the literature.

Data are gathered from five sources: (1) the patient; (2) family members, friends, and associates; (3) other members of the health care team; (4) records of the patient's present and past health status; and (5) written information regarding the problem or problems and treatment facing the patient.

Interview

While you are making general observations and doing a nursing physical examination, you must also interview the patient. Ask specific questions about the patient's health status, health history, and responses to illness. The information stated by the patient is *subjective data.* These data may lead you to further observation or examination of the patient. Note that a nursing history is a formalized tool for interviewing patients. Module 14, Admission, Transfer, and Discharge, provides an example of an initial patient interview. (See page 288.)

[2]You will note that rationale for action is emphasized throughout this module by the use of italics.

Observation

Observational skills improve with experience. Whenever you contact a patient, be sure to observe very carefully, paying close attention to detail.

When we speak of general observation, we mean what is seen, heard, and smelled. Look at both the patient and the environment. (Maintaining an environment that is therapeutic for the patient is a nursing responsibility.) Note the general symmetry of the body, posture, and movement, as well as facial expressions and gestures, which are especially important. Listen for the characteristic sounds of ordinary life, among them the sound of breathing. Check out thoroughly any differences from the norm. Smells are often difficult to describe, but comparing them to something familiar can help. For example, there are odors associated with wounds and drainage, with the breath, and sometimes with the body itself. Be familiar with these smells; they are all important.

Physical Examination

After you have made a general survey, perform a physical examination. Take temperature and blood pressure; measure height, weight, and fluid intake and output; palpate, count, and describe the pulse.

You will need a stethoscope for *auscultation* (listening to body sounds) of the lungs, the bowel, and other organs. Although at first you may not recognize what you hear, you will quickly learn to identify normal sounds. You can consult someone else when you hear a sound that is unfamiliar. Palpate soft areas of the body to check for solid masses or abnormal rigidity. (See Module 13 for specific information on auscultation and palpation.)

You can do some parts of a nursing physical examination while bathing a patient or during other contact. You can examine the skin closely, check any dressings, and observe the patient's response to activities. All information gathered by observation and examination is *objective data.*

A physical examination is a complex task involving many components, and here too experience improves skill. Still, even at the beginning you can identify normal and abnormal characteristics in general ways. Later, as you study each system of the body in physiology and learn disease entities and nursing care, you will develop new skills to use in physical examinations. Below is a summary of items included in a complete physical examination. A discussion of all the specific skills needed for a complete physical examination is beyond the scope of these modules. Many excellent texts on physical examination are available.

1. *Head and neck*
   a. *Head* The cranium is palpated with the fingers for lumps, abrasions, and asymmetry. The condition of the hair is noted.
   b. *Neck* The neck is palpated for asymmetry, distended veins, abnormal lymph nodes, and enlarged thyroid. Range of motion of the neck is performed to detect any limitations. The stethoscope is placed over the carotid artery to listen for bruits (abnormal sounds resulting from circulatory turbulence).
   c. *Face* The face is inspected for asymmetry, ptosis (drooping of the eyelids), and skin condition.
   d. *Eyes* Using a flashlight or ophthalmoscope (see Figure 19.1), the eyes are observed for pupillary response (accommodation in a darkened room). (For further information on observation of the eye, see Module 13, Inspection, Palpation, Auscultation, and Percussion.) With the ophthalmoscope, each eye is inspected, while the patient gazes straight ahead, for corneal, lens, or vitreous abnormalities. The optic disc is assessed for size and color; each lower eyelid is pulled down for observation of the color and condition of the conjunctiva. Visual acuity is tested using a Snellen chart. If corrective lenses (glasses or contact lenses) are worn, vision is checked with and without the corrective lenses in place.
   e. *Nose* With the patient's head tilted slightly back, each inner nostril is inspected using a nasal speculum (see Figure 19.2). Some examiners use the light from the ophthalmoscope instead of room light or a flashlight. The nares are inspected for color and condition of the mucosa, bleeding, and the presence of foreign bodies or masses.
   f. *Ears* With the head turned, each ear is examined with the otoscope for evidence of excess cerumen (earwax), growths, or redness (see Figures 19.3 and 19.4). The eardrum (tympanic membrane) is assessed for signs of swelling or color change and for perforations. The area around the outer ear is palpated for tenderness. To test for hearing, a tuning fork is struck and held an equal distance from each ear to test for air conduction (see Figure 19.5). The struck tuning fork is then placed on each mastoid process, just below and behind the ears, and on the center top of the cranium to test for bone conduction of sound. A more definitive hearing test may be performed using electronic equipment. Hearing aids, if used, are checked to see that they are in place and functioning.
   g. *Mouth* With a flashlight and tongue blade, the back of the throat is examined for swelling, redness, bacterial or viral patches, and the position and size of the uvula. When the patient says "Ah," the tonsils are checked. The teeth are inspected for looseness and the presence of caries. The mucosa of the inner mouth are observed for color and the presence of lesions. The patient is asked to clench the teeth and smile, which helps in assessing bite and facial musculature. The color and smoothness of the lips are noted.
2. *Arms, hands, and fingers* The patient is asked to extend both arms out in front of the body. The musculature is examined for asymmetry and palpated for turgor. The arms, hands, and fingers are ranged to assess agility. The skin is observed for lesions, spotting, and general color. Joints are palpated and observed for nodules

and enlargements. The hands and fingers are observed for color and palpated for temperature. The hands are observed for any tremors. Any deviation of alignment in the fingers is noted. The nails are observed for hardness and general condition. The grip of each hand is tested.

3. *Back*   The patient either is placed in the prone position or sits in bed with the back facing the examiner. After the back is exposed, the skin is examined for spots or lesions. The curvature of the spine is noted, and the vertebral column is palpated. School-age children are checked for scoliosis (lateral curvature of the spine) by (1) looking for asymmetry of shoulders and hips while observing the standing child from behind, and (2) observing for asymmetry or prominence of the rib cage while watching the child bend over so that the back is parallel to the floor. With the stethoscope, the examiner listens to the lower lobes of the lungs. (See Module 13 for specific information on examination of the lungs.)

4. *Chest*   A male patient will have the gown removed. Because a female patient may feel modest about exposing the breasts, her gown can be untied and parted for the chest examination. If more exposure is needed, the gown can be dropped to the waist. With either a male or female patient, the levels of the shoulders are observed for equality while the patient is sitting and facing the examiner. The pectoralis muscles of each side of the chest are observed for symmetry as the patient presses the palms together and lifts the hands over the head. Any abnormal dimpling, color, or discharge of the nipples is noted.

   A female patient is then asked to lie in the supine position. Each breast is examined, and a small folded towel is placed under its outer side. With the flat of the fingers, each breast is palpated for masses or lumps from the nipple outward and then around the periphery.

5. *Heart*   With the patient in the supine position, the neck veins are palpated for normal filling, and the cardiac margins

(outline of the heart) are percussed. A stethoscope is used to listen to the heart sounds. Then the gown is replaced.

6. *Abdomen*   The patient remains in the supine position. The abdomen is observed for general contour, distention, and asymmetry. The skin is grasped between the fingers to test for turgor. A stethoscope is used to listen to bowel sounds. The area is then palpated and percussed for areas of tenderness, for the presence of fluid, and for the loss of normal dullness of tone. With the patient breathing deeply and with the knees flexed, the abdomen is palpated for organs and masses. On expiration, the examiner's fingers can feel for the position of abdominal structures. (For further information on examination of the abdomen, see Module 13.)

7. *Legs, feet, and toes*   With the patient still in the supine position, each leg is palpated for muscle bulk and observed for color, temperature, and skin condition. Each foot is dorsiflexed to check for calf pain, which is a possible sign of thrombo-phlebitis (Homan's sign). Pedal pulses are taken on each foot and compared. The ankles are palpated with the fingers to assess for edema. Strength is tested by having the patient press the sole of the foot against the examiner's palm. The joints are inspected for enlargement.

8. *Reflexes*   Depending on the situation, the examiner may test only a few of the more prominent reflexes or may proceed with an abbreviated neurological exam. Many of the measurements of neurological functioning will have been tested when the other systems or areas were examined. For example, an examination of the optic discs with the ophthalmoscope can reveal a neurological deficit or disease. If the examiner wants to check the cranial nerves, this is usually accomplished during the examination of the face by having the patient protrude the tongue, smile, and resist supraorbital pressure. (For a detailed description of a complete neurological examination, refer to a medical-surgical text or a neurological nursing text.)

61

Reflexes are usually recorded using the following symbols: 0 (no response), 1+ (hypoactive), 2+ (normal), 3+ (hyperactive), 4+ (very hyperactive).

a. *Corneal reflex (blink)* When the cornea is touched with a soft, small wad of cotton, the patient should blink.

b. *Biceps reflex* The examiner places his or her thumb on the biceps tendon, which is located just above the antecubital fossa. Striking the thumb should cause flexion of the forearm.

c. *Triceps reflex* The upper arm is supported at a right angle to the body, and the forearm is allowed to hang freely. The triceps tendon is struck with the reflex hammer (see Figure 19.6) just above the elbow. Extension of the forearm should occur.

d. *Brachioradial reflex* Striking the radius slightly above the wrist with the reflex hammer should cause flexion and supination of the forearm.

e. *Knee reflex* The patient's lower leg must be relaxed and hanging freely from the knee. When the patellar tendon, which is just below the knee, is struck with the reflex hammer, extension of the lower leg should occur.

f. *Ankle reflex* The foot is held in a position of dorsiflexion by the examiner. Striking the Achilles tendon at the back of the ankle with the reflex hammer should cause plantar flexion of the foot (the toes bending downward).

g. *Babinski reflex* Using the end of the reflex hammer or the sharper edge of a tongue blade, the sole of the foot is stroked from heel to toe. The negative response is plantar flexion. This is normal from the age of six months on.

h. *Skin sensation* The examiner may choose to test sensation by using a pinwheel that can be rolled over broad skin areas (see Figure 19.7). The patient is asked to state, without looking at the pinwheel, whether the sensation is sharp or dull.

9. *Genitalia*

a. *Male patients* Male patients are examined in the standing position, if at all possible, so that the inguinal ring can be palpated for herniation. The foreskin of the penis is retracted and inspected for irritation, ulceration, and the presence of lesions. The testes are palpated to assess for size, position, and the presence of masses.

b. *Female patients* Female patients are examined in the lithotomy position with the knees flexed. Drape the patient as you would for catheterization, using a clean sheet or bath blanket. Cover both legs, exposing only the perineum. An examination table with stirrups is preferred, but the patient can be examined in bed. Provide a gooseneck lamp. The examiner puts on clean gloves and lubricates the outside of a vaginal speculum (see Figure 19.8). The inside is not lubricated because the presence of the lubricating jelly interferes with the accuracy of the Papanicolaou (Pap) test. This test is done by obtaining secretions from the cervical os on a swab. The secretions are put on a glass slide, preserved with a fixative, and sent to the lab to be examined for the presence of abnormal cells. After the cervix is inspected with the speculum, the speculum is withdrawn and the examiner lubricates the index and middle fingers of one hand. By inserting these fingers into the vagina and pushing downward on the patient's abdomen with the other hand, the examiner can palpate the uterus and ovaries. These organs are assessed for location, size, outline, masses, and tenderness.

10. *Rectum* In female patients, this examination is usually done after the genital exam has been completed. With the hand gloved and lubricated, the examiner inserts the middle finger and palpates for size of lumen, masses, internal hemorrhoids, and tenderness. The anal area is evaluated for the presence of external hemorrhoids. The same exam is performed on the male patient, with the patient either bending over the side of the bed or positioned in lithotomy with the penis and testes held aside. The knee-chest position can also be used. In the male exam, the prostate gland is also assessed for size and tenderness.

Consultation with Other Members of the Health Care Team

A patient's record contains essential information regarding identified problems. Consult the physician's history and physical examination records, the results of laboratory and diagnostic studies, the various nursing records, and the records of other specialists working with the patient. It is not always possible to review a record completely before your initial patient contact, but a thorough nursing assessment cannot be made without reference to the data contained in the record. Records of previous hospitalizations may also be useful. Module 6, Documentation, gives more information on using the patient's record.

In addition to reviewing the record, you may wish to consult verbally with other individuals who are or have been involved in the care of the patient. Depending on the individual situation, the physician, dietitian, chaplain, or physical therapist are among those who may be able to share useful information regarding the patient.

Review of the Literature

Consulting textbooks and journals to gain more information about the patient's medical diagnosis, common problems related to that diagnosis, usual diagnostic tests, medications, and other forms of treatment can be an invaluable part of the data gathering process. Although your patient will probably not fit the "textbook picture" in every way, you will be better able to plan care if you have refreshed or expanded your knowledge in this way.

Basic Data Gathering Guides

The Guides on pages 70–75 give you a basic, systematic way to approach assessment. Still, they are only tools and should not become too confining. You should consider the major categories of assessment in their order of importance for the individual patient.

As you study the physiology and pathophysiology related to each of the categories listed, you will recognize the complexity of assessment. This discussion does not begin to cover all the data relating to specific areas. Rather, it is an outline of major components to give you a beginning framework. Some components relate to skills and knowledge you have now. Others require skills you will learn in the weeks ahead. As you learn, you will add more and more detail to your assessments of patients.

Because a person is a whole entity, not simply a collection of parts, you may find it difficult to determine whether certain data are more applicable to one area or to another. In such cases, note the data under two or more categories. At other times, the problem may be very clear, in which case list the data in the area that pertains to the known problem. Remember that the location of data is not so critical as your ability to relate facts to one another in order to recognize problems.

Two systems for organizing your assessment will be presented. It is important that you understand that, whichever system you use, the total patient is to be assessed. The same data are required in both, but the organization will differ. The differences in the data gathering systems stem from differing approaches to the organization of concepts relating to people and nursing. Your instructor may specify that you are to use a particular data gathering system. In that case, you may not need to read the section on the other system. If you are to choose your own system, read through both, comparing and contrasting the terminology and the organization of the data. Be aware that the information contained in both systems is identical: it is the organization of that information that differs. Consider both systems in the light of your own approach to nursing and to people, and identify the one that will work more comfortably for you. Remember that only an overview of each area is presented. You will need to study your theory text for a complete discussion.

Human Needs Approach

This system for data gathering is based on organizing data around human needs. It is used most often by those who approach nursing with the objective of meeting human needs or preventing interference with the meeting of needs. The physical needs are identified separately, and the psychosocial needs are grouped together.

Physical Needs

Activity   This component pertains to the patient's ability to move and exercise for optimal functioning. Consider the patient's usual exercise at home, diversional choices, and the effects of exercise. Any recent variation from the norm, such as joint or muscle pain or disability, is important. The individual's posture and positioning and the level of activity ordered by the physician are other items of concern. Note the pathophysiology of bones, joints, and muscles, as well as the use of traction, bedboards, or assistive devices. Note also any medications prescribed for the patient that relate to this area.

Circulation   Under this category, collect all data that relate to the delivery of nutrients and oxygen to the cells and the removal of wastes from the cells. Objective data include pulses and blood pressure; color and warmth of the skin; medications taken for heart, blood pressure, or other cardiovascular problems; and any symptoms that are specific to cardiovascular problems. Include laboratory data that relate to hematology and blood chemistry in this category.

During your interview, try to elicit the patient's perception of any current cardiovascular problem, understanding of previous problems, and medications prescribed.

Elimination   This category covers the excretion of wastes from the large intestine and the urinary system. Observe the patient's bowel habits and the type and frequency of stools. Listen for bowel tones. Ask about the patient's normal pattern of bowel movements and characteristics of the stool, noting those that are unusual. Elicit any history of constipation or diarrhea, along with pertinent information about medication. Be aware of the pathophysiology of the GI system, and of any relevant medications or laboratory tests ordered by the physician.

The urinary system handles the excretion of waste products by the kidneys via the urethra and bladder. Note usual patterns of urination and the appearance and odor of the urine. Note whether a catheter of any kind is present. Measure urinary output and compare it to fluid intake. Note any problems with incontinence, any urinary pathophysiology, and any medications taken for urinary problems.

Fluid and Electrolyte Balance/Hydration   This category deals with keeping the proper fluid and electrolyte composition within the body. Observe fluid intake and output, including the type and amount of intravenous fluids being given. Note changes in alertness or mental capacity and changes in muscle tone. Observe for changes in respiration that are not related to exertion, and also for changes in cardiac rate and rhythm that are not due to heart disease. Alteration in the amount of fluid present in the tissues may be demonstrated by poor skin turgor or edema, as well as by observation of daily weight. Note serum electrolyte levels and any medications being received that might affect fluid and electrolyte balance.

Nutrition   This category deals with getting nutrients into the body. Observe the patient's eating habits (the amount of food taken and the kinds of foods preferred). Ask the patient about food likes and dislikes, dietary modification, and history in regard to food intake. Consider the patient's knowledge of proper nutrition as well as his or her understanding of any special dietary restrictions.

Oxygenation   This category includes all data concerned with getting oxygen into the lungs and carbon dioxide out of the lungs. Gather information on breathing patterns and changes in breathing patterns. Include observations of chest symmetry and of the rate, depth, and rhythm of respirations. Check breath sounds. Look for indications of impaired airways and for signs or symptoms of difficulty in respiration. Note the patient's need for oxygen. Note whether the patient coughs, whether suction is being applied, and what medications the patient used at home as well as those currently in use. Note any pathophysiology present.

Protection from Infection/Safety   These data are concerned with the effect of the total environment on the patient. Consider the environment both in light of the patient's ability to respond to it and in terms of safety from microorganisms for the patient and others. Include data concerning the care of equipment, the position of side rails, procedures for handwashing, and provisions for isolation. Consider also such factors as room temperature, cleanliness, drafts, lighting, and noise. Note whether the patient is able to reach the call light. Also note the accommodations (private or nonprivate room), the impact of other patients on your patient, and the location of the patient's room in relation to the nurses' station.

The ability to communicate with others is essential to maintaining safety and must be investigated. Can the person speak? If speech is not possible, is another method of communication being used? For a young child, find out what words are used for communicating body functions such as urination and defecation. Try to determine the extent of the child's vocabulary and the general pattern of speech.

Regulation and Sensation/Comfort   This category includes all characteristics associated with both the central nervous system and the autonomic nervous system, including special senses and pain. It also includes levels or states of consciousness. Special senses include visual and auditory acuity or lack of it and sensitivity to touch or lack of it. The pain component includes the nature of pain and its location, its duration, the patient's perception of its intensity, the pathophysiology involved, the length of time pain has been present, and all medications used to control it. Sometimes it is more appropriate to list pain under another area—when the pain is known to relate to a specific problem, for example. Be sure to include any pathophysiology of the nervous system (unconsciousness, tremor, and the like) and any related observations you have made.

Vision might be checked by asking the patient to read a name tag or a menu. You might ask whether he or she regularly wears glasses. Hearing may be checked by noting the patient's response to your questions and comments. If you suspect a problem, always validate your assumptions by asking the patient if he or she feels that there is a vision or hearing problem.

Rest and Sleep   Included in this category are data related to the patient's normal sleep and rest patterns and data that reflect how illness and/or hospitalization may have affected those patterns. Observe the patient's appearance. Does the patient appear tired or rested? What amount of sleep does the patient normally need, and what is the usual bedtime? Does the patient use any sleep aids (warm milk, medications) or need any special equipment (special mattress, extra pillows)? Both the patient's physical and psychological status are important. Identify factors that might be interfering with the amount and/or quality of sleep the patient is getting. Include such items as pain, equipment (noise, interference with comfort or normal position), other unusual noises, and the like. Consider the patient's diagnosis and what that means in terms of extra sleep and rest periods needed.

Skin Integrity/Hygiene   The condition of the skin—its turgor, hydration, color, lesions, wounds, rashes, scars, tattoos, and needle injection scars—should be noted. It is also important to list any sensitivity of the skin to soaps or lotions. Finally, include hygienic needs, among them the care of mouth, hair, and nails.

Psychosocial Needs

Psychosocial assessment is very complex and involves many different components. You will need to investigate the patient's development; mental health; sexuality; social, cultural, and ethnic identity; and values and beliefs.

Development   A person's life stage reflects that person's stage of development. To clearly understand a person's life stage, it is important to know his or her age, gender, occupation, and role in the family. For example, one client may be a 28-year-old woman who has a full-time job, a husband, and two children. This woman's response to hospitalization will be different from that of a 68-year-old retired man who lives alone. The problems surrounding adaptation to illness will be quite different. Try to learn people's perceptions of how well they meet the expectations related to their stage in life.

Mental Health (Self-Esteem, Love, and Belongingness)   Look for behavior and record any statements that indicate how the patient feels about himself or herself and his or her own life situation. What kind of immediate family or close support does the patient have? Is assistance available at home? Will the patient have visitors? How do the patient and significant others interact? What statements does the patient make regarding feelings about others and their support and about his or her relationship with them? Note eye contact, tone of voice, affect, and level of anxiety.

Sexuality Gather information about sexual difficulties, menstruation, and menopause. Note medications taken or pathophysiology that relates to the reproductive system.

It is especially important to gather information about sexuality when the person has had an illness that affects the reproductive system or gynecological, breast, or urological surgery. Sexuality is a very sensitive area for most people, so word your inquiries carefully and take care not to offend the patient or make him or her feel that you are prying into matters that do not concern you.

Social, Cultural, and Ethnic Identity You will need to assess each person within the context of his or her own cultural or ethnic environment, and how this affects the reaction to illness and/or hospitalization. Is the patient able to speak and understand English? Will general care customs, dietary restrictions or preferences, and/or religious practices make a difference in the way you approach the care of this patient? What are the expectations of the family regarding their participation in care? They may be accustomed to visiting in large groups, providing much of the care (especially any intimate aspects), and providing food for the patient. Does the patient have insurance or the ability to pay for care?

Values and Beliefs These may be based on an organized religion or on a general philosophical system. Note any religious preference listed on the hospital admission form. Ask the patient whether a religious advisor, pastor, or church should be notified. Observe religious or philosophical reading materials and conversation. Consult your hospital chaplain or written materials about any religious group with which you are not familiar, or ask the patient if there is any way in which you can be of help.

Body Systems Approach

In the body systems approach to assessment, data are organized according to the anatomic-

physiologic divisions of the body. Those who favor this approach often see it as fitting more easily into the systems used by other health care professionals; data, therefore, are more easily communicated throughout the health care system. This approach to nursing is based on dealing with imbalances or disturbances in basic body systems. In order to encompass the whole person, psychosocial concerns and the patient's environment are also included.

Circulatory Data Under this category, collect all data that relate to the delivery of nutrients and oxygen to the cells and removal of wastes from the cells. Objective data include pulse and blood pressure; color and warmth of the skin; medications taken for heart, blood pressure, or other cardiovascular problems; and any symptoms that are specific to cardiovascular problems. Include laboratory data that relate to hematology and blood chemistry in this category.

During your interview, try to elicit the patient's perception of any current cardiovascular problem, his or her understanding of any previous problems, and medications prescribed.

Fluid and electrolyte balance are very important components of circulatory data. Observe fluid intake and output, including the type and amount of intravenous fluids being given and the status of any site of entry into the circulatory system. Note changes in alertness or mental capacity and changes in muscle tone. Observe for changes in respiration that are not related to exertion and for changes in cardiac rate and rhythm that are not due to heart disease. Alteration in the amount of fluid present in the tissues may be demonstrated by poor skin turgor or edema, as well as by observation of daily weight. Note serum electrolyte levels and any medication being taken that might affect fluid and electrolyte balance.

Environmental Data These data are concerned with the total environment and its effect on the patient. Consider the environment both in light of the patient's ability to respond to it and in terms of safety from microorganisms for the patient and others. Include data concerning the care of equipment, the position of side rails, procedures for handwashing, and provisions for isolation. Consider also such factors as room temperature, cleanliness, drafts, lighting, and noise. Note whether the patient is able to reach the call light. Also note the accommodations (private or nonprivate room), the impact of other patients on your patient, and the location of the patient's room in relation to the nurses' station.

Gastrointestinal Data This category deals with getting nutrients into the body and excreting wastes from the large intestine. Observe the patient's eating habits (the amount of food taken and the kinds of foods preferred). Interview the patient about food likes and dislikes, dietary modification, and history in regard to food intake. Observe the patient's bowel habits and the type and frequency of stools. Listen for bowel tones. Ask about the patient's normal pattern of bowel movements and characteristics of the stool, noting those that are unusual. Elicit any history of constipation or diarrhea, along with pertinent information about medication. Be aware of the pathophysiology of the GI system, and of any relevant medications or laboratory tests ordered by the physician.

Genito-Urinary Data This approach combines the genital and urinary systems because of their close proximity in the female and their interrelationship in the male. In the genital or reproductive area, gather information about sexual difficulties, menstruation, and menopause. Note medications taken and pathophysiology or surgery that relates to the reproductive system.

The urinary system handles the excretion of waste products by the kidneys via the bladder and urethra. Note usual patterns of urination and the appearance and odor of the urine. Note whether a catheter of any kind is present. Measure urinary output and compare it to fluid intake. Note any problems with incontinence, any urinary pathophysiology, and any medications taken for urinary problems.

Integumentary Data Integument involves the condition of the skin and mucous membranes. The condition of the skin—its turgor, hydration, color, lesions, wounds, rashes, scars, tattoos, and needle injection scars—should be noted. It is also important to list any sensitivity of the skin to soaps or lotions. Finally, include hygienic needs, among them the care of mouth, hair, and nails.

Musculoskeletal Data This component pertains to the patient's ability to move and exercise for optimal functioning. Consider the patient's usual exercise at home, diversional choices, and the effects of exercise. Any recent variation from the norm, such as joint or muscle pain or disability, is important. The individual's posture and positioning and the level of activity ordered by the physician are other items of concern. Note the pathophysiology of bones, joints, and muscles, as well as the use of traction, bedboards, or assistive devices. Note also any medications prescribed for the patient that relate to this area.

Neural Data The nervous system includes all characteristics associated with both the central nervous system and the autonomic nervous system, including special senses and pain. Levels or states of consciousness and sleep patterns are included in these data. Special senses include visual and auditory acuity or lack of it, and sensitivity to touch or lack of it. The pain component includes the nature of pain and its location, its duration, the patient's perception of its intensity, the pathophysiology involved, the length of time pain has been present, and all medications used to control it. Sometimes it is more appropriate to list pain under another area—when the pain is known to relate to a specific problem, for example. Be sure to include any pathophysiology of the nervous system (unconsciousness, tremor, and the like) and any related observations you have made.

Vision might be checked by asking the patient to read a name tag or a menu. You might ask whether the patient regularly wears glasses. Hearing may be checked by noting the patient's response to your questions and comments. If you suspect a problem, always validate your assumptions by asking the patient if he or she feels that there is a vision or hearing problem.

Psychosocial Data Psychosocial assessment is very complex and involves many different components. You will need to investigate the patient's development; mental health; social, cultural, and ethnic identity; and values and beliefs.

Development A person's life stage reflects that person's stage of development. To clearly understand a person's life stage, it is important to know his or her age, gender, occupation, and role in the family. For example, one client may be a 28-year-old woman who has a full-time job, a husband, and two children. This woman's response to hospitalization will be different from that of a 68-year-old retired man who lives alone. The problems surrounding adaptation to illness will be quite different. Try to learn people's perceptions of how well they meet the expectations related to their stage in life.

Mental Health (Self-Esteem, Love, and Belongingness) Look for behavior and record any statements that indicate how the patient feels about himself or herself and his or her own life situation. What kind of immediate family or close support does the patient have? Is assistance available at home? Will the patient have visitors? How do the patient and significant others interact? What statements does the patient make regarding feelings about others and their support and about his or her relationship with them? Note eye contact, tone of voice, affect, and level of anxiety.

Social, Cultural, and Ethnic Identity You will need to assess each person within the context of his or her own cultural or ethnic environment, and how this affects his or her reactions to illness and/or hospitalization. Is the patient able to speak and understand English? Will general care customs, dietary restrictions or preferences, and/or religious practices make a difference in the way you approach the care of this patient? What are the expectations of the family regarding their participation in care? They may be accustomed to visiting in large groups, providing much of the care (especially any intimate aspects), and providing food for the patient. Does the patient have insurance or the ability to pay for care?

Values and Beliefs These may be based on an organized religion or on a general philosophical system. Note any religious preference listed on the hospital admission form. Ask the patient whether a religious advisor, pastor, or church should be notified. Observe religious or philosophical reading materials and conversation. Consult your hospital chaplain or written materials about any religious group with which you are not familiar, or ask the patient if there is any way in which you can be of help.

Respiratory Data This category includes all data concerned with getting oxygen into the lungs and carbon dioxide out of the lungs. Gather information on breathing patterns and changes in breathing patterns. Include observations of chest symmetry and of the rate, depth, and rhythm of respirations. Check breath sounds. Look for indications of impaired airways and for signs or symptoms of difficulty in respiration. Note the patient's need for oxygen. Note whether the patient coughs, whether suction is being applied, and what medications the patient used at home as well as those currently in use. Note any pathophysiology present.

Identifying the Patient's Problems: Nursing Diagnosis

After you have gathered data related to your patient, you will need to analyze the data and write nursing diagnoses. Nursing diagnoses are conclusions you reach based on the data you have collected. A nursing diagnosis includes a statement of an actual or potential problem and a statement indicating the etiology or etiologies of that problem.

One definition of a nursing diagnosis is as follows: "A nursing diagnosis is anything that requires nursing intervention and management, interferes with the quality of life the patient is used to or desires, and/or deals with concerns that the patient, significant others, and/or the nurse identify. The nursing diagnosis focuses attention on . . . a current or a potential problem . . . (and) provides direction for nursing care." (Doenges and Moorhouse, 1985)

A number of specific nursing diagnoses have been identified and approved by NANDA, the North American Nursing Diagnosis Association, and the list continues to be expanded every two years when that group meets. Etiology and defining characteristics have also been identified. You can find a current listing in any fundamentals text or in one of the many books available on nursing diagnosis. Again, a nursing diagnosis includes both a statement of the problem and a statement indicating the etiology of that problem. The etiology of the problem is especially important because your nursing intervention could well vary depending on the cause or causes of the problem. To illustrate, your nursing diagnosis might be "Bowel Elimination, Alteration in: Constipation related to lack of privacy." Change the etiology to "medications," however, and the appropriate intervention would be quite different.

Nursing diagnosis provides a common language for nurses to use in the identification of patient problems. With frequent use, you will begin to feel comfortable with this "new language." The use of nursing diagnoses helps to assure continuity of care for the patient who moves from one area of a health care setting to another or who must change facilities.

REFERENCES

Doenges, Marilynn, and Mary Moorhouse. *Nurse's Pocket Guide: Nursing Diagnosis with Interventions.* Philadelphia: F. A. Davis Company, 1985, p. 8.

BASIC DATA GATHERING GUIDE

Human Needs Approach

Patient Initials _____ Room _____ Major Health Problem _____

Physical Needs

I. Activity

  A. Posture

  B. Ability to move

  C. Gait

  D. Activity ordered

  E. Abnormalities

  F. Assistive devices

  G. Medications

II. Circulation

  A. Blood pressure

  B. Pulse

    1. Radial

    2. Apical

    3. Pedal

    4. Rhythm

  C. Skin and mucous membrane color

  D. Nailbed color

  E. Skin temperature

  F. Diagnostic/lab.

  G. Medications

III. Elimination

  A. Bowel

    1. Date of last B.M.

      a. Description

      b. Stool specimen?

    2. Control?

    3. Bowel sounds

    4. Medications

  B. Bladder

    1. Amount

    2. Appearance/odor

    3. Urinary control?

    4. Urinalysis results

    5. Medications

IV. Fluid and Electrolyte Balance/ Hydration

  A. Intake and output

  B. Intravenous fluids

    1. Type

    2. Amount

  C. Abnormalities

  D. Daily weight?

  E. Serum electrolytes

  F. Medications

V. Nutrition
  A. Diet

  B. Height and weight

  C. Amount eaten

  D. Abnormalities

  E. Medications

VI. Oxygenation
  A. Respiration
    1. Rate

    2. Rhythm

    3. Depth

    4. Chest movement

  B. Breath sounds

  C. Secretions
    1. Amount

    2. Appearance

  D. Cough?

  E. Diagnostic/lab.

  F. Medications

VII. Protection from Infection/Safety
  A. Temperature

  B. Speech

  C. Environment
    1. Side rails

    2. Call light

    3. Accommodations

  D. Gait

  E. Medications

VIII. Regulation and Sensation/Comfort
  A. Level of consciousness

  B. Special senses
    1. Vision

    2. Hearing

    3. Tactile sense

  C. Pain
    1. Description

    2. Location

    3. Duration

    4. Medications

IX. Rest and Sleep
  A. Normal sleep patterns

  B. Sleep aids?

  C. Appearance

  D. Factors interfering with rest/ sleep

X. Skin Integrity/Hygiene
  A. Skin temperature

  B. Color

  C. Integrity

  D. Lesions/wounds/scars?

  E. Rash?

  F. Hydration

  G. Sensitivity to soap/lotion?

  H. Hygiene

  I. Medications

Psychosocial Needs

XI. Development

    A. Age

    B. Life stage

    C. Occupation

    D. Position in family unit

XII. Mental Health

    A. Self-esteem

      1. Feelings about self

      2. Behaviors exhibited

    B. Love and belongingness

      1. Immediate family

      2. Help at home

      3. Feelings about relationships

      4. Behaviors exhibited

XIII. Sexuality

    A. Gender

    B. Last menstrual period (LMP)—menstrual history

    C. Gravida; para?

    D. Significant other

    E. Concerns expressed

    F. Diagnostic/lab.

    G. Medications

XIV. Social, Cultural, and Ethnic Identity

    A. Country of origin

    B. Language?

    C. Special needs?

    D. Insurance/financial support?

XV. Values and Beliefs

    A. Religious preference

    B. Notification desired?

    C. Special needs?

BASIC DATA GATHERING GUIDE

Body Systems Approach

Patient Initials _____ Room _____ Major Health Problem _____

I. Circulatory
   A. Blood pressure

   B. Pulse
     1. Radial

     2. Apical

     3. Pedal

     4. Rhythm

   C. Skin/mucous membrane color

   D. Nailbed color

   E. Skin temperature

   F. Intravenous fluids
     1. Type

     2. Amount

   G. Diagnostic/lab.

   H. Medications

II. Environmental
   A. Side rails

   B. Bed position

   C. Equipment

III. Gastrointestinal
   A. Diet

   B. Height and weight

   C. Amount eaten

   D. Bowel function
     1. Date of last B.M.

     2. Description

     3. Bowel sounds

   E. Abnormalities

   F. Medications

   G. Diagnostic/lab.

IV. Genito-Urinary
   A. Gender

   B. Last menstrual period (LMP)—menstrual history

   C. Gravida; para?

   D. Significant other

   E. Concerns expressed

   F. Urination
     1. Amount

     2. Appearance/odor

   G. Urinary control?

   H. Urinalysis results

   I. Medications

V. Integumentary
   A. Skin temperature

   B. Color

   C. Integrity

D. Hydration

E. Rash?

F. Lesions/wounds/scars?

G. Sensitivity to soap/lotion?

H. Hygiene

I. Medications

VI. Musculoskeletal
   A. Posture

   B. Ability to move

   C. Activity ordered

   D. Abnormalities

   E. Assistive devices

   F. Medications

   G. Diagnostic/lab.

VII. Neural
   A. Temperature

   B. Speech

   C. Vision

   D. Hearing

   E. Tactile sense

   F. Sleep pattern

   G. Gait

   H. Pain
      1. Location

      2. Duration

      3. Cause

      4. Patient description

I. Medications

J. Diagnostic/lab.

VIII. Psychosocial
   A. Development
      1. Age

      2. Life stage

      3. Occupation

      4. Position in family unit

   B. Mental health
      1. Self-esteem
         a. Feelings about self

         b. Behaviors exhibited
      2. Love and belongingness
         a. Immediate family

         b. Help at home

         c. Feelings about relationships

         d. Behaviors exhibited

   C. Social, cultural, and ethnic identity
      1. Country of origin

      2. Language?

      3. Special needs?

      4. Insurance/financial support?

   D. Values and beliefs
      1. Religious preference

      2. Notification desired?

      3. Special needs?

IX. Respiratory
 A. Respiration
  1. Rate

  2. Rhythm

  3. Depth

  4. Chest movement

 B. Breath sounds

C. Secretions
 1. Amount

 2. Appearance

D. Cough?

E. Diagnostic/lab.

F. Medications

QUIZ

Short-Answer Questions

For questions 1–3, provide answers for (a) the human needs approach and (b) the body systems approach.

1. Respiratory rate is included in which assessment category?

   a. _____

   b. _____

2. Chest pain could be listed under which assessment category?

   a. _____

   b. _____

3. A patient tells you that he or she can breathe comfortably at night only if resting on two pillows. Under which assessment category should this information be listed?

   a. _____

   b. _____

Multiple-Choice Questions

For questions 4–7, indicate which data gathering method would be most useful in acquiring the information indicated: (a) interview, (b) observation, (c) physical examination, (d) consultation with other members of the health care team, or (e) review of the literature.

_____ 4. The best way to learn whether a patient has had a bowel movement during your shift.

_____ 5. The best way to learn whether a patient is developing edema (tissue swelling from retained fluid).

_____ 6. For a night nurse, the best way to learn the sleeping patterns of a patient.

_____ 7. The best way to learn the potential side effects of a medication the patient is taking.

For questions 8–12, mark *O* if the data are objective and *S* if they are subjective.

_____ 8. The patient says he or she has severe nausea.

_____ 9. After ambulation, the patient is pale and has a pulse rate of 100.

_____ 10. The patient feels depressed.

_____ 11. The patient is breathing shallowly at a rate of 30 respirations per minute.

_____ 12. The laboratory report indicates that the patient has a hemoglobin level of 8.

MODULE 6

Documentation

PREREQUISITES

Successful completion of the following modules:

OVERALL OBJECTIVE

To use patients' records to communicate effectively with other health care team members and provide a legal record of the nursing aspect of patients' care.

SPECIFIC LEARNING OBJECTIVES

	Know Facts and Principles	Apply Facts and Principles	Demonstrate Ability	Evaluate Performance
1. *Purposes*	Explain rationale for use of chart as a legal record, for determining quality of care, and for communication	Given a situation in which someone wants information from a chart, determine whether that should be permitted	Maintain privacy of patient's record. Use record to gain information regarding patient.	Evaluate own performance
2. *Content*	List types of information to be recorded. Give rationale for use of objective terminology. State situations in which subjective terminology is appropriate.	Given a situation, do sample charting containing all appropriate information. . Given a situation, describe it in objective terminology.	Record all needed information as outlined on Performance Checklist. Use objective terminology for all observations. Identify subjective material clearly. State problems correctly. Describe nursing actions taken. Record evaluation of patient response.	Evaluate own performance using Performance Checklist
3. *Methods of organization of content*	List two methods of organization of contents of chart	Given a sample chart, identify method of organization in use	Document appropriately given method of organization	Evaluate with instructor
4. *Styles of progress notes*	List two styles of writing progress notes	Given a situation, write progress notes using either style	Document in style appropriate to facility	Evaluate documentation with instructor

LEARNING ACTIVITIES	VOCABULARY

LEARNING ACTIVITIES

1. Review the Specific Learning Objectives.
2. Review the abbreviations in Ellis and Nowlis, *Nursing: A Human Needs Approach*, or those in the procedure manual of your facility and those in Tables 6.1, 6.2, 6.3, and 6.4 in this module.
3. Read the section on written communication in Ellis and Nowlis, *Nursing: A Human Needs Approach*, or comparable material in another textbook.
4. Look up the module vocabulary terms in the Glossary.
5. Read through the module.
6. If samples of charting are available in your practice setting, review them.
7. Practice charting using the situations provided in the module. Make a sample form for practice charting that is similar to the one used in your facility.
8. Exchange your practice charting with another student and check each other's work. Review and rewrite your own charting based on this critique.
9. Have your instructor review your practice charting.
10. Review your instructor's comments and rewrite your practice charting if necessary.
11. Chart data regarding a patient to whom you are assigned. Make a first draft on a piece of paper and have it reviewed by your clinical instructor before you write in the patient's record.
12. Continue to chart on patients assigned in the clinical area. Have your first draft reviewed before writing in patients' records until your instructor directs you to do otherwise.

VOCABULARY

assessment
data
excretion
flow sheet
graphic
infused
ingested
legibility
military (24-hour) clock
narrative charting
objective
problem-oriented medical record (POMR)
problem-oriented record (POR)
subjective

DOCUMENTATION

Rationale for the Use of This Skill

The chart, or patient's record, is used by all members of the health care team to follow the patient's progress and to learn what is being done concerning that progress by members of the team. Therefore, entries into the record must be clear. The chart serves as a legal record of care and is used to determine the quality of care being given; therefore accuracy, legibility, and clarity are very important. Finally, each health care facility establishes its own format for patients' records. This format must be used for all documentation in the facility.[1]

Types of Records

All health care agencies keep many different records. All recording systems, however, share characteristics that, if you understand them, will make it easier for you to adapt to any system you find.

Temporary Records

A nursing unit will almost always have a variety of temporary records that are used to facilitate communication or to maintain information for easy accessibility. These are valuable, but they must be recognized as temporary and should not be used as the only record of important information about the patient. Although they are temporary, these records do need to be accurate.

A "Vital Signs List" is often maintained. This list may include the temperature, pulse, respiration, and blood pressure of every patient on the unit. If one person is assigned to take all these measurements, the list is a convenient way to record the data as they are obtained. The list may also serve as a quick reference for a nurse in charge of the unit. The list may be used for immediate access, with the information being transferred to the individual patient's permanent record at a later time by the nurse responsible for care or by a unit secretary.

Many nursing units maintain a chalk board or other list for noting patients' special needs. This board might, for example, list patients who are not allowed to take oral food and fluids, those to be weighed daily, those with intravenous infusions, and those going for special tests or surgery. This allows a staff member to obtain information quickly and conveniently. It is important that these lists be updated whenever a change in the patient's plan of care occurs.

Temporary records may also be placed at the bedside to facilitate carrying out specific measures for the patient. An example would be a "turning record" that specifies when the patient is to be turned and to which position. Having the information at the bedside makes it easier for the staff person to keep track of what is needed.

Another common temporary record is a fluid intake and output worksheet. This is used to keep track of all fluids taken by a patient and all fluid losses that occur. (See Module 15, Intake and Output, for further instructions.)

In some facilities, the Nursing Care Plan is kept on a card file (such as a Kardex) and changed as the patient's care needs change. This record may be written in pencil and considered a temporary record. In many settings, however, the Nursing Care Plan is now considered a permanent part of the record and is written in ink and retained along with the other permanent parts of the chart.

The Patient's Chart

The permanent record of the patient's health care is called the "chart." This record is the *legal* record of care. During the patient's stay in a health care facility, the chart serves as a means of communication among members of the health care team. It is also used to evaluate the quality of care given. In addition, data from the chart are used for teaching and research.

Charting Content

In order to provide a complete record, you must determine what information to include in your charting. This is a complex responsibility, and one in which you will become more skilled with experience. The Joint Commission on Accredi-

---

[1]You will note that the rationale for action is emphasized throughout the module by the use of italics.

tation of Hospitals states, "Documentation of nursing care shall be pertinent and concise and shall reflect the patient's status. Nursing documentation shall reflect the patient's needs, problems, capabilities, and limitations. Nursing intervention and patient response must be noted" (JCAH, 1983). Basically, you should try to provide a clear and concise record of the nursing process in relation to the individual patient. This includes aspects of assessment, planning, intervention, and evaluation.

Assessment data include both subjective and objective information. You will have to decide which assessment data are relevant in a particular situation. As a general guideline, record assessment data when they reflect (1) findings that relate to the patient's reason for being hospitalized, (2) any abnormal findings, and (3) normal findings that relate to previously noted problems. In addition to these data, you also must record any new problems that you have identified.

Depending on the policies of your facility, *planning data* may or may not be included in the chart. In some institutions, planning is recorded on a separate nursing care plan, which is then included with the rest of a patient's record at the time of discharge.

Intervention data include nursing actions that are taken in response to an existing problem, as well as measures that are planned to prevent problems. Even actions that are part of routine care, such as those related to hygiene, are usually noted in some manner.

Evaluation data, which gauge the effectiveness of nursing actions and therapies, are also important. They are a vital aspect of planning future care.

Methods of Organization of Content

Although you will see a variety of chart forms and styles of documentation, there are currently two methods of organizing the information in a patient's record: the source-oriented method and the problem-oriented record (POR or POMR). Both methods contain the following elements:

1. *Data base*   This includes the initial history and physical examination, original labora-tory and diagnostic test results, the social and financial data, and the admission nursing interview. The particular term *data base* may not be used, but this type of information will be part of the record.

2. *Flow sheets*   These are charts or graphs that allow information to be recorded quickly and progress to be monitored with ease. Some facilities use many different flow sheets; others, only a few. Usually, you will use flow sheets to record vital signs, intake and output, medications given, and routine nursing care, although a more complex parameter such as patient teaching may also be recorded on flow sheets. Again, the term *flow sheet* may not be used, but you will easily recognize the charts and graphs that compose this element.

3. *Progress notes*   The most important difference between the methods of charting is the structure of the progress notes. In source-oriented records, these are separated: there is one form for the physician's progress notes, another for the nurses' notes, and still others for the notes of other health care groups (physical therapists, respiratory therapists, occupational therapists). Since source-oriented records may use fewer flow sheets, you may find most information in the various progress notes. With problem-oriented records, all progress notes (from all sources) use the same form. The notes may have a formal, specific structure (page 95), which makes them easier to use in finding information.

4. *Problem list*   A fourth feature—the problem list—was once seen as unique to POR, but it is now found in other documentation systems as well. This list serves as a combination table of contents and index to the patient's condition and progress. Each problem is numbered and titled for easy reference. Titles may be done according to medical diagnoses, patient problems, or nursing diagnoses, depending on the setting. The date when the problem was initially identified is included, and once the problem is resolved, that fact and the date of resolution are added.

Mechanics of Charting

Legal Standards

As a legal record, a chart must conform to certain legal standards. All entries must be in ink *so that changes are noticeable and the record is permanent.* Your facility may specify a particular color of ink to be used. If it has no policy, remember that black or dark blue ink reproduces especially well on microfilm. Legibility is critical; obviously, *statements that are not legible are not usable.*

Errors If you make an error, draw a line through the incorrect entry so that it remains legible. In the space above, write "error" and your initials. This practice is traditional. Recently, attorneys have recommended adding a brief note as to the nature of the error, which would be helpful if the chart were needed in a legal proceeding. Such a note might read "charted on wrong chart" and your initials. This notation and the traditional "error" notation are both legally correct, so follow the policy of your facility. If it has no policy, we recommend the second type of notation.

Spaces If you are using the narrative form of charting, do not leave blank spaces. Draw a straight line through any empty space *to prevent later entries from being made above your signature.*

Signature When you sign a notation on a patient's record, use your first initial and full last name followed by the abbreviation of your position. If you were a student nurse named Jane Smith, you would sign the record "J. Smith SN" (unless your facility required that you sign your full name). Traditionally, student nurses have used the abbreviation *SN* (student nurse) to designate their position. In some areas, the current practice is to use the abbreviation *NS* (nursing student). Your instructor will indicate the notation your facility prefers.

You must use the designation appropriate to your current position. For instance, a licensed practical nurse who is currently enrolled in a program preparing registered nurses would use the SN or NS designation while working as a student. The nurse would use the LPN designation only when employed by and working for the facility as an LPN.

Time Notations of time and date are important *for health care reasons as well as for legal reasons. Time sequences can be crucial in certain problems.*

You can note time in conventional notation or according to the 24-hour clock, or military clock. The 24-hour clock works as follows: when the time reaches 12:00 noon (or 1200), instead of returning to 1:00 p.m., the time goes on to 1300, continuing until 2400 is reached, at midnight. The hours before noon are recorded as 0100, 0200, 0300, and so on. (See Figure 6.1.) The 24-hour clock eliminates confusion as to whether something took place before noon (a.m.) or after noon (p.m.). In some facilities this confusion is lessened by using different ink colors for different shifts or different times of day. This method is quite effective in the original, but when records are photocopied or microfilmed, the color distinction is lost, and certain colors do not reproduce as well as others.

Right to Privacy A chart is a legally protected, private record of a patient's care. Access to a chart is restricted to those in the facility using it for care and, in some instances, for research or teaching. A chart may not be photocopied except following careful procedures designed to protect the patient's privacy. If you, as a student, are using a chart as a learning tool, it is your responsibility to protect the patient's privacy by not using his or her name or any identifying statements in any notations you make for your own use. Papers or case studies based on a patient's care should likewise protect the anonymity of the patient.

The "chart," or medical record, is the *property* of the hospital, but patients *do* have a right to the *information* contained in that record. Usually, however, there is a procedure that the patient must follow to obtain this information, and you must know what that procedure is. Clear and timely explanations and progress reports to patients and families may result in fewer requests to see the chart.

Special Terminology and Abbreviations

Traditionally, a great deal of specialized medical terminology has been used in charting. In addition, there are traditional patterns of word usage. As a beginner, concentrate on describing

Conventional Time	24-hour Clock	Conventional Time	24-hour Clock
1 A.M.	0100	1 P.M.	1300
2 A.M.	0200	2 P.M.	1400
3 A.M.	0300	3 P.M.	1500
4 A.M.	0400	4 P.M.	1600
5 A.M.	0500	5 P.M.	1700
6 A.M.	0600	6 P.M.	1800
7 A.M.	0700	7 P.M.	1900
8 A.M.	0800	8 P.M.	2000
9 A.M.	0900	9 P.M.	2100
10 A.M.	1000	10 P.M.	2200
11 A.M.	1100	11 P.M.	2300
12 noon	1200	12 midnight	2400

FIGURE 6.1 *TIME NOTATION*

what you see. Even if you do not know the medical terminology, you will be understood if you clearly describe the situation.

As you progress in your nursing and related studies, you will pick up a large medical vocabulary. Then, you must be careful to use this vocabulary effectively and correctly, as needed. For example, a false belief is called a delusion. Rather than charting that a patient has a delusion, chart the exact nature of his or her belief. *This is certainly more informative to others using the chart. (It can also save you from jumping to conclusions: sometimes what appears to be a false belief is true.)*

Abbreviations are used in charting *to save time and space.* Most nursing texts include a list of common abbreviations, and health care facilities often have their own lists of approved abbreviations. Although certain abbreviations are in general usage, others are used only in one geographic area. When in doubt, use the full term, which will be understood regardless of local custom. This is particularly true for simple initial-type abbreviations. (See Tables 6.1, 6.2, 6.3, and 6.4 for special terminology and abbreviations.)

In charting, sentences are typically reduced to their essential components *in order to lessen work and decrease the space used.* Thus articles (*a, an, the*) and even verbs may be omitted. *Because the entire chart is about an individual patient,* the subject of a sentence is omitted when it represents the patient (see Example 1). Do not omit the subject if it represents someone other than the patient. Also, when you omit words, be careful that your meaning remains clear. Be sure to begin each statement with a capital letter and end it with a period, even if the statement is not a complete sentence. *This helps to clarify meaning.*

Chart Forms

Many different chart forms are in use. It is important that you become familiar with all the forms used in your facility, *so that you know where to look for information you need as well as where to record your own data.* The ones to concentrate on initially are those that it is the nurses' responsibility to maintain. These usually include a graphic chart for vital signs, an intake and output record, a checklist for routine care, a medication record, and the nursing progress notes. Other forms that may be your responsibility are the parenteral fluid record, the diabetic record (for recording urine testing, blood sugar results, and insulin given), the blood pressure graph, and the patient teaching flow sheet.

Example 1 Using the Minimum Number of Words

Thought: The patient ate all of the soft diet.
Charted: Ate all of soft diet.

Thought: Bedbath was given to the patient by the nurse.
Charted: Bedbath given.

TABLE 6.1 DESCRIPTIVE CHARTING TERMS

1. *Body location* Use specific anatomical terms. For example:
      Right upper quadrant
      Left upper quadrant
      Right lower quadrant
      Left lower quadrant
      Distal/proximal

2. *Body functions* Urinate—void
      Have a bowel movement—defecate
      Profuse sweating—diaphoresis
      Walk—ambulate

3. *Skin description* Intact—not open, broken, or blemished
      Moist/dry
      Smooth, rough, cracked
      Warm, brown (light, medium, dark): describes healthy color of the
          black- or brown-skinned person
      Warm, pink: describes healthy color of what is usually termed white
          skin
      Warm, tan: healthy color of most Asians and those termed dark-
          complected
      Dull, ash brown: black person's skin without adequate blood supply
      Dull, gray-brown: black or dark-complected person's skin with
          unoxygenated blood apparent
      Pale, pallor: white person's skin without adequate blood supply
      Cyanotic: blue-gray color in skin of white person and in conjunctiva,
          mucous membranes, and nailbeds of all people

4. *Nutrition* List proportion of meal eaten:
      ¼, ½, ¾; all (*not* poor or good)
      Specify types of foods eaten when more specific information needed

5. *Urine description* Color: pale, yellow, amber, dark amber
      Clarity: clear, cloudy, smokey
      Contents: mucus, clots, sediment

6. *Stool description* Color: black, brown, clay-colored (gray)
      Consistency: liquid, watery, semiformed, soft, formed, hard
      Tarry: indicates black, sticky
      Mucoid: indicates contains mucus

7. *Drainage or secretions* Quantity: Exact measurement preferred
          Estimate milliliters if you have a standard to compare.
          Specify number of dressings saturated.
          Other terms: slight, scanty, small, moderate, large, copious,
              profuse.
      Character: Watery, thin
          Thick, tenacious
          Stringy
          Mucoid (like mucus)
          Serous (like serum)
          Sanguineous (with blood)

TABLE 6.1   DESCRIPTIVE CHARTING TERMS *continued*

Serosanguineous (serum and blood mixed)
Purulent—containing pus

8. *Mental attitude or mood*	When you observe behavior, ask the patient for an appraisal of his or her own feelings. Chart both your description of the patient's behavior and the patient's statement of feelings.

Patient's statement of feelings	*Behaviors observed*
a. "I feel depressed." "I feel sad."	Does not smile. Avoids eye contact. Drooping posture. Cries when alone.
b. "I am glad to go home." "I am happy."	Speaks with animation. Smiles and jokes. Moves about room briskly.
c. "I am worried." "I feel anxious."	Asks many questions. Paces the floor. In constant movement. Short attention span. Worried look on face.
d. "I am mad." "I feel angry."	Loud and belligerent. Frown on face. Vigorous movements.

TABLE 6.2 COMMON ABBREVIATIONS

Abbreviation	Latin Meaning	English Meaning
@		at
abd.		abdomen
a.c.	ante cibum	before meals
A.D.L.		activities of daily living
ad lib.	ad libitum	at will
ax.		axillary
b.i.d.	bis in die	twice a day
B.M.		bowel movement
B.P.		blood pressure
B.R.P.		bathroom privileges
c̄	cum	with
cap.		capsule
c/o		complains of
D.O.A.		dead on arrival
et	et	and
Frax., Fx.		fractional, fracture
gtt.	gutta	drop
h.	hora	hour
H/P		history and physical
h.s.	hora somni	hour of sleep (bedtime)
I.M.		intramuscular
I.V.		intravenous
K.V.O.		keep vein open (with intravenous infusion)
L.L.Q.		left lower quadrant (of abdomen)
L.U.Q.		left upper quadrant (of abdomen)
N.P.O.	non per ora	nothing by mouth
n.r.	non repetatur	not to be repeated
"o"		orally
o.d.	omne die	every day
O.D.	oculus dexter	right eye
O.S.	oculus sinister	left eye
O.T.		occupational therapy
O.U.	oculi uterque	each eye
p.c.	post cibum	after meals
p.o.	per ora	by mouth
p.r.n.	pro re nata	when needed
P.T.		physical therapy
q.s.	quantum sufficiat	sufficient quantity
q.d.	quaque die	each day
q.h.	quaque hora	every hour
q.2h.		every two hours
q.3h., etc.		every three hours, etc.
q.i.d.	quater in die	four times a day
q.o.d.	quaque alto die	every other day
R.L.Q.		right lower quadrant (of abdomen)
R.O.M.		range of motion
R.U.Q.		right upper quadrant (of abdomen)

TABLE 6.2   COMMON ABBREVIATIONS *continued*

Abbreviation	Latin Meaning	English Meaning
s̄	sine	without
s.o.b.		short of breath
s.o.s.	si opus sit	if necessary
spec.		specimen
stat.	statim	immediately
sub q.		subcutaneous
tab.		tablet
t.i.d.	ter in dies	three times a day
T.K.O.		to keep open (intravenous infusion)
T.L.C.		tender loving care
T.P.R.		temperature, pulse, and respiration
U.A.		urine analysis
ung.	unguent	ointment

TABLE 6.3   ABBREVIATIONS OF MEDICAL CONDITIONS

Abbreviation	Condition
A.R.D.S.	adult respiratory distress syndrome
A.K. Amp.	above-knee amputation
A.S.C.V.D.	arteriosclerotic cardiovascular disease
A.S.H.D.	arteriosclerotic heart disease
B.E.	bacterial endocarditis
B.K. Amp.	below-knee amputation
B.P.H.	benign prostatic hypertrophy
Ca.	cancer (carcinoma)
C.F.	cystic fibrosis
C.H.D.	coronary heart disease
C.H.F.	congestive heart failure
C.O.P.D.	chronic obstructive pulmonary disease
C.V.A.	cerebral vascular accident
D.&C.	dilation and curettage (of uterus)
D.I.C.	disseminated intravascular coagulation
D.T.'s	delirium tremens
F.U.O.	fever of undetermined origin
G.B.	gall bladder
G.C.	gonococcal infection
H.C.V.D.	hypertensive cardiovascular disease
L.T.B.	laryngo-tracheobronchitis
M.I.	myocardial infarction, mitral insufficiency
M.S.	multiple sclerosis
P.A.P.	primary atypical pneumonia
P.I.D.	pelvic inflammatory disease
P.V.D.	peripheral vascular disease
R.D.S.	respiratory distress syndrome
R.F.	rheumatic fever
R.H.D.	rheumatic heart disease
S.B.E.	subacute bacterial endocarditis
S.I.D.S.	sudden infant death syndrome
T.&A.	tonsillectomy and adenoidectomy
T.B. or T.B.C.	tuberculosis
T.I.A.	transient ischemic attacks
T.U.R.B.	transurethral resection of the bladder
T.U.R.P.	transurethral resection of the prostate
U.R.I.	upper respiratory infection
U.T.I.	urinary tract infection

TABLE 6.4   COMBINING FORMS

The combining form may appear at the beginning of, within, or at the end of a term. By identifying the meaning of each combining form contained in a word, it is possible to discern the meaning of the word. A dash preceding the form indicates that it is most commonly a suffix (appearing at the end of a term); a dash following the form indicates that it is most commonly a prefix (appearing at the beginning of a term).

Form	Meaning
a-, an-	without
ab-	away from
ad-	to, toward
adeno-	gland
-algia	pain
ambi-	on two sides
angio-	vessel
ano-	anus
ante-	before, forward
arterio-	artery
arthro-	joint
bis-	two
broncho-	bronchus
cardi-, cardio-	heart
-cele	hernia, tumor, protrusion
-centesis	puncture
cepha-, cephalo-	head
cerebro-	cerebrum of brain
cervico-	neck
chole-	bile
cholecysto-	gall bladder
chondro-	cartilage
circum-	around
cranio-	head
cysto-	sac, cyst, bladder (most often urinary bladder)
-cyte	cell
derm-	skin
dys-	abnormal, painful
-ectasis	expansion, dilation
-ectomy	excision
-emia	blood
encephalo-	brain
endo-	within, inner layer
entero-	intestines
ex-	out, out of, away from
exo-	outside, outer layer
gastro-	stomach
hem-, hema-, hemo-, hemato-	blood
hemi-	half

TABLE 6.4 COMBINING FORMS *continued*

Form	Meaning
hepato-	liver
histo-	tissue
hyper-	excessive
hypo-	low, lesser
hystero-	uterus
-iasis	condition, formation of, presence of
ileo-	ileum (part of small intestine)
ilio-	ilium (part of pelvic bones)
intra-	within
-itis	inflammation of
laparo-	loin, flank, abdomen
laryngo-	larynx
latero-	side
lith-	stone
lympho-	lymph
-lysis	dissolution, breaking down
macro-	large
mal-	bad, poor
-malacia	softening
masto-	breast
medio-	middle
-megaly	enlargement
meningo-	meninges
micro-	small, microscopic
mono-	single
myelo-	bone marrow, spinal cord
myo-	muscle
naso-	nose
neo-	new
nephro-	kidney
neuro-	nerve
non-	not
oculo-	eye
odonto-	tooth
-oma	tumor
oophoro-	ovary
ophthalmo-	eye
orchio-, orchido-	testes
oro-	mouth
-orrhaphy	suture/repair of
os-	bone, mouth
-osis	condition, disease, increase
osteo-	bone
-ostomy	artificially created opening into an organ
oto-	ear
-otomy	incision into
ovario-	ovary
para-	beside, along with

TABLE 6.4 COMBINING FORMS *continued*

Form	Meaning
-pathy	disease
-penia	deficiency, decrease
peri-	around
-pexy	suspension, fixation
pharyngo-	pharynx
phlebo-	vein
-plasty	surgical correction, plastic repair of
-plegia	paralysis
pneumo-	lungs, breath
post-	after
pro-	in front of, before
procto-	rectum
pseudo-	false
-ptosis	falling, drooping
pyo-	pus
retro-	behind
rhino-	nose
salpingo-	Fallopian tube
sclero-	hard
-spasm	involuntary contraction
spleno-	spleen
sterno-	sternum
super-, supra-	above, more than
teno-	tendon
thoraco-	thorax, chest
thyro-	thyroid
tracheo-	trachea
trans-	across, throughout
urethro-	urethra
uro-	urine, urinary
utero-	uterus
vaso-	blood vessel
veno-	vein

Using Flow Sheets

Flow sheets allow information to be recorded in tables or graphs. This facilitates charting in that *it takes less time to record information on a table than to write it in a paragraph.* In most instances, *it is also easier to review data when they appear in a table or graph.*

All systems of charting use some standard flow sheets, such as a graph for temperature, pulse, and respirations, and a table for intake and output. Some facilities have more flow sheets than others. In the narrative system of charting, anything that does not fit onto one of the existing forms is written into the progress notes. In the Problem-Oriented Record system, you are encouraged to initiate flow sheets whenever you will be collecting data or performing actions on a regular basis. Blank forms are usually available for this purpose. Thus, it will be your responsibility to figure out how best to represent the information in a table. Be sure you provide a place to note the date and time of each item in your table.

Writing Progress Notes

Narrative Charting

Narrative charting, as the name indicates, is a narration, or telling, of information. Most narrative charting is time-sequenced. You begin your statement with the data that were observed or that occurred first, and move forward in time (see Example 2). This type of narration is easy to follow, and most persons find that it traces thought patterns well. Finding relevant data regarding a single problem can be difficult, however, since a great deal of material must be read to gather a small amount of data. Thus, individual hospitals have made some modifications to narrative charting. Checklists and graphs are sometimes used for routine information, and the narration itself may be organized according to anatomical systems or assessment categories. In this case, you would chart, in a time sequence, all the information available on one area before going on to another category (see Examples 3 and 4).

Problem-Oriented Medical Records

In this style, progress notes are written for significant data regarding any problem, and detailed data may be entered by any member of the health care team. The following format is frequently used (sometimes not all components are included).

Problem   Identified by number and title
Subjective data   The patient's perception or statements regarding the problem
Objective data   Your observation regarding the problem and data from the chart that are relevant (for example, temperature and blood pressure)
Assessment   The conclusions you reach based on the data gathered. (This is slightly different from the common meaning of assessment. Some persons call this *analysis.*)
Plan   Your plan of action to deal with the problem

This format is commonly called *SOAP notation,* and the process has been called *SOAPing* (see Examples 5–7), from the terms *Subjective, Objective, Assessment,* and *Plan.* Although the SOAP format was developed for use with POR,

*Example 2 Simple Narrative Progress Note

1/1/88

7:00 a.m.	a.m. care. Up in chair c̄ assistance for 30 minutes. No c/o weakness or fatigue. IV running @ 22 gtt/min into R. forearm. Abd. dressing dry and intact.
7:30 a.m.	Assisted back to bed. Voided 250 ml clear straw-colored urine. Moderate-sized, soft, dark brown BM. Demerol 75 mg. IM given for moderate abd. incisional pain. Stated relief in 20 min.
8:30 a.m.	Complete bedbath given. ROM done.
9:00–10:30 a.m.	Rested quietly in bed. No further c/o pain.

J. Jones, R.N.

*Example 3 Modified Narrative Progress Note

1/1/88

| 7:00–10:30 a.m. | Hygiene: a.m. care ā bkft. Complete bedbath.
Activity: Up in chair c̄ assistance for bkft. No c/o fatigue or weakness. ROM p̄ bath.
Nutrition: Ate all of soft diet.
Elimination: Voided 250 ml clear amber urine @ 8:00. Moderate amt soft dark brown BM @ 8:00.
Pain: c/o moderate abd. incisional pain @ 8:00. Demerol 75 mg. IM given. Stated relief in 20 minutes. No further pain in a.m.
Fluids and Elec.: IV running at 22 gtt/min into R forearm. Site s̄ redness, pain, swelling. |

J. Jones, R.N.

*Flow sheets are commonly used for the IV, the abd. dressing, and pain med (prn meds), making less detail necessary in the progress notes.

*Example 4 Modified Narrative Progress Note

1/1/88

7:00–
10:30
a.m.

Circ: IV running at 22 gtt/min into R. forearm. Abd. drg. dry and intact.
GI: Ate all of soft diet. Mod. amt. soft, dark brown BM @ 8:00.
GU: Voided 250 ml clear amber urine @ 8:00.
Musc-Skel: Up in chair c̄ assistance for 30 minutes. No c/o weakness or fatigue. ROM p̄ bath. Rested p̄ ROM.
Neur: c/o moderate abd incisional pain @ 8:00. Demerol 75 mg. IM given. Stated relief in 20 min. No further pain in a.m.

J. Jones, R.N.

Example 5 POMR Progress Note Using Nursing Diagnosis Title (SOAPing)

1/22/88
7:00–3:30 p.m.

3. Alteration in comfort: Abd. pain related to retained gas
S States pain relieved by passing flatus but has not been able to pass flatus.
O Abd. feels tense and hard. Guards when moving.
A Has retained gas.
P Increase ambulation. Encourage movement in bed.

J. Jones, R.N.

it may be used for progress notes even when the record is not entirely problem-oriented.

On occasion, facilities modify the POMR and use a more traditional style for progress notes. It is also common for facilities to make individual modifications in charting style. You should consult the procedure book in your clinical setting for specific policies and procedures related to documentation.

Special Notes At times, information must be recorded that does not seem to fit within

Example 6 POMR Progress Note Using Medical Diagnosis Title (SOAPing)

12/21/88
7:00–3:30 p.m.

4. Congestive Heart Failure
S States cannot walk farther than doorway without shortness of breath. Feels as if cannot get enough air.
O Resp. 24, shallow, rales over both lung bases. Became cyanotic when moving to chair.
A Fluid in lungs causing decreased aerating surface. Not enough O_2 exchange for activity.
P Minimize activity. Provide supportive care to lessen O_2 need. Encourage coughing and deep breathing and turning to remove secretions.

J. Jones, R.N.

Example 7 POMR Progress Note Using Patient Problem Title (SOAPing)

12/28/88
3:00–11:30 p.m.

3. Pain related to developing wound infection.
S Has c/o of "increased pain" in incisional area.
O Had pain med. q4h yesterday and q3h today (see Med. Record). Temp. increasing steadily to 101.6 (see graphic). Wound drainage has increased from scant serosanguineous to moderate and odorous (see Drsg. Flow Sheet).
A Wound infection developing.
P Notify Dr. Jones immediately. Culture wound drainage. Increase fluid intake to a minimum of 3,000 ml./24 hrs. Change drsg. at frequent intervals. Establish dressing isolation.

John Stuart, R.N.

the scope of a single problem, and, therefore, SOAPing may not be appropriate. Information of this kind is placed in the progress notes and identified as a special note. Some types of special notes used are Temporary Problems, Discharge Planning, Family Involvement, and Interim Notes. Temporary problems are concerns that could be SOAPed but that are so quickly resolved that it is inappropriate to place them on the problem list. An example might be a misplaced valuable that is found or urinary reten-

tion that is resolved through nursing action. (See Example 8.)

Discharge planning is very important for a patient, but it often encompasses many problems and therefore cannot be SOAPed in the conventional manner. A section of the progress notes is titled Discharge Planning, and then the relevant information is recorded. (See Example 9.)

Recognition of the role that the family plays in the patient's life is leading to an increased emphasis on including the family in care. This may be done by teaching family members and discussing the patient's care needs with them. When family involvement occurs, it is appropriate to make a legal record of it. This is done by writing a note titled Family Involvement in the progress notes. (See Examples 10 and 11.)

Interim Notes Still another type of special note is the Interim Note. This note is most often used to provide a legal record of nursing action that is not directly related to observations of the patient. For example, if a patient's condition is becoming worse and you are unable to locate the physician, your interim note might be a series of entries recording your attempts to contact the physician, your conferences with the nursing supervisor, and your subsequent contacting of another physician. This provides the necessary legal record that appropriate nursing action was taken. Your observations of the patient would, of course, be recorded in a conventional SOAP note. An interim note might also be used to record the time of departure and return of a pa-

---

Example 8 Sample SOAPing Notation for POMR

3/10/88
1600

Temporary problem: Missing hearing aid

S Wife thought it was with patient when he entered through Emergency Room.

O Hearing aid not listed in initial personal effects list and not found in belongings.

A _____

P 1. Emergency Room to be contacted.
  2. Wife to search at home for hearing aid.
  3. Recheck tomorrow evening when wife visits.

J. Jones, R.N.

3/11/88
1700

Temporary problem: missing hearing aid, resolved:

Wife brought in hearing aid this evening.

J. Jones, R.N.

3/11/88
2000

3. Urinary incontinence

S States: "I think I'm doing better. I was only wet once today."

O Voiding when offered urinal on q2h schedule. See flow sheet.

A Current program successful.

P Continue bladder rehab. program without change.

J. Jones, R.N.

Example 9 Discharge Planning

12/30/88
7:00–3:30 p.m.

Discharge Planning

S Mrs. E. wishes to go to her own home for convalescence.

O Resources for home care equipment and assistance with care discussed. Expected activity limitations reviewed.

A Pt. will be able to manage home care only with some outside assistance.

P Contact social services.

M. Rosen, R.N.

Example 10 Family Involvement

1/15/88
2100   Family Involvement
Rules regarding visiting hours
discussed with relatives (2
brothers, mother, aunt, and
cousin). Family asked to arrange
for not more than two people at the
patient's bedside at any one time,
to allow adequate rest for both
patients in room. Special
arrangements will be made for a
larger number to be with the
patient when the grandfather
arrives to visit. Other family
members may wait in lounge area.
Family agreed to make these
arrangements. Nurses will give the
family notice when procedures are
to be done so that an appropriate
family member can be present to
offer support to the patient.
            M. Sanchez, R.N.

Example 11 Family Involvement

1/15/88
2200   Family Involvement
Growth and development
information regarding common
2-yr.-old behavior discussed with
mother. Mother encouraged to let
nurse know when she must leave
and to be direct with Robbie and
not sneak out. Reassured mother
that nurses understand why he
cries when she leaves and this is
O.K.
            R. Filipi, S.N.

tient leaving a facility on a temporary pass. (See Examples 12 and 13.)

Choosing Which Problems to SOAP In most facilities, there is a policy that states the minimum intervals for SOAPing the active problems on the problem list. A common policy is that a SOAP note should be written if there are any significant changes, new data, or new insights, or if there is a new plan of care. Additionally, the

Example 12 Interim Note

1/23/88   Interim Note
11:30 p.m. Phone call to Dr.
Johnson regarding patient's
condition. His answering service
was notified that immediate contact
is needed.   C. Chang, R.N.
11:45 p.m. Call to Dr. Johnson has
not been returned. Nursing
Supervisor notified of pt.'s
condition and of call placed to
physician.   C. Chang, R.N.
12:00 midnight. Supervisor here.
Dr. Johnson's answering service
contacted again. Unable to reach
him. E.R. doctor contacted and
arrived at 12:10 p.m.
            C. Chang, R.N.

Example 13 Interim Note

1/27/88   Interim Note
Pt. left on pass at 1:00 p.m.
Plans to return at 7:00 p.m.
            P. Jensen, N.S.

facility may require that each problem on the problem list be SOAPed at least once in every 24-hour period even if there are no significant changes. In some facilities the Nursing Care Plan indicates how often a problem must be SOAPed if it is not necessary to SOAP it every 24 hours (for example, "document on Mondays and Thursdays" or "document every Wednesday").

As a student, you should review the problems listed for the patient as you review your assessment data. Identify those problems in which there are changes to report. If you have not identified any changes, then identify the problems that were of the most significance for the patient during the time you were there and that have not been noted within the previous 24 hours. Plan to do a SOAP note on these problems if the facility policy requires it.

Remember that your SOAP note should not just duplicate information that is on the flow sheets. You will want to summarize data and may even refer to a flow sheet for specific data.

Charting Procedure

When you are ready to chart, review all the activities in which you have engaged and the assessments you have made. Consider your plans for the future and your evaluation of the patient's response to care. Be sure to consider such things as drainage and excretions; substances ingested or infused; the condition of all devices, tubes, and dressings; the feelings and concerns of the patient; and all the patient's activities.

Start with the specialized checklists and graphs in the chart. Fill each one in appropriately. The forms will help you to remember what data need to be recorded. Go over each form thoroughly to make sure you have not forgotten anything. Then sign each form as required by your facility.

Next, turn to the form on which you will record your nursing progress notes (the nurses' notes or progress notes). Chart your relevant assessment data, both objective and subjective, and new problems. Then, using the narrative style, record the actions you have taken—this is not necessarily done in the POR style. If you are using the POR style, record future plans in the chart. If you are using the narrative style, check where plans are recorded (perhaps in a separate nursing care plan) and, if necessary, make a note to yourself to add to or alter the nursing plan. Record your evaluation of the patient's response to care. Be sure that you organize your information in the style required by your facility. Do not duplicate information that has already been recorded on a checklist or flow sheet unless your facility expressly requires duplication. Not only does duplicating records waste time, it also makes the record more cumbersome. Finally, sign your charting as required.

After you have finished, go back and double-check all that you have done to make sure that dates, times, and signatures are present and correct. Reread your progress notes to make sure that they are legible and understandable. Although as a student you will be expected to write out your charting on a separate piece of paper for approval before putting it in the actual record, you should develop the habit of double-checking yourself. It is very easy to forget a time or a signature. Although it may make the record less neat in appearance, correcting errors or adding information that was omitted may be essential to the accuracy and clarity of the record.

Computer-Generated Records

Computerized information systems are currently in place in many health care facilities. In some, the system may be limited to only one or two functions, such as patient location and laboratory or diagnostic test results. In others, there are comprehensive patient care information systems that provide a complete "paperless" record and include all aspects of nursing assessment, care planning, charting, scheduling, and patient information input and retrieval.

The components of these systems will vary, but they generally include a keyboard and a screen, or monitor, and possibly a light pen and a printer. The keyboard allows you to input information, although some systems use hospital-defined menus to reduce typing to a minimum. The screen allows you to read information and, in many cases, respond to computer-generated questions. You may respond by typing in words, phrases, or actual narrative, or the system may include a light pen, which, when touched to the screen, inputs information. A printer can provide printouts of patient information that become a part of the patient's record.

In any event, the information constitutes a legal and confidential record, whether it is on paper or somewhere in a computer system. In most health care facilities, staff members must use a special "password" of some kind to access patient information. Access to system functions may be limited by job category and level of authorization.

Computerized patient information systems are often unique to the setting in which they are found. You will learn the specifics necessary to use a particular system effectively in that setting.

PRACTICE SITUATIONS

The following is a series of clinical "situations" designed to be used as documentation exercises. You can use them on your own to practice writing various styles of progress notes, filling in forms used in your facility, or designing flow sheets. Alternatively, your instructor may direct you to other specific activities based on these situations.

Situation 1

You worked as a student nurse from 7:00 a.m. until 10:30 a.m. During that time you cared for Mr. Oscar Johanson. He is 66 years old and is in the hospital for bronchial pneumonia. This is his third hospital day. You assisted him with a bedbath; you washed his back and legs and he did the rest. He sat in a chair while you made his bed. At the end of 15 minutes, he felt tired and asked to return to bed. For breakfast he was served and ate hot cereal with cream, toast with butter and jelly, orange juice, and coffee. His blood pressure was 146/84, his pulse was 78, and his respirations were 22. He coughed intermittently, but the cough was nonproductive.

Situation 2

You worked as a student nurse from 4:30 p.m. to 8:30 p.m., caring for Mrs. Effie Sturdevan. She is 45 years old and had a hysterectomy five days ago. Her post-op course has proceeded smoothly. She had a soft diet for dinner and had a large, soft bowel movement after dinner. She complained of abdominal pain and was given a pain pill by the medication nurse at 7:00 p.m. During visiting hours her husband and daughter were present. After they left you observed that she was quiet, did not speak, and had tear-stained cheeks.

You helped her to ambulate at 4:30 p.m. and again at 8:00 p.m. Then you helped her get ready for bed and gave her a back rub. While you were giving her the back rub, she said that she knew the surgery had been necessary, but she somehow felt like a different person. After you had listened to her for ten minutes she seemed more relaxed and said she felt she would be able to sleep.

Situation 3

You worked as a student nurse from 0700 to 1200, caring for Mr. John Steiner, age 36. He is recovering from surgery to repair a right inguinal hernia. This is his second post-op day, and you helped him bathe himself and gave him back care. For breakfast he ate one egg and a slice of toast and drank a cup of coffee. You assisted him in ambulating the length of the hall and back, after which he asked for and was given his pain medication. His vital signs were T, 98⁸F(o); P, 78; R, 14; BP, 134/86. His pulse and respiration were unchanged after ambulation.

Situation 4

During clinical laboratory practice, from 1300 to 1600, you cared for Mrs. Jennie Johnson, age 77. She had a mild stroke two weeks ago, has some difficulty speaking, and cannot use her right arm. You washed her hair and set it, read a newspaper article to her, and helped her select her menu for the next day. She understood what you asked her about the menu and nodded yes or no about food selection. She could not comb her hair with her left hand; she held the comb awkwardly and kept dropping it. Her speech was not clear, but with enough time, she made some appropriate verbal responses. She said, "Toilet," and urinated when taken to the bathroom. Her right arm was in a supportive sling. When you took her arm out to exercise it, her elbow flexed easily but her shoulder was stiff.

Situation 5

Your clinical time was from 0700 to 1100. You were assigned to care for Mrs. Dorothy Wu, age 88. Mrs. Wu was transferred from a nursing home for diagnostic studies. She is totally dependent and on complete bed rest. You did complete morning hygiene, including a bedbath and oral, nail, and hair care. You turned her every two hours and gave her a back massage each time you turned her. At 0800 you fed her breakfast. She took a bowl of oatmeal, a dish of applesauce, and a glass of milk (240 ml); she would not take coffee and could not chew toast because she had no dentures. She was incontinent of urine twice and had an incontinent stool after breakfast.

Situation 6

Between the hours of 3:00 p.m. and 7:00 p.m., you cared for Mr. Joseph Gonzales, age 38. He had surgery for repair of a right inguinal hernia at 8:00 a.m. today. He returned to the surgical nursing unit from the postanesthesia room at 12:00 noon.

You took his blood pressure, pulse, and respiration every two hours, and they were as follows: 4:00 p.m. 130/82, 68, 14; 6:00 p.m. 128/82, 66, 16. He took 200 ml liquid during the four hours you were present and had no nausea. You helped him to walk to the bathroom and stand to void. He voided 150 ml. When you examined his dressing, you noted that there was no drainage and the dressing was clean. He had pain in the incisional area, and you gave him Demerol 50 mg IM at 6:00 p.m. He stated this relieved his pain. He moved about in bed with ease and deep-breathed well when directed to do so.

Situation 7

From 7:00 a.m. to 3:30 p.m. you were on a general medical unit as a nursing student. You cared for Mr. Thomas Brown. Mr. Brown, age 32, has been diagnosed as having hypertension and is hospitalized to establish control of his blood pressure through an appropriate medication regime. He is on a 500 mg sodium diet and allowed up ad lib. He had routine a.m. care. He ate all of his breakfast and borrowed salt from his roommate, which he used liberally on his eggs. He complained that the food was tasteless. He was dizzy when he got up to go to the shower. His blood pressure at 9:00 a.m. was 180/100 while lying, 130/80 while sitting, and 118/70 when standing. His pulse was 72, respirations 20, and temperature 98.4F. At noon he ate all of his lunch plus some potato chips brought in by a friend. He rested in the afternoon. At 1:00 p.m. his blood pressure was 176/98 lying, 128/76 sitting, and 122/70 standing.

Situation 8

You cared for Mr. Wayne Jefferson this morning. He is 60 years old and had a right inguinal hernia repair. He ate all of a general diet for breakfast. He has been constipated, and you gave him a Fleet's enema at 8:30 a.m. He then had a large, formed, brown stool. He bathed himself at the bedside. You washed his back and gave him a back rub. Vitals checked at 7:30 were: T, 97^8F(o); P, 62; R, 18; BP, 144/90. He has had no incisional pain. He walked about the room and down the hall twice. He napped for an hour from 11:00 a.m. until noon, when you left.

Situation 9

During the evening, from 3:00 p.m. to 7:00 p.m., you cared for Mrs. Bessie McDonald, who was admitted four days ago with mild heart failure. At 4:00 p.m. you assisted her to walk to the bathroom, where she urinated 250 ml clear urine. She then sat in a chair until after she had eaten all of her dinner. She said, "I'm so glad I can get around some now. I was so short of breath when I came in." You noted that there was no shortness of breath and that she did not seem fatigued from her activity. She returned to bed after dinner and rested quietly. As you were leaving at 7:00 p.m., her husband arrived to visit.

REFERENCES

Accreditation Manual for Hospitals. Chicago: Joint Commission on Accreditation of Hospitals, 1983, p. 115.

PERFORMANCE CHECKLIST

Mechanics	Unsatisfactory	Needs More Practice	Satisfactory	Comments
1. Ink used/correct color				
2. Legible				
3. No erasures—errors drawn through and identified				
4. Dated				
5. Time noted				
6. Material not duplicated unnecessarily				
7. Brief				
8. Correct abbreviations used				
9. Signature with correct designation				
Type of charting				
1. Correct method of charting used				
2. Correct location or form used for each category of information				
Content				
1. Data clear to another person				
2. Terms used are objective, descriptive				
3. Subjective material clearly identified as such				
4. All appropriate data included				
a. Assessment				
(1) Complete assessment for initial data base if needed				
(2) Assessments related to presenting or existing problem				
(3) Drainage and excretions				
(4) Substances ingested or infused				
(5) Condition of all devices, tubes, and dressings				
(6) Feelings and concerns of patient				
(7) Activities of patient				
b. Identification of problems				
c. Nursing actions taken				

	Unsatisfactory	Needs More Practice	Satisfactory	Comments
d. Evaluation of effectiveness of nursing actions				
e. Routine items noted (baths and the like) (1) Checklist (if applicable)				
(2) On notes (if applicable)				

QUIZ

Multiple-Choice Questions

_____ 1. Ink is used for all charting because (1) it looks neater; (2) it is more permanent; (3) changes or erasures can be seen; (4) it is a custom.

    a. 1 and 2
    b. 2 and 3
    c. 3 and 4
    d. 1 and 4

_____ 2. If a 24-hour clock is in use, the correct term for 4:00 p.m. would be

    a. 0400.
    b. 0800.
    c. 1600.
    d. 2000.

_____ 3. In problem-oriented medical records, the progress notes are often written in a standard form. This form is abbreviated

    a. SOAP.
    b. SOLD.
    c. COAP.
    d. PROP.

Short-Answer Questions

4. List two methods of organizing the contents of the chart.

    a. _____

    b. _____

5. What are two methods of writing progress notes?

    a. _____

    b. _____

6. Why should objective terminology be used in charting?

_____

7. In the following sample, underline the subjective terms:

Crying. States upset over
upcoming surgery. Paced the room
for an hour before bedtime.

8. On the following charting sample, an error was made in the quantity of urine. The correct amount was 175 ml. Correct the sample as if it were a real chart.

Up in chair for 30 min. No sign of
fatigue. Assisted to BR to urinate. 225
ml clear yellow urine.

9. To whom does the chart or medical record belong?

_____

10. Discuss the patient's right to the information contained in his or her chart.

_____

_____

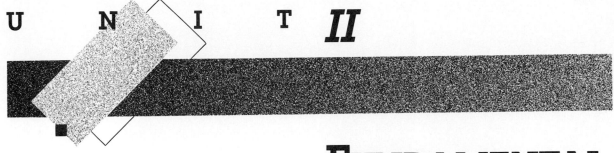

U N I T *II*

FUNDAMENTAL PERSONAL CARE SKILLS

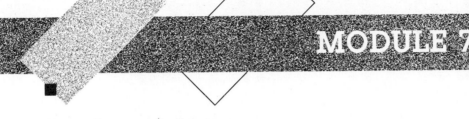

MODULE 7

Bedmaking

PREREQUISITES

Successful completion of the following modules:

VOLUME 1
Module 1 / An Approach to Nursing Skills
Module 2 / Medical Asepsis
Module 3 / Safety
Module 4 / Basic Body Mechanics
Module 25 / Special Mattresses, Frames, and
　Beds

OVERALL OBJECTIVE

To make beds correctly for hospitalized patients.

SPECIFIC LEARNING OBJECTIVES

	Know Facts and Principles	Apply Facts and Principles	Demonstrate Ability	Evaluate Performance
1. *Related principles* 　*a. Medical asepsis* 　*b. Body mechanics*	State principles of medical asepsis and body mechanics related to bedmaking	Apply principles of medical asepsis and body mechanics when making beds	Use principles of medical asepsis and body mechanics in making hospital beds	Evaluate own performance with instructor
2. *Types of beds* 　*a. Closed (unoccupied)* 　*b. Open* 　*c. Occupied* 　*d. Post-op*	Describe types of beds	Given a patient situation, identify appropriate type of bed to be made	In the clinical setting, identify type of bed to be made for particular patient	Evaluate own performance with instructor
3. *Linen*	Identify individual pieces of linen used in making hospital beds	Given a patient situation, identify appropriate pieces of linen to use in correct order	In the clinical setting, identify appropriate pieces of linen to use in correct order for particular patient	Evaluate own performance with instructor
4. *Procedures* 　*a. Closed (unoccupied)* 　*b. Open* 　*c. Occupied* 　*d. Post-op*	Describe correct procedures for making closed (unoccupied), open, occupied, and post-op beds	Initiate appropriate bedmaking activities in patient settings	Demonstrate ability to correctly make closed (unoccupied), open, occupied, and post-op beds	Evaluate own bedmaking ability with instructor using Performance Checklist

5. *Accessory devices*
  a. *Cradle*
  b. *Footboard*
  c. *Bedboard*
  d. *Special mattresses*
	Identify cradle, footboard, bedboard, and special mattresses	Given a patient situation, identify appropriate accessory device to use	Initiate use of accessory devices in appropriate situations	Evaluate appropriateness of choice with instructor

LEARNING ACTIVITIES

1. Review the Specific Learning Objectives.
2. Read the section on care of the patient's bed (in the chapter on hygiene) in Ellis and Nowlis, *Nursing: A Human Needs Approach,* or comparable material in another textbook.
3. Look up the module vocabulary terms in the Glossary.
4. Read through the module.
5. In the practice setting:
   a. Identify the various pieces of linen used in making beds in the facility to which you are assigned.
   b. Make a closed bed, using the Performance Checklist as a guide. When you are satisfied with your performance, have a fellow student evaluate you. Compare your own evaluation with that of the other student. Perfect your technique. Have your instructor evaluate your performance.
   c. Demonstrate how to convert a closed bed to an open bed.
   d. Demonstrate how to make a post-op bed from a closed bed.
   e. Make an occupied bed, using a fellow student as a patient. Pretend that it is a real situation, complete with patient explanation. Have the student comment on his or her comfort. When you are satisfied with your performance, have your instructor evaluate you.
   f. Identify the bedboard, footboard, and cradle, and incorporate them in the making of an unoccupied bed.
6. In the clinical setting:
   Make an unoccupied bed, an occupied bed, and a post-op bed to your instructor's satisfaction.

VOCABULARY

bedboard
cradle
edema
fan-fold
footboard
footdrop
mitered corner
toe pleat

110

BEDMAKING

Rationale for the Use of This Skill

One of the most important parts of the environment of a hospitalized patient is the bed. Knowing how to make various types of beds and how to modify them for special situations is of paramount importance for the nurse. A clean bed that is wrinkle-free and that remains intact when a patient moves around does a great deal for the patient's physical and psychological comfort.[1]

Asepsis in Bedmaking

Apply these principles of asepsis to all bedmaking procedures:

1. *Microorganisms move through space on air currents.* Therefore, handle linen carefully. Avoid shaking it or tossing it into the laundry hamper (it should be *placed* in the hamper). In addition, avoid throwing it on the floor *to prevent the spread of any bacteria present either on the linen or on the floor.*

2. *Microorganisms are transferred from one surface to another whenever one object touches another.* Therefore, hold both soiled and clean linen away from your uniform *to prevent contamination of the clean linen by the uniform and contamination of the uniform by the soiled linen.*

3. *Proper handwashing removes many of the microorganisms that would be transferred by the hands from one item to another.* Therefore, wash your hands before you begin and after you finish bedmaking.

Body Mechanics in Bedmaking

Apply these principles of body mechanics to all bedmaking procedures:

1. *A person or an object is more stable if the center of gravity is close to the base of support.* Therefore, when you must bend, bend your knees, not your back, *in order to keep the center of gravity directly above and close to the base of support and to help prevent fatigue* (see Figure 7.1).

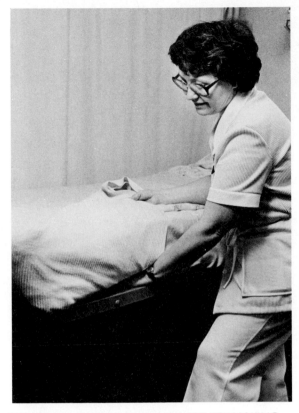

FIGURE 7.1 CORRECT POSTURE FOR BEDMAKING
Courtesy Ivan Ellis

2. *Facing in the direction of the task to be performed and turning the entire body in one plane (rather than twisting) lessens the susceptibility of the back to injury.* Therefore, face your entire body in the direction that you are moving and avoid twisting *in order to prevent back strain or injury.*

3. *Smooth, rhythmical movements at moderate speed require less energy.* Therefore, organize your work. Conserve steps by making as few trips around the bed as possible.

Procedure for Making the Unoccupied Bed

☐ *Assessment*

1. Check the activity order for the patient *to confirm whether it is possible for the patient to be out of bed during the bedmaking procedure.*

2. Assess the patient *to determine whether there are factors present that might affect the ability of the patient to be out of bed during the bedmaking procedure (fatigue or pain, for example).*

---

[1]You will note that rationale for action is emphasized throughout the module by the use of italics.

111

3. Check the condition of the linen on the bed to *determine which items need to be replaced or added to complete the bedmaking procedure.*

4. Check for any special needs of the patient that might require extra linen or special equipment.

Planning

5. Wash your hands *for asepsis.*
6. Obtain a laundry or hamper bag.
7. Gather the linen to be used and place it in order, so that the first item to be used will be on the bottom, the second item next, and so on.
   a. Mattress pad (not used in all facilities)
   b. Bottom sheet (some facilities will have fitted bottom sheets)
   c. 1 rubber or plastic drawsheet (may be optional)
   d. 1 cloth drawsheet (a top sheet folded in half may be used in some settings)
   e. 1 top sheet
   f. 1 blanket
   g. 1 spread
   h. 1 pillowcase for each pillow on the bed.

   If linen is stacked in this order, the stack need merely be turned over for it to be in the correct order for use.

8. Obtain any other needed items or equipment.

Implementation

9. Raise the bed to an appropriate working height to *help prevent fatigue.* Be certain the wheels are locked *to keep the bed from moving.*
10. Remove attached equipment (call light, waste bag, personal items). Side rails should be in the down position.
11. Remove cases from pillows and place the pillows on a chair or bedside table.
12. Loosen the top and the bottom linen from the mattress, moving around the bed from head to foot on one side and from foot to head on the opposite side.
13. Remove items to be reused (spread, blankets, sheets), fold them in quarters, and place them across the back of a chair.
14. Remove the remaining linen and place it in a laundry hamper.
15. If the mattress is to be turned, do so at

this point by grasping it, pulling it toward you, and turning it.

16. Move the mattress to the head of the bed.
17. Wash your hands after handling the soiled bed linens.
18. Place a mattress pad on the mattress, and secure it smoothly.
19. Place a bottom sheet on the bed, with the center fold at the center of the bed, the lower hem even with the edge of the mattress at the foot of the bed, and the seam toward the mattress. Spread the sheet, tucking it under at the head of the bed.

   Some facilities use fitted sheets. If your facility does, you may find that it is easier to fit diagonal corners over the mattress. If the facility does not use fitted sheets, mitered or square corners are used. Sheets with either mitered or square corners remain tucked in better and appear neater than sheets that are simply tucked under the mattress.

20. To make a mitered corner:
    a. Pick up the side edge of the sheet, holding it straight up and down, parallel to the side of the mattress.
    b. Lay the upper part of the sheet on the bed as shown in Figure 7.2, part B.
    c. Tuck the part of the sheet that is hanging below the mattress smoothly under the mattress.
    d. Holding the sheet in place against the mattress with one hand, use your other hand to lift the folded part of the sheet lying on the bed and bring it down. Tuck it under the mattress.

    To make a square corner:
    In step a, pick up the sheet to form a 45-degree angle, so that when the folded edge is placed on the top of the mattress before tucking, it is even with the bottom edge of the mattress.

21. Tuck the remainder of the sheet under the side of the mattress all the way to the foot of the bed.
22. If a rubber or plastic drawsheet is to be used, place it over the middle part of the bed, with the center fold at the center. Unfold the drawsheet toward the far side of the bed, tucking the near edge smoothly under the mattress.

112

23. Place the cloth drawsheet over the plastic drawsheet, and place it on the bed as in step 21, making sure that the rubber or plastic drawsheet is completely covered. It is easier to make one entire side of the bed (both bottom and top linen) before moving to the other side *in order to save time and energy.* If you do this, omit steps 24–27 and finish the first side, beginning with step 28.

24. Go to the other side of the bed. Tuck the bottom sheet under the head of the mattress and make a mitered or square corner.

25. Tuck the bottom sheet along the side of

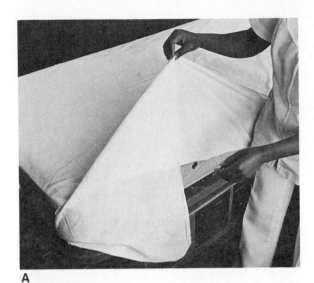

A

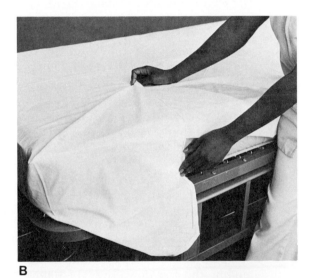

B

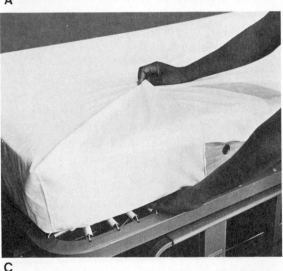

C

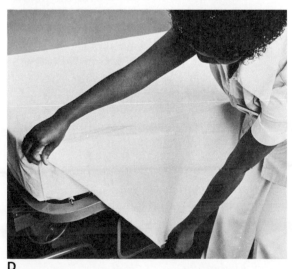

D

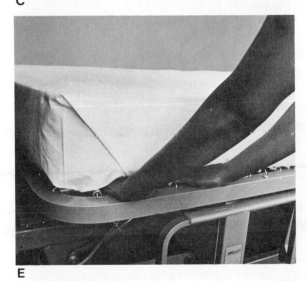

E

FIGURE 7.2 MITERING A CORNER   *A and B:* Pull sheet up at corner and fold back; *C:* tuck sheet under at corner; *D and E:* fold rest of sheet down and tuck under
Courtesy Ivan Ellis

the bed, pulling and straightening, moving toward the foot of the bed.

26. Pull the plastic drawsheet toward you from the center. With palms down, tuck it under the mattress, as snugly as possible. Grasp the top corner of the drawsheet, pull it diagonally, and tuck it under the mattress snugly. Repeat this activity with the lower corner of the drawsheet *in order to obtain an absolutely wrinkle-free surface.*

27. Tuck the cloth drawsheet under the mattress along the side of the bed, pulling and straightening, moving toward foot of the bed.

28. Place the top sheet on the bed with the center fold at the center of the bed, seam side up. Align the top edge of the sheet with the top edge of the mattress. Unfold it toward the far side of the bed.

29. Make a toe pleat (optional—follow the procedure at your clinical facility) by folding a 2-inch pleat across the sheet about 6 to 8 inches from the foot of the bed. Then tuck the end of the sheet under the mattress. This is more comfortable for the patient in that *it prevents impingement of the top linen upon the patient's toes.*

30. Place the blanket on the bed, center fold at the center of the bed, so that the top edge of the blanket is about 6 inches from the top of the mattress. Unfold the blanket toward the far side of the bed. Tuck it under the foot of the mattress, making a toe pleat if that is used. *In warm weather, or at the patient's request,* a blanket may be omitted.

31. Place the bedspread on the bed, with the center fold at the center of the bed. The top edge of the spread should be about 6 inches from the top of the mattress. Unfold the remainder of the spread toward the far side of the bed. Tuck it under at the foot of the mattress, making a toe pleat if that is used. Some nurses prefer to tuck all three—top sheet, blanket, and spread—together.

32. Miter the corner of the top linen at the foot of the bed. Do not tuck in the upper portion; allow it to hang down smoothly and freely.

33. Move to the other side of the bed.

Straighten and tuck the top sheet, blanket, and spread at the foot of the bed. Miter the corner.

34. Fold the top sheet back over the top edge of the blanket and the spread. If there is more spread than blanket at the top of the bed, fold the excess spread back over the blanket to form an even line. Then fold the top sheet over as described. In some facilities the upper edge of the spread is left even with the upper edge of the mattress to designate a *closed* bed (one not currently assigned to a patient). *Open* beds are usually made *when patients are up for a brief period in the room or out of the unit, perhaps for x-ray or lab procedures. If beds are left open,* it is easier to assist patients back to bed when they are ready.

Opening a bed is usually done by grasping the upper edge of the top linen with both hands, bringing it all the way to the foot of the bed, then folding it back toward the center of the bed. This is known as *fan-folding* (see Figure 7.3).

35. Put a pillowcase on the pillow. One way to do this is as follows:

a. Grasp the pillowcase at the center of the closed end of the case (see Figure 7.4).

b. Gather the case up over that hand and grasp the zipper, or open end of the pillow cover, with the same hand, pulling the case down over the pillow with the other hand.

c. Straighten and smooth the case over the pillow and place it at the head of the bed with the open end away from the door (*for neater appearance*).

d. Keep the pillow and case away from your uniform as you apply the case.

36. Replace the call light in an appropriate place and leave the bed in low position, *ready for the patient.*

When a patient is to be transferred from a stretcher to the bed, the bed is sometimes left in the high position *for easier access.* In some facilities, unassigned beds are left in the high position.

☐ *Evaluation*

37. Evaluate the unoccupied bed, using the following criteria:

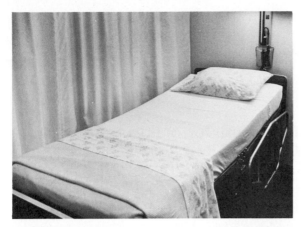

FIGURE 7.3 OPEN BED (top linen fan-folded back)
Courtesy Ivan Ellis

a. Smooth, wrinkle-free surface
b. Tight corners
c. Low position
d. Call light attached in appropriate place

Procedure for Making the Post-Op, or Surgical, Bed

The post-op bed is also called the anesthetic or surgical bed. It is made *so that the patient can be transferred from a stretcher to the bed with a minimum of motion and discomfort, then covered with the top linen, which is easily within reach* (see Figure 7.5), *to prevent chilling.*

☐ *Implementation*

1. Follow steps 5–27 of the Procedure for Making the Unoccupied Bed.

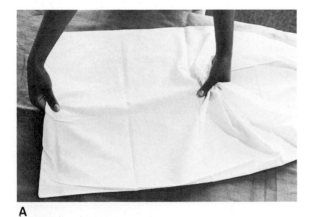

A

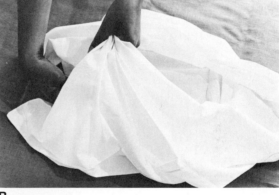

B

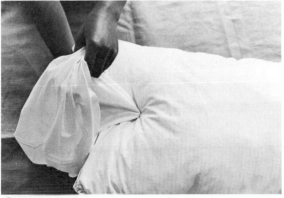

C

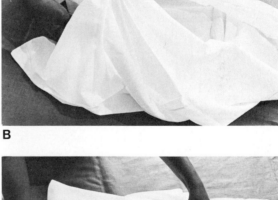

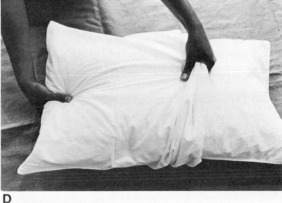

D

FIGURE 7.4 PUTTING A CASE ON A PILLOW *A:* Hold pillowcase at closed end, from outside; *B:* gather pillowcase over your hand, inside out; *C:* with pillowcase in hand, grasp pillow at center of one end; *D:* holding pillow, pull case over pillow, right side out.
Courtesy Ivan Ellis

2. Place a bath blanket over the base of the bed if policy in your facility so indicates. *This is sometimes done to provide extra warmth.*

3. Follow steps 28–31 of the Procedure for Making the Unoccupied Bed, but *do not* tuck at bottom.

4. Fold back top linen toward head of bed to make a cuff.

5. Fan-fold top linen to the far side of the bed or to the foot of the bed, as indicated by facility policy.

6. Place each pillow in a pillowcase.

7. Place pillow(s) on a table or chair, or on top of the fan-folded top linen.

8. Leave the bed in high position *to receive the patient.*

9. Place emesis basin, tissues, IV standard, call light, and any other necessary items conveniently in the unit.

10. Evaluate, using the following criteria:
    a. Smooth, wrinkle-free surface
    b. Top covers folded back out of the way
    c. Necessary items at bedside
    d. Bed in high position *to receive patient*

Procedure for Making the Occupied Bed

There are many instances in which a bed must be wholly or partially made with a patient in it. In most cases this is *because the patient is too ill or disabled to get out of bed.*

Practice making an occupied bed, keeping the safety and comfort of the patient foremost in your mind, and taking care to avoid bumping the bed or exposing the patient. The order of activities remains the same; the procedure differs only *because a patient is in the bed.*

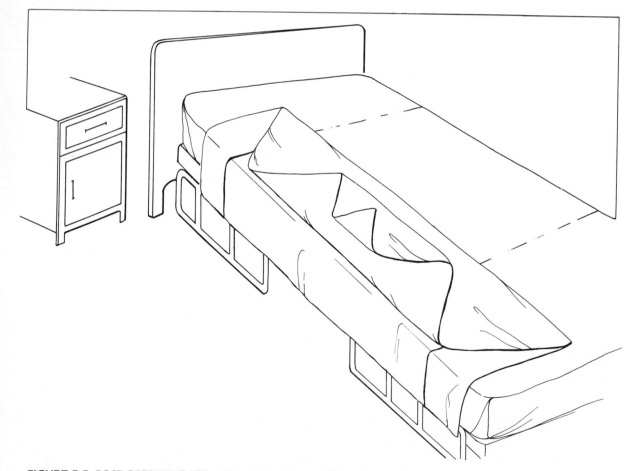

FIGURE 7.5 POST-OPERATIVE BED   Top sheet, blanket, and spread are fan-folded for convenient transfer of patient from stretcher to bed.

116

Assessment

1. Check activity orders for the patient *to be sure that he or she must stay in bed.*
2. Check orders for any restrictions related to position. Also check for any position that *must* be maintained (for example, head of bed elevated 30 degrees).
3. Assess the patient *to determine whether any factors are present that might affect the ability of the patient to undergo the bedmaking activity at the present time* (such as fatigue, shortness of breath, or pain, for example).
4. Check the condition of the linen on the bed *to determine which items of linen you will need to complete the bedmaking procedure.*
5. Check for any special needs of the patient that might require extra linen or special equipment.

Planning

6. Wash your hands *for asepsis.*
7. Gather linen as if you were making the unoccupied bed. You will need a laundry hamper or bag *for soiled linen.*
8. Obtain any other needed items or equipment.

Implementation

9. Explain what you plan to do. *The cooperation of the patient will be a great help to you.* Provide for the privacy of the patient by closing the door to the room or pulling the curtain around the patient.
10. Raise the bed to an appropriate height for you *to help prevent fatigue.* Be certain the wheels are locked.
11. Remove the call light and other equipment, spread, and blanket from the bed. If the spread and the blanket are to be reused, fold them.
12. Before removing the top sheet, place a bath blanket over it. Ask the patient to hold the top edge of the bath blanket while you pull the sheet out from under it. Discard the top sheet. The bath blanket will remain *to provide privacy and warmth for the patient.* In some facilities the top sheet is saved and used as a bottom sheet; follow the procedure used in your facility. If the mattress must be moved toward the head of the bed, you will probably need the assistance of another person.
13. Move the patient to the far side of the bed, making sure that the pillow is moved also. If possible, the patient should be side-lying, facing away from you. The side rail on the far side of the bed should be up *for safety and comfort.*
14. Loosen the foundation (bottom linen) of the bed on the near side, leaving the mattress pad in place unless it is wet or soiled.
15. Fan-fold each piece toward the center of the bed, with the last fold toward the opposite side of the bed and tucked under the patient's back and buttocks *to make it easier to reach.*
16. Straighten the mattress pad.
17. Lay the bottom sheet lengthwise on the bed and unfold it so that the center fold of the sheet is at the center of the bed, the bottom hem is at the bottom edge of the mattress, and the top hem of the sheet is over the top of the mattress. Fan-fold half the sheet lengthwise toward the center of the bed, allowing the other half to drape.
18. Tuck the sheet under at the top, miter the top corner, and tuck it in along the side of the mattress to the foot of the bed.
19. Place the fan-folded sheet under the patient as far as possible, tucking it under the soiled bottom sheet so that it is not against the soiled upper surface.
20. If a rubber or plastic drawsheet is in use, unfold it at this point, pull it over the folded bottom sheets, and tuck it in snugly and smoothly.
21. Place the cloth drawsheet on the bed in position in similar fashion as you did the bottom sheet.
22. Tuck the near side under the mattress. Fan-fold the other half toward the center of the bed, tucking it under the patient's back and buttocks. Help the patient roll over the folded linen and onto the clean linen. Adjust the pillow. Put up the side rail *for safety and comfort.*
23. Move to the other side of the bed. Lower the side rail.
24. Loosen the bottom linen of the bed. Remove the soiled linen (bottom sheet and cloth drawsheet) and place it in a laundry hamper or bag.
25. Pull the fan-folded bottom sheet, plastic drawsheet, and cloth drawsheet out from under the patient. Straighten the mattress

pad. Straighten, pull, and tuck the bottom sheet as if making an unoccupied bed. Pull the sheet tight by bracing against the bed and pulling with both hands to make the sheet smooth and tight under the patient before tucking it in.

26. Pull and tuck the plastic drawsheet as you did previously.

27. Pull and tuck the cloth drawsheet snugly and smoothly. Pulling and tucking the center of the drawsheet first and then the top and bottom edges will result in a tighter drawsheet.

28. Now move the patient to the center of the bed in a position of comfort.

29. Place the top sheet on the bed over the bath blanket. Remove the bath blanket, instructing the patient to hold the sheet as you pull the blanket from the top to the bottom. Place the bath blanket in the laundry hamper or (if it is unsoiled and dry) fold it and leave it in the patient's unit *for future use.*

30. Add the blanket and the spread as in the Procedure for Making the Unoccupied Bed. Instead of making a toe pleat, you may have the patient point his or her toes up, *which allows room for the toes after the bed has been made.*

31. Remove the pillow and put on a clean pillowcase.

32. Reattach the call light and any other equipment you removed.

33. Place the bed in the low position, adjusting the side rails according to your facility's policies and the individual situation.

☐ **Evaluation**

34. Evaluate the occupied bed using the following criteria:
    a. Patient comfort
    b. Smooth, wrinkle-free surface
    c. Tight corners
    d. Bed and side rails in correct position
    e. Call light within patient's reach.

Accessories for the Bed

Among the devices often added to the bed are the bedboard, the footboard, and the cradle.

These devices may be ordered by a physician, but in many facilities they are added at the nurse's discretion.

Bedboards

A bedboard is used *when the patient needs an especially firm bed;* it is placed directly under the mattress. Bedboards are often *used for orthopedic patients or for those who have a history of back problems. Some patients are simply more comfortable sleeping on a firm surface.*

Footboards

A footboard may be placed at the foot of the bed for a variety of reasons, *most commonly to keep the patient from sliding to the foot of the bed or to provide a firm surface for the patient to exercise against.* A footboard can also *help prevent footdrop,* since it allows the patient's feet to rest flat against it. (See Figure 7.6.) Some physicians routinely order a footboard for their patients. Linen is tucked in around the footboard and is held up off the patient's feet, although this is not the primary function of the device.

Not all footboards are alike. Some are merely boards that fit at the foot of the mattress. Some require that a box or "block" be added, *so*

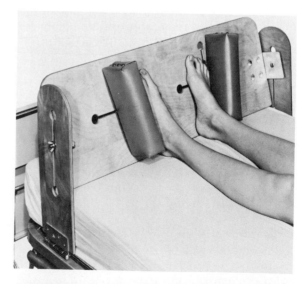

FIGURE 7.6 FOOTBOARD The footboard holds the linen off the feet and provides a firm surface to hold the feet at a right angle. Footboards are usually padded.
Courtesy J. T. Posey Company, Arcadia, California

that the feet of a shorter patient can reach the board. Other footboards fit under the mattress and slide up to the appropriate point on the bed. Only footboards that allow the patient's feet to rest flat against them *help to prevent footdrop.*

Special Mattresses

A variety of special mattresses have been manufactured *to diminish pressure on the patient's skin and thus help prevent the formation of pressure sores (decubitus ulcers).* These include egg-crate, inflatable, and alternating-pressure mattresses. A more detailed description of these special mattresses is given in Module 25, Special Mattresses, Frames, and Beds. When making a bed that has one of these mattresses, the linen should not be tucked tightly under the mattress, *as this would not allow the mattress to expand and would defeat the purpose of the special mattress.*

Cradles

A cradle is a device designed specifically *to keep linen up off the feet and lower legs of patients when necessary, as in cases of edema, leg ulcers, and burns.* Arrange the top linen over the device and pin it in place. Some facilities do not allow pinning *be-*

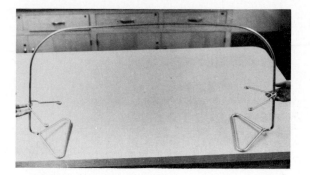

FIGURE 7.7 CRADLE   The triangles at the base of the cradle slide under the mattress; the V-shaped parts just above fit over the top of the mattress.
Courtesy Ivan Ellis

cause it can tear the linen. In these situations, linen must simply be tucked as securely as possible around the frame.

There are several kinds of cradles, including one called the Anderson frame, which is a simple rod that arches over the bed and is held in place by the mattress (see Figure 7.7), and a lattice-work affair that is also arch-shaped and that sometimes includes a socket for light treatments (see Module 27, Applying Heat and Cold, Figure 27.4). If your facility has no cradle, you can make one by simply cutting one side out of a strong cardboard box.

PERFORMANCE CHECKLIST

	Unsatisfactory	Needs More Practice	Satisfactory	Comments
Asepsis in bedmaking				
1. Handle linen carefully.				
2. Hold both soiled and clean linen away from your uniform.				
3. Wash hands before and after bedmaking.				
Body mechanics				
1. When you must bend, bend your knees, not your back.				
2. Face your entire body in the direction in which you are moving and avoid twisting.				
3. Organize your work and conserve steps.				
Procedure for making the unoccupied bed				
☐ *Assessment*				
1. Check activity order for patient.				
2. Assess patient.				
3. Check condition of linen on bed.				
4. Check for special needs of patient.				
☐ *Planning*				
5. Wash your hands.				
6. Obtain laundry hamper or bag.				
7. Gather linen to be used.				
8. Obtain other needed items or equipment.				
☐ *Implementation*				
9. Raise bed to appropriate working height. Be certain wheels are locked.				
10. Remove attached equipment.				
11. Remove cases from pillows.				
12. Loosen top and bottom linen from mattress.				
13. Remove items to be reused, fold, and place across back of chair.				

	Unsatisfactory	Needs More Practice	Satisfactory	Comments
14. Remove remaining linen and place in hamper.				
15. Turn mattress if necessary.				
16. Move mattress to head of bed.				
17. Wash your hands.				
18. Place mattress pad on mattress.				
19. Place bottom sheet on bed.				
20. Miter top corners of bottom sheet.				
21. Tuck remainder of sheet under.				
22. Place rubber or plastic drawsheet on bed, using center fold as guide. Tuck near edge.				
23. Place cloth drawsheet over rubber drawsheet. Tuck near edge.				
24. Go to other side of bed. Tuck bottom sheet under head of bed and miter corner.				
25. Tuck bottom sheet along side of bed.				
26. Tuck plastic drawsheet snugly.				
27. Tuck cloth drawsheet snugly.				
28. Place top sheet on bed, using center fold as guide.				
29. Make toe pleat if facility policy so indicates.				
30. Place blanket on bed, using center fold as guide.				
31. Place bedspread on bed, using center fold as guide. Tuck sheet, blanket, and spread separately or together.				
32. Miter corner of top linen at foot of bed. Allow upper portion to hang freely.				
33. Move to other side of bed, straighten and tuck top linen at foot of bed, and miter corner.				
34. Fold top sheet back over top edge of blanket and spread.				
35. Apply pillowcase, taking care to keep pillow and case away from uniform.				
36. Replace call light and leave bed in appropriate position.				

	Unsatisfactory	Needs More Practice	Satisfactory	Comments
Evaluation				
37. Evaluate using the following criteria: a. Smooth, wrinkle-free surface				
b. Tight corners				
c. Low position				
d. Call light attached in appropriate place				

Procedure for making the post-op, or surgical, bed

	Unsatisfactory	Needs More Practice	Satisfactory	Comments
Assessment				
1. Assess as in Checklist steps 1–3 of Procedure for Making the Unoccupied Bed (check activity order and condition of patient and assess bed linen).				
Planning				
2. Follow Checklist steps 5–8 of Procedure for Making the Unoccupied Bed (wash hands and obtain laundry bag, linen, and other needed equipment).				
Implementation				
3. Follow Checklist steps 9–14 of Procedure for Making the Unoccupied Bed (raise bed, remove attached equipment, and remove cases from pillows and bottom soiled linen). Turn and move mattress if needed. Wash your hands. Place mattress pad and other linen on bed as before.				
4. Follow Checklist steps 28–34 of procedure for placing top linen on bed as when making an unoccupied bed (top sheet, blanket, spread).				
5. Fold top linen away from head and foot of bed to form a cuff.				
6. Fan-fold top linen to far side of bed.				
7. Place pillow(s) on chair and put bed in raised position.				
8. Put IV stand, emesis basin, tissues, and other needed items at bedside.				

122

	Unsatisfactory	Needs More Practice	Satisfactory	Comments
Evaluation				
9. Evaluate using the following criteria: a. Smooth, wrinkle-free surface				
b. Top covers folded back out of the way				
c. Necessary items at bedside				
d. High position				

Procedure for making the occupied bed

Assessment				
1. Check activity order for patient.				
2. Check orders for restrictions related to position.				
3. Assess patient.				
4. Check condition of linen on bed.				
5. Check for special needs of patient.				
Planning				
6. Follow Checklist steps 5–8 of Procedure for Making the Unoccupied Bed (wash hands and obtain laundry bag, linen, and other needed equipment).				
Implementation				
7. Explain what you plan to do and provide for privacy of patient.				
8. Raise bed to appropriate height and lock wheels.				
9. Remove attached equipment, spread, and blanket from bed. Fold spread and blanket if they are to be reused.				
10. Place bath blanket over top sheet and pull sheet out from under it.				
11. Move patient to far side of bed.				
12. Loosen bottom linen on near side.				
13. Fan-fold each piece toward center of bed and tuck under patient's back and buttocks.				
14. Straighten mattress pad.				

	Unsatisfactory	Needs More Practice	Satisfactory	Comments
15. Place bottom sheet on bed.				
16. Tuck sheet under at top, miter top corner, and tuck along side of mattress.				
17. Fan-fold other half of sheet toward center of bed, tucking it *under* the soiled bottom sheet.				
18. If rubber or plastic drawsheet is in use, unfold and pull over the folded bottom sheets. Tuck in.				
19. Place cloth drawsheet on bed.				
20. Tuck near side under mattress and fan-fold other half toward center of bed, tucking it under patient's back and buttocks. Help patient roll over folded linen and onto clean linen, adjust pillow, and put up side rail.				
21. Move to other side of bed and lower side rail.				
22. Loosen bottom linen, remove soiled linen, and place it in laundry hamper or bag.				
23. Straighten mattress pad and straighten, pull, and tuck bottom sheet.				
24. Pull and tuck plastic drawsheet.				
25. Pull and tuck cloth drawsheet.				
26. Move patient to center of bed.				
27. Place top sheet on bed and remove bath blanket from beneath it.				
28. Add blanket and spread.				
29. Remove pillow, put on clean pillowcase, and replace pillow under patient's head.				
30. Reattach call light and any other equipment removed.				
31. Place bed in low position and adjust side rails appropriately.				
☐ *Evaluation*				
32. Evaluate using the following criteria: a. patient comfort				
b. Smooth, wrinkle-free surface				
c. Tight corners				

	Unsatisfactory	Needs More Practice	Satisfactory	Comments
d. Bed and side rails in correct position				
e. Call light within patient's reach				

QUIZ

Short-Answer Questions

1. Because the bed is the bedridden patient's environment, beds should be made with two goals, which are _____ _____ and _____ _____.

2. The reason for completely finishing one side of the unoccupied bed and then moving to the other side is that this _____ _____.

3. Two important differences between the post-op bed and the unoccupied bed are _____ _____ and _____.

4. The most important safety step when making an occupied bed is to remember to _____.

5. Linen is never tucked tightly over special mattresses because doing this _____.

Multiple-Choice Questions

_____ 6. Mr. Green is to be up in a chair each morning for 30 minutes. Given this information, what type of bed would be most appropriate for you to make for him?

   a. Closed bed
   b. Open bed
   c. Occupied bed
   d. Post-op bed

_____ 7. Mrs. Pine is going to x-ray for some special tests. She will arrive back on the floor via stretcher. Under these circumstances, what type of bed would be most appropriate for you to make?

   a. Closed bed
   b. Open bed
   c. Occupied bed
   d. Post-op bed

_____ 8. A patient who has severe edema of the lower legs should be provided with which accessory device?

   a. Cradle
   b. Bedboard

    c. Footboard
    d. Mattress pad

_____ **9.** Patients who are confined to bed should be provided with which accessory device to help prevent footdrop?

    a. Cradle
    b. Bedboard
    c. Footboard
    d. Mattress pad

_____ **10.** Which of the following beds may be left in the high position on completion: (1) closed bed; (2) open bed; (3) occupied bed; (4) post-op bed?

    a. 1 only
    b. 4 only
    c. 2 and 3
    d. 1 and 4

Short-Answer Question

_____ **11.** Number the following pieces of linen in the order in which they would be used in the usual unoccupied hospital bed.

    _____ Blanket

    _____ Pillowcase

    _____ Top sheet

    _____ Bottom sheet

    _____ Mattress pad

    _____ Cloth drawsheet

    _____ Spread

    _____ Rubber or plastic drawsheet

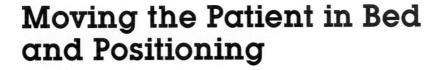

MODULE 8

Moving the Patient in Bed and Positioning

OVERALL OBJECTIVES

To move patients in bed, using good body mechanics. To place patients in positions that are anatomically correct as well as comfortable. To place patients in the special positions required for examination and therapy.

SPECIFIC LEARNING OBJECTIVES

	Know Facts and Principles	Apply Facts and Principles	Demonstrate Ability	Evaluate Performance
Moving the patient in bed				
1. General procedure	Give assessment factors and safety precautions for both nurse and patient	State rationale for assessment and safety	Adapt procedure to individual patient	Evaluate own performance with instructor
2. Moving patient closer to one side of bed				
3. Moving patient up in bed: one-person assist				
4. Moving patient up in bed: two- or three-person assist	Describe each move in detail	Choose best movement procedure for particular patient	In clinical setting, perform each move with patient if possible	Using the Performance Checklist, evaluate moves performed with help of instructor
5. Turning patient in bed: back to side				
6. Turning patient in bed: back to abdomen				

7. Turning patient: logrolling				
8. Using turn sheet with any of above				
Documentation			Record plan for turning on care plan as well as on chart	
Positioning				
1. Reasons for frequent and proper positioning	Give three reasons for frequent and proper positioning	State rationale underlying each reason	Make adaptations for individual patients	
2. Positioning aids	List available aids that are used for positioning	From list, select appropriate aids for each body position	In clinical setting, use aids correctly for patient situation	Evaluate own performance with help of instructor
3. Supine position				
4. Side-lying position				
5. Prone position				
6. Sitting position	Describe each	Choose best position for particular patient	In clinical setting, place at least one patient in each position if possible	Using the Performance Checklist, critically evaluate patient's body alignment and comfort
7. Fowler's position				
8. High-Fowler's position				
9. Orthopneic position				
10. Dorsal recumbent position				
11. Lithotomy position				

Know Facts and Principles	Apply Facts and Principles	Demonstrate Ability	Evaluate Performance
12. *Sims's position* 13. *Knee-chest position* 14. *Trendelenburg position* } Describe each	Choose best position for particular patient	In clinical setting, place at least one patient in each position if possible	Using the Performance Checklist, critically evaluate patient's body alignment and comfort
Documentation		Record plan for positioning in nursing care plan. Chart on record, using proper format.	

LEARNING ACTIVITIES

1. Review the Specific Learning Objectives.
2. Read the section on the effects of immobility (in the chapter on activity and rest) in Ellis and Nowlis, *Nursing: A Human Needs Approach,* or comparable material in another textbook.
3. Look up the module vocabulary terms in the Glossary.
4. Read through the module.
5. In the practice setting, select three other students and form a group of four.
   a. Changing so that each has the opportunity to play the role of the patient, perform each of the following procedures for moving the patient in bed. Use the Performance Checklist for guidance. Those who are not participating at a given time can observe and evaluate the performances of the others.
      (1) Move the "patient" closer to one side of the bed.
      (2) Move the "patient" up in bed: one-person assist.
      (3) Move the "patient" up in bed: two- or three-person assist.
      (4) Turn the "patient" in bed: back to side.
      (5) Turn the "patient" in bed: back to abdomen.
      (6) Turn the "patient" in bed: logrolling.
      (7) Perform two of the above using a pull sheet. Does this make the task easier? How?
   b. With the same group, change roles as you did before and position the "patient" in the following ways:
      (1) Supine position
      (2) Side-lying position
      (3) Prone position
      (4) Sitting position (in a chair)
      (5) Fowler's position
      (6) High-Fowler's position
      (7) Orthopneic position
      (8) Dorsal recumbent position
      (9) Lithotomy position
      (10) Sims's position
      (11) Knee-chest position
      (12) Trendelenburg position
   c. Note the different positions you assume during a normal night's sleep. Is one particular position more comfortable for you than others? How often do you estimate you change your position during the night?
6. In the clinical setting:
   a. Consult with your instructor regarding the opportunity to move patients using a variety of techniques. Evaluate your performance with the instructor.
   b. Consult with your instructor regarding the opportunity to position patients in a variety of appropriate positions. Evaluate your performance with the instructor.

VOCABULARY

alignment
anatomical position
axilla
dorsiflexion
extension
external rotation
flaccid
flexion
footdrop
gravity
orthopneic
paralysis
plantar flexion
pronation
trapeze
trochanter

MOVING THE PATIENT IN BED AND POSITIONING

Rationale for the Use of This Skill

A very important nursing function is moving and positioning patients. To do this properly, the nurse must have a knowledge of anatomy and good body alignment. The nurse should learn a number of positions, so that patients can be repositioned approximately every two hours. A regimen of good positioning prevents pressure sores (decubitus ulcers) and joint contractures. Frequent movement also improves muscle tone, respiration, and circulation.

Many examinations and procedures use special positions to improve visibility. It is usually the nurse's responsibility to assist patients into these positions and to make them as comfortable as possible.

When you must move a patient in bed, correct body mechanics are essential for both you and the patient. If you do not use correct body mechanics and moving techniques, you may injure your back. You may also put excessive stress on a patient's joints and cause him or her severe discomfort.

The aim in moving the patient is to put the least possible stress on his or her joints and skin. Patient positioning is designed to maintain body parts in correct alignment so that they remain functional and unstressed.[1]

General Procedure for Moving a Patient in Bed and Positioning

☐ Assessment
1. Assess the patient's need to move.
2. Assess the patient's ability to move unaided.
3. Check on the assistive devices that are available.

☐ Planning
4. Plan the moving technique.
5. Wash your hands.
6. Obtain any needed supportive devices or assistance.

[1]You will note that rationale for action is emphasized throughout the module by the use of italics.

☐ Implementation
7. Identify the patient *to be sure you are carrying out the procedure for the correct patient.*
8. Raise the bed to the high position. *This lets you use correct body mechanics and protects you from back injury.*
9. Put the bed in the flat position, if possible. In this way *you will not be working against gravity.* If the patient is medically unable to lie flat, you will have to adjust to the altered position, possibly with the help of an assistant.
10. Move the patient in one of the ways indicated in the following pages. Remember to use smooth, coordinated movements for all of them.
11. Correctly position the patient, using one of the positions described in the following pages.
12. Make sure all safety devices (side rails, pillows, protective restraints, call lights) are in place *to protect the patient.*
13. Wash your hands.

☐ Evaluation
14. Examine the patient's position for correct alignment.
15. If the patient is able to respond, ask about comfort.

☐ Documentation
16. Record the patient's activity as required by your facility. Usually position changes from side to side or from back to abdomen are noted on a flow sheet. If your facility does not use a flow sheet, record this activity in the narrative nurses' notes. Simply assisting a patient to move up in bed is not usually recorded.
17. *To help other nursing personnel,* you may note the techniques used for moving the patient on a nursing care plan. If the patient's ability to move is a significant part of the general assessment, you may have to write a progress note about his or her activity.

Specific Procedures for Moving Patients

For each procedure discussed, some steps in the General Procedure may be modified. The com-

134

plete procedures, which include all the steps of the General Procedure as well as the steps that have been modified, are found in the Performance Checklist.

Moving a Patient Closer to One Side of the Bed

This activity is needed in many other moves; therefore, it is being presented separately. Most of the time, you will use this technique in conjunction with another type of movement.

10. Implementation
    a. Slide your hands and arms under the patient's head and shoulders, and pull them toward you. Be sure you bend from the hips and knees, keeping your back straight *to protect your back.*
    b. Move your hands and arms down under the patient's hips, and pull that section of the body toward you. Keep your back straight and your hips and knees flexed. Keep one foot forward to give you a broad base of support that can withstand a shift in weight as the patient is pulled toward the side of the bed.
    c. Slide your hands and arms under the patient's legs, and pull them toward you.
    d. Repeat steps a–c above in sequence until the patient is in the desired location on the bed.

If two people are available, the same general technique is used, but two sections of the body are moved at the same time. One nurse slides hands and arms under the patient's shoulders; the other nurse slides hands and arms under the patient's hips. *To make sure they work together,* one of the nurses signals the move by saying, "One, two, three, *pull!*" (See Figure 8.1.)

Moving a Patient Up in Bed: One-Person Assist

The following technique is used for the patient who is alert and able to cooperate and help. Encourage independence, *both to benefit the patient's physical progress and to support feelings of self-esteem.*

10. Implementation
    a. Have the patient bend the knees and

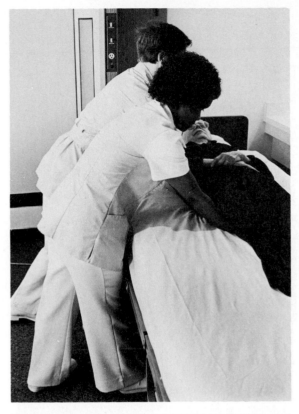

FIGURE 8.1 MOVING A PATIENT TO ONE SIDE OF A BED: TWO-PERSON ASSIST   *The nurses slide their arms under the patient (one at the shoulders, one at the hips) and pull toward themselves.*
Courtesy Ivan Ellis

place the soles of the feet firmly on the surface of the bed. *This reduces the drag of the legs.* He or she may need some assistance with this procedure.
    b. Have the patient grasp the overhead trapeze, if one is in place, or the side rails at shoulder level. Some patients may be able to grasp the headboard and pull themselves up.
    c. Slide your hands and arms under the patient's hips. You should be turned slightly toward the foot of the bed with your outside foot slightly ahead of your inside foot (see Figure 8.2). Keep your back straight, bend at the hips and the knees, and keep your elbows bent *so that you are using your strong leg muscles to pull.*
    d. Instruct the patient to move with you on the count "One, two, three, *up!*" All effort should be simultaneous *to*

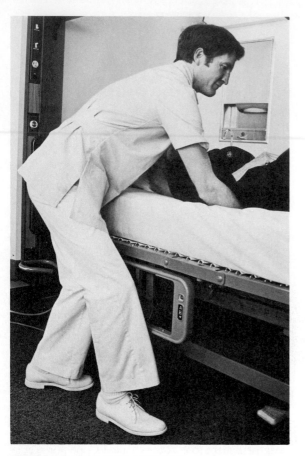

FIGURE 8.2 *MOVING A PATIENT UP IN BED: ONE-PERSON ASSIST* The patient pushes with feet flat on the bed. The side rails and trapeze have been omitted to clarify the nurse's position. If they are not available, the patient pushes on the bed with the palms of the hands to further assist in moving.
Courtesy Ivan Ellis

supply the most combined energy to the task.

e. Count, "One, two, three, *up!*" The patient should pull with the arms and push with the feet. From your position, you will *pull* the patient up in bed. *In pulling, you use your strong flexor muscles most effectively.* Many people carry out this maneuver facing the head of the bed, pushing the patient up. This method has two drawbacks: first, *you cannot move as much weight this way; second, you meet greater resistance from the bed surface in pushing along it than in pulling along it.*

Moving a Patient Up in Bed: Two- or Three-Person Assist

When you must move a heavy patient or one who is unable to help, you will find an assistant useful. Two people are sufficient for most patients, but for exceptionally heavy patients, three people may be necessary.

10. Implementation

a. Move the patient close to one side of the bed.

b. If possible, have the patient bend the knees and plant the soles of the feet firmly on the bed. Even if the patient is unable to push with the feet and legs, *this positioning of the knees and soles eliminates the need to drag the weight of the legs as well as the weight of the trunk.*

c. The first nurse (nurse 1) slides his or her arms under the patient's head and shoulders. This nurse faces the foot of the bed. *This puts him or her in a position to pull strongly.*

d. The second nurse (nurse 2) slides his or her arms under the patient's hips from the same side of the bed. This nurse also faces the foot of the bed (see Figure 8.3).

e. The nurse with the heavier burden (usually nurse 2) counts, "One, two, three, up!" *so that both pull the patient up in bed at the same time.*

This procedure can be repeated several times until the patient is in the correct position.

If a third nurse is needed, all three should position themselves on the same side of the bed, distributing the weight among them. Since the patient is close to the side of the bed where the nurses are standing, it is possible for each *to maintain firm support with the legs, keeping the center of gravity over that base of support and working close to the body. This is an efficient way to use muscles.* On occasion, it will be necessary to leave a patient in the middle of the bed. In that case, the lifters should position themselves on each side of the bed, paying close attention to their body mechanics. *It is very easy to bend from the waist and put strain on the back.*

Under no circumstances should a nurse pull a patient up in bed by grasping the patient under the axillae and pulling. This may work well

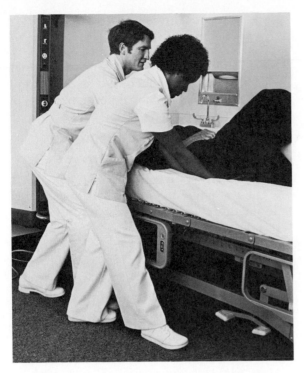

FIGURE 8.3 *MOVING A PATIENT UP IN BED: TWO-PERSON ASSIST* The nurses face toward the foot of the bed. The outside foot (right, in this instance) is placed more toward the foot of the bed to provide a wide stance. The back is straight, and knees and hips are slightly bent.
Courtesy Ivan Ellis

for the nurse, but it is very uncomfortable for the patient and can cause a shoulder dislocation, especially for a person with extremely weak muscles or paralysis.

Turning a Patient in Bed: Back to Side

10. Implementation
   a. Move the patient so that the side the patient is to lie on is close to the center of the bed. *This will help the patient to end up in the correct place in the bed and will also help to prevent falls from the bed.*
   b. Raise the side rail and move to the other side of the bed. You will be rolling the patient toward you.
   c. Prepare the pillows needed for support. (See Side-Lying Position, page 141.)
   d. Two different methods are used to

turn the lower body. The one you use will depend on your preference and the patient's ability.
   (1) Cross the patient's far ankle over the near ankle *so that the weight of the legs will help to turn the body.* Then grasp the patient with one hand behind the far hip.
   (2) Raise the knee on the far leg. Then reach over and grasp the far side of the knee. *This also allows the weight of the legs to help in the turn.*
   e. Move the patient's near arm out away from the patient's body, *so that it is not trapped under the body.*
   f. Place the patient's far arm across the chest. *This allows the arm to be used as leverage for the body.*
   g. Grasp the patient behind the far shoulder.
   h. Roll the patient toward you (see Figure 8.4).
   i. Adjust the patient until he or she is in the correct side-lying position.

Turning a Patient in Bed: Back to Abdomen

10. Implementation
   a. Move the patient to the extreme edge of the bed.
   b. Raise the side rail on that side and move to the other side of the bed.
   c. Prepare the pillows needed for support. *Frequently, a heavy-breasted patient will need a pillow under the abdomen for comfort. A very thin patient might be more comfortable with a small pillow under the iliac crests.*
   d. Place the patient's near arm over the head *so that it is out of the way as the patient rolls.*
   e. Turn the patient's face away from you *so that the patient will not roll onto his or her face during the turning procedure* (see Figure 8.5).
   f. Roll the patient onto his or her side, using the technique noted in the last section.
   g. Once the patient is on his or her side,

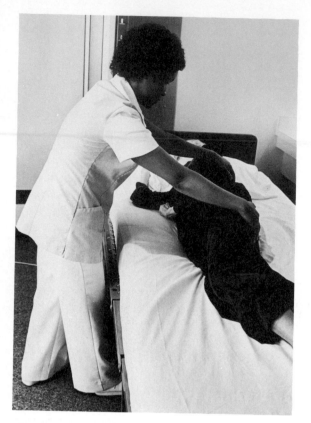

check the arm and face carefully *to see that they are correctly positioned.*

h. Roll the patient over onto the abdomen.

i. Adjust the patient until he or she is in a correct abdominal position.

Turning a Patient in Bed: Logrolling

Patients who must maintain a straight alignment at all times are turned by a technique called *logrolling.* The technique requires at least two nurses, and sometimes three if the patient is very large.

10. Implementation

a. Move the patient to one side of the bed as a single unit. Each person assisting with the turn slides his or her arms under the patient. At a signal ("One, two, three, *move!*"), all pull the patient, making sure that the patient's body stays correctly aligned at all times.

b. Raise the side rail on that side of the bed *for safety.*

c. All assistants move to the other side of the bed.

d. Place the pillows where they will be needed for support after the patient has been turned. One is needed *to*

FIGURE 8.4 TURNING A PATIENT FROM BACK TO SIDE   The nurse uses a wide base of support, with back straight and knees slightly bent. The nurse rocks backward, using the entire weight of the body to turn the heavy patient. (Side rails have been omitted for clarity.)
Courtesy Ivan Ellis

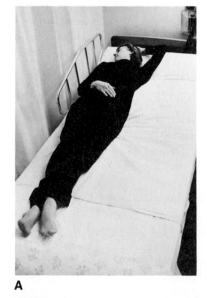

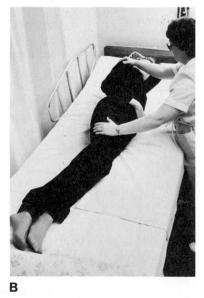

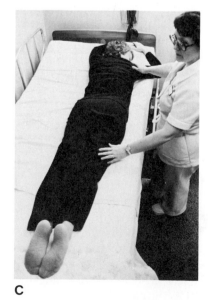

A   **B**   **C**

FIGURE 8.5 TURNING A PATIENT TO THE ABDOMEN   *A:* Patient positioned for turn; *B:* turning the patient; *C:* patient positioned on abdomen.
Courtesy Ivan Ellis

138

support the head with the spine straight.
Another is needed between the legs
(in fact, two may be needed here) *to
support the legs and prevent twisting of
the hips.*

e. All assistants reach across and grasp
the far side of the patient's body.

f. At the signal ("One, two, three,
turn!"), all turn the patient smoothly,
keeping the patient's body perfectly
straight, like a log (see Figure 8.6).

*A turn sheet under the patient makes
the turn smoother and easier.* Proceed as
outlined above, but instead of
grasping the patient's body, grasp the
turn sheet on the far side of the
patient and pull it toward you. *The
turn sheet supports the patient's entire body
and makes it easier to keep the patient
straight.* (See next section.)

Moving a Patient in Bed: Using a Turn Sheet or Pull Sheet

A sheet can be used as an aid in turning and
moving a patient in bed. Place the turn sheet, or
pull sheet, under the patient's trunk, with the
bottom edge below the patient's buttocks and
the top edge at the top of the patient's shoulders. *The sheet will then support the heaviest part of
the patient's body.* Do not tuck in the sides; fan-
fold or roll them along the patient on each side.
To move the patient up in bed or to turn the
patient, grasp the fan-folded edges of the sheet
instead of the patient's body (see Figures 8.7 and
8.8).

One advantage of using a turn or pull sheet
is that *the movement takes place between two layers of
dry cloth, which produces less friction than does skin
on cloth. Another advantage is that it is much easier*

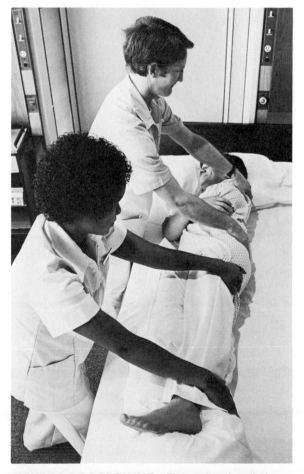

FIGURE 8.6 LOGROLLING   The patient is rolled as a
unit. The legs remain parallel, and a pillow is placed
between them to keep the upper leg from dropping
and twisting the spine. A pillow is placed under the
head so that the head does not drop down. At least
two nurses are essential for this procedure.
Courtesy Ivan Ellis

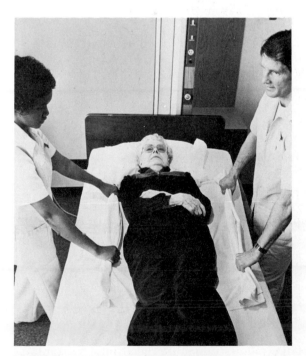

FIGURE 8.7 TURN SHEET (PULL SHEET) IN
PLACE   The sheet extends from the shoulders to below
the hips and is rolled or fan-folded at each side of the
patient's body.
Courtesy Ivan Ellis

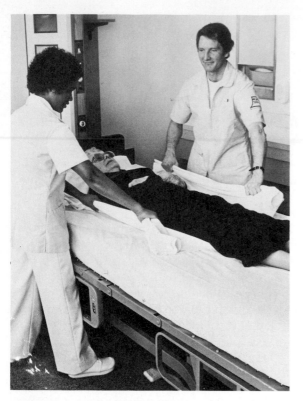

FIGURE 8.8 MOVING A PATIENT UP IN BED USING A TURN SHEET   Both nurses face the foot of the bed. Knees and hips are slightly bent and backs are straight. Feet are spread to form a wide base of support.
Courtesy Ivan Ellis

to grasp a sheet firmly than it is to hold a patient's body. Your hands can slip off the patient if you do not grasp hard enough; and if you grasp too hard, you can cause discomfort or even bruising. Do not lift the patient with the pull sheet; always slide the patient *to lessen strain on your back.*

Positioning a Patient in Bed

Positioning patients in bed in proper body alignment and changing their positions frequently are important nursing functions. Many alert patients automatically reposition themselves and readily move about in bed. They may not need special attention, but they often need a reminder that comfort and good body alignment are sometimes not the same. For example, two large pillows under the head may be comfortable, *but when the neck is in constant flexion, it can develop spasms and even contracture.* Patients' bodies must be repositioned during the night as well. Keep in mind that healthy people turn

many times and adopt many positions during sleep. Repositioning is usually done every two hours. For some patients more frequent turning is needed *to prevent skin breakdown. Without a 24-hour repositioning schedule, patients will develop pressure sores readily.* It is helpful to give range-of-motion exercises (ROM) to patients when they are repositioned *to maintain joint flexibility* (see Module 24).

You can make positioning aids easily from ordinary items found in your facility. Pillows, towels, washcloths, sandbags, footboards, and strong cardboard cartons can all be used to help maintain a position (see Figure 8.9).

The following directions can be used to position the patient (step 11 of the General Procedure).

Supine Position

The patient should lie on his or her back, with the spine in straight alignment. Place a low pillow under the head *to prevent neck extension.* The arms may be at the patient's side with the hands pronated. The forearms can also be elevated on pillows. In either position, if the patient's hands are paralyzed, handrolls should be in place. Handrolls can be made of several washcloths (or other linen) that have been rolled and taped. Place the handroll in the palm of the patient's hand. The fingers and thumb should be flexed around it. The roll should be large enough so that the fingers are only slightly flexed. A handroll may have to be secured to the hand with paper tape (see Figure 8.10). This *maintains the hands in a functional position.*

When the body is lying flat on the bed, position the legs so that external rotation does not occur. *A trochanter roll is effective in preventing external hip rotation.* This roll can be made from a sheet, bath towel, or pad. Place one end flat under the patient's hip (*trochanter*) and roll the linen under to form a roll *that stabilizes the leg and prevents it from turning outward.* An ankle roll, which is made in the same way but is smaller than a trochanter roll, can accomplish the same purpose. If both legs are paralyzed, place a roll on either side at the hip or the ankle.

The foot should be supported so that the toes point upward in anatomical position and do not fall into plantar flexion. *When plantar flexion is maintained for a long time, a permanent deformity called footdrop develops. The foot becomes unable to*

140

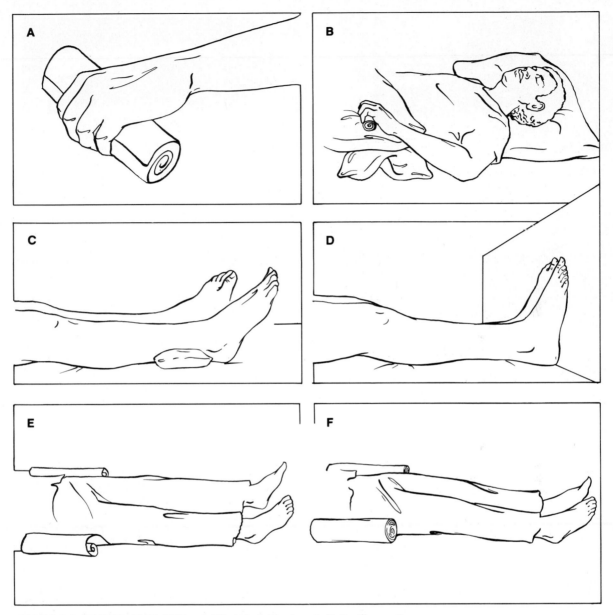

FIGURE 8.9 POSITIONING AIDS   *A:* Washcloth in a handroll; *B:* pillows; *C:* sandbag; *D:* footboard; *E and F:* bath blanket in a trochanter roll.

dorsiflex and ceases to be functional. A manufactured footboard, sandbags, or a strong cardboard carton can be used *to maintain the feet at right angles to the legs.*

Side-Lying Position

If adopted properly, the side-lying position can be particularly comfortable for the patient (see Figure 8.11). A patient who is paralyzed on one side can be placed on that side as well as on the unaffected side unless this is uncomfortable. Give special attention to body alignment, however.

In this position, the patient is on the side with the head supported on a low pillow. Undertuck a pillow along the patient's back *to both support the back and hold the position.* Bring the underlying arm forward and flex it onto the pillow used for the head. Bring the top arm forward, flex it, and rest it on a pillow in front of the body. Put handrolls in place if needed. The

141

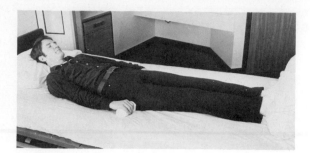

FIGURE 8.10 SUPINE POSITION   A small pillow and a footboard help put the patient in correct supine position. Handrolls are used for patients whose hands are paralyzed.
Courtesy Ivan Ellis

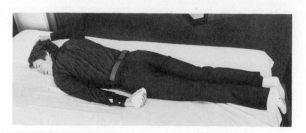

FIGURE 8.12 PRONE POSITION   A small pillow supports the patient's ankles. The patient's arms bend upward toward the shoulders. A small pillow may be used under the head.
Courtesy Ivan Ellis

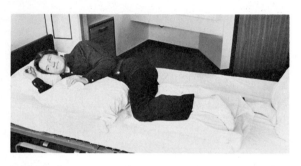

FIGURE 8.11 SIDE-LYING POSITION   Two pillows support the upper leg and arm; the lower leg lies straight.
Courtesy Ivan Ellis

top leg should be flexed and brought slightly forward *to help provide balance.*

A pillow placed lengthwise under the top leg *keeps the legs separated and supports the top leg. Take care to support the feet to prevent plantar flexion and footdrop.*

Prone Position

The prone position (see Figure 8.12) is used infrequently by nurses *because respirations may be compromised in this position.* However, if it is done properly, a great number of patients can tolerate it. The position can be used very effectively with a patient who has pressure sores because it *relieves the pressure on the buttocks and both hips.*

With the patient on the abdomen, turn the head to one side. Usually you do not use a pillow, but sometimes a small pillow or a folded bath towel *may provide added comfort for the patient.*

Be sure that the spine is straight. Place a folded towel under each shoulder. Put a flat pillow under the abdomen of a female patient who

has large breasts. *This should add to her comfort without defeating the principles of good alignment.* The arms may be flat at the patient's side or flexed at the elbow with the hands near the patient's head. Place handrolls if needed. With tall patients, the feet should extend beyond the end of the mattress, so that they are pointing down in the space between the mattress and the footboard. With shorter patients, place a roll under the ankles. *This will keep the feet in proper alignment, preventing plantar flexion.*

Positioning a Patient in a Chair

In a chair, a patient's feet should be flat against the floor with the knees and hips at right angles. The buttocks should rest firmly against the back of the chair, and the spine should be in straight alignment *to provide proper support and comfort* (see Figure 8.13). Avoid placing pillows at the back *because they may interfere with proper alignment.* Support the patient's elbows with armrests. If needed, place handrolls in the patient's hands. A footrest of some type may be needed for shorter patients.

Therapeutic Positions

In addition to the resting positions described above, a variety of special positions are used for therapeutic reasons. The reasons for their use can be found in a medical-surgical text.

Fowler's Position

The patient is in the supine position with the head elevated 18 to 20 inches (approximately 45 degrees). (See Figure 8.14.)

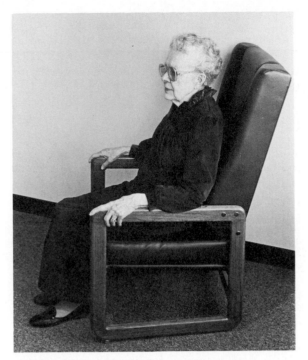

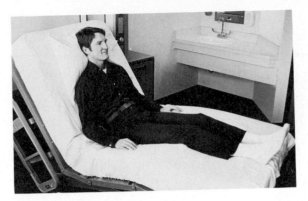

FIGURE 8.15 HIGH-FOWLER'S POSITION
Courtesy Ivan Ellis

FIGURE 8.13 POSITIONING A PATIENT IN A
CHAIR   The patient's buttocks should fit well back into
the seat of the chair. The back is straight, the knees are
bent, and the feet are flat on the floor. The elbows are
supported by armrests.
Courtesy Ivan Ellis

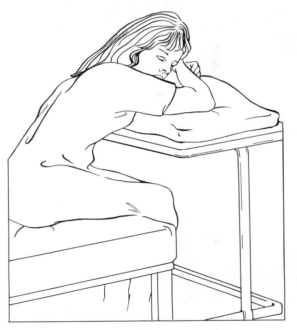

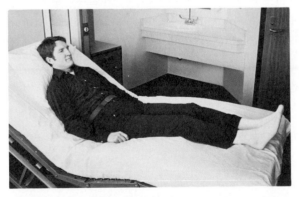

FIGURE 8.14 FOWLER'S POSITION   In the traditional
Fowler's position, the knees were also elevated. This is
seldom done today because of potential pressure on
the popliteal areas.
Courtesy Ivan Ellis

FIGURE 8.16 ORTHOPNEIC POSITION   The patient
rests the elbows on a pillow on the overbed table.

Semi-Fowler's Position

The patient is in the supine position with the
head of the bed elevated to an angle of less than
45 degrees (often 20–30 degrees).

Orthopneic Position

The patient sits up in or at the edge of the bed
with an overbed table across his or her lap. The
table is padded with a pillow and elevated to a
comfortable height. The patient leans forward
and rests head and arms on the table *for support*.
(See Figure 8.16.)

High-Fowler's Position

The patient is in the supine position with the
head of the bed elevated to an angle of more
than 45 degrees. (See Figure 8.15.)

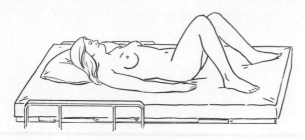

FIGURE 8.17 DORSAL RECUMBANT POSITION (Draping omitted for clarity.)

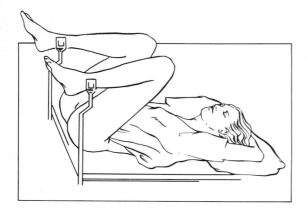

FIGURE 8.18 LITHOTOMY POSITION (Draping omitted for clarity.)

Dorsal Recumbent Position

The dorsal recumbent position is often used as a position of comfort for patients with back strain. The patient is in the supine position with the knees flexed. (See Figure 8.17.)

Lithotomy Position

The patient is supine. Both knees are flexed simultaneously so that the feet are brought close to the hips. The legs are then separated widely, maintaining the flexed position. When the patient is on the examining table, the feet are placed in stirrups. (See Figure 8.18.) The patient is then draped *to provide for visibility of the perineal area and coverage of the legs and body.*

Sims's Position

This is a side-lying position that uses only a single supporting pillow—that under the head. The patient is turned far enough onto the abdomen that the lower arm is extended behind the back and both knees are slightly flexed. (See Figure 8.19.)

Knee-Chest Position (Genupectoral)

The patient kneels on the bed or table, then leans forward with the hips in the air and the chest and arms on the bed or table. A pillow can be placed under the patient's head. (See Figure 8.20.) There are special examination tables that

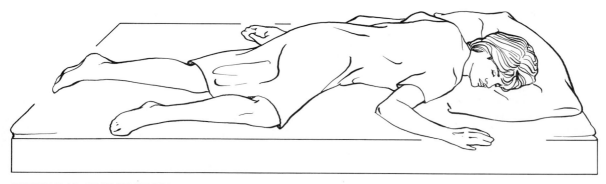

FIGURE 8.19 SIM'S POSITION

144

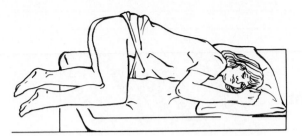

FIGURE 8.20 KNEE-CHEST POSITION (Draping omitted for clarity.)

are constructed to allow a patient to kneel on a platform and lean on the table. The patient is draped *to allow visibility of the rectal area and coverage of the rest of the body.*

Trendelenburg Position

In this position, the patient lies on the back. The head is lowered at a 30-degree angle below horizontal level. (See Figure 8.21.)

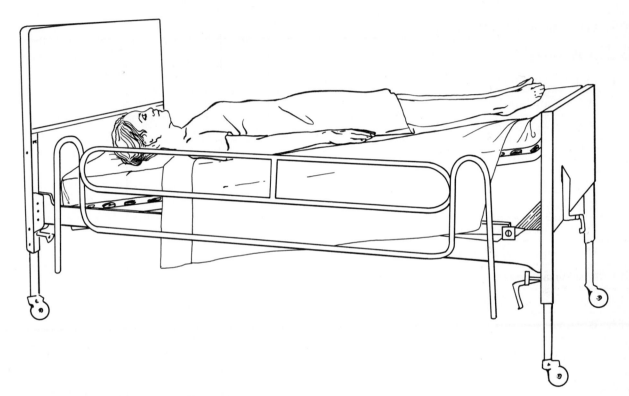

FIGURE 8.21 TRENDELENBURG POSITION

PERFORMANCE CHECKLIST

General procedure for moving a patient in bed

	Unsatisfactory	Needs More Practice	Satisfactory	Comments
Assessment				
1. Assess patient's need.				
2. Assess patient's ability.				
3. Check on assistive devices available.				
Planning				
4. Plan moving technique.				
5. Wash your hands.				
6. Obtain assistive devices.				
Implementation				
7. Identify patient.				
8. Raise bed to high position.				
9. Put bed in flat position.				
10. Move patient according to specific procedure.				
11. Position patient correctly.				
12. Make sure safety devices are in place.				
13. Wash your hands.				
Evaluation				
14. Evaluate position for alignment.				
15. Evaluate patient comfort.				
Documentation				
16. Record time and position on flow sheet or nurses' notes.				
17. Record technique for moving on nursing care plan.				

Moving a patient closer to one side of a bed

	Unsatisfactory	Needs More Practice	Satisfactory	Comments
Assessment				
1. Follow Checklist steps 1–3 of the General Procedure for Moving a Patient in Bed (assess patient's need to move and ability to move unaided, and check on available assistive devices).				

	Unsatisfactory	Needs More Practice	Satisfactory	Comments
☐ *Planning*				
2. Follow Checklist steps 4–6 of the General Procedure (plan moving technique, wash your hands, and obtain assistive devices or assistance).				
☐ *Implementation*				
3. Follow Checklist steps 7–9 of the General Procedure (identify patient, raise bed, and put bed in flat position).				
4. Slide your hands and arms under patient's head and shoulders, and pull toward you.				
5. Move your hands and arms under patient's hips, and pull toward you.				
6. Slide your hands and arms under patient's legs, and pull toward you.				
7. Repeat in sequence until patient is in correct position.				
8. Follow Checklist steps 11–13 of the General Procedure (correctly position patient, have safety devices in place, and wash your hands).				
☐ *Evaluation*				
9. Follow Checklist steps 14 and 15 of the General Procedure (assess for correct alignment and ask patient about comfort).				
☐ *Documentation*				
10. Follow Checklist steps 16 and 17 of the General Procedure (record as required by your facility and add to care plan if appropriate).				

Moving a patient up in bed: One-person assist

	Unsatisfactory	Needs More Practice	Satisfactory	Comments
☐ *Assessment*				
1. Follow Checklist steps 1–3 of the General Procedure for Moving a Patient in Bed (assess patient's need to move and ability to move unaided, and check on available assistive devices).				

147

	Unsatisfactory	Needs More Practice	Satisfactory	Comments
Planning				
2. Follow Checklist steps 4–6 of the General Procedure (plan moving technique, wash your hands, and obtain assistive devices or assistance).				
Implementation				
3. Follow Checklist steps 7–9 of the General Procedure (identify patient, raise bed, and put bed in flat position).				
4. Have patient bend knees and place soles firmly on bed.				
5. Have patient grasp overhead trapeze, side rails, or headboard.				
6. Slide your hands and arms under patient's hips, facing foot of bed, with outside foot ahead of inside foot.				
7. Instruct patient to move with you at count.				
8. On count, patient pulls with arms and pushes with feet as you pull.				
9. Follow Checklist steps 11–13 of the General Procedure (correctly position patient, have safety devices in place, and wash your hands).				
Evaluation				
10. Follow Checklist steps 14 and 15 of the General Procedure (assess for correct alignment and ask patient about comfort).				
Documentation				
11. Follow Checklist steps 16 and 17 of the General Procedure (record as required by your facility and add to care plan if appropriate).				

Moving a patient up in bed: Two- or three-person assist

Assessment				
1. Follow Checklist steps 1–3 of the General Procedure for Moving a Patient in Bed (assess patient's need to				

	Unsatisfactory	Needs More Practice	Satisfactory	Comments
move and ability to move unaided, and check on available assistive devices).				
☐ *Planning*				
2. Follow Checklist steps 4–6 of the General Procedure (plan moving technique, wash your hands, and obtain assistive devices or assistance).				
☐ *Implementation*				
3. Follow Checklist steps 7–9 of the General Procedure (identify patient, raise bed, and put bed in flat position).				
4. Move patient close to one side of bed.				
5. If possible, have patient's knees bent and soles firmly on bed.				
6. Nurse 1 slides arms under patient's head and shoulders.				
7. Nurse 2 slides arms under patient's hips.				
8. Nurse 2 counts, and both move patient.				
9. Follow Checklist steps 11–13 of the General Procedure (correctly position patient, have safety devices in place, and wash your hands).				
☐ *Evaluation*				
10. Follow Checklist steps 14 and 15 of the General Procedure (assess for correct alignment and ask patient about comfort).				
☐ *Documentation*				
11. Follow Checklist steps 16 and 17 of the General Procedure (record as required by your facility and add to care plan if appropriate).				

Turning a patient in bed: Back to side

	Unsatisfactory	Needs More Practice	Satisfactory	Comments
☐ *Assessment*				
1. Follow Checklist steps 1–3 of the General Procedure for Moving a Patient in Bed (assess patient's need to move and ability to move unaided, and check on available assistive devices).				

	Unsatisfactory	Needs More Practice	Satisfactory	Comments
☐ *Planning*				
2. Follow Checklist steps 4–6 of the General Procedure (plan moving technique, wash your hands, and obtain assistive devices or assistance).				
☐ *Implementation*				
3. Follow Checklist steps 7–9 of the General Procedure (identify patient, raise bed, and put bed in flat position).				
4. Move patient to one side of bed.				
5. Raise rail and move to other side.				
6. Prepare pillows for support.				
7. Turn lower body, using one of two methods described.				
8. Move patient's near arm out of patient's way.				
9. Place patient's far arm across chest.				
10. Grasp patient behind far shoulder.				
11. Roll patient toward you.				
12. Adjust position as needed.				
13. Follow Checklist steps 11–13 of the General Procedure (correctly position patient, have safety devices in place, and wash your hands).				
☐ *Evaluation*				
14. Follow Checklist steps 14 and 15 of the General Procedure (assess for correct alignment and ask patient about comfort).				
☐ *Documentation*				
15. Follow Checklist steps 16 and 17 of the General Procedure (record as required by your facility and add to care plan if appropriate).				

Turning a patient in bed: Back to abdomen

☐ *Assessment*				
1. Follow Checklist steps 1–3 of the General Procedure for Moving a Patient in Bed (assess patient's need to				

	Unsatisfactory	Needs More Practice	Satisfactory	Comments
move and ability to move unaided, and check on available assistive devices).				
☐ *Planning*				
2. Follow Checklist steps 4–6 of the General Procedure (plan moving technique, wash your hands, and obtain assistive devices or assistance).				
☐ *Implementation*				
3. Follow Checklist steps 7–9 of the General Procedure (identify patient, raise bed, and put bed in flat position).				
4. Move patient to edge of bed.				
5. Raise side rail and move to other side of bed.				
6. Prepare pillows for support.				
7. Place patient's near arm close to body.				
8. Turn patient's face away from you.				
9. Roll patient onto side.				
10. Check arm and face positioning.				
11. Roll patient further onto abdomen.				
12. Adjust position as needed.				
13. Follow Checklist steps 11–13 of the General Procedure (correctly position patient, have safety devices in place, and wash your hands).				
☐ *Evaluation*				
14. Follow Checklist steps 14 and 15 of the General Procedure (assess for correct alignment and ask patient about comfort).				
☐ *Documentation*				
15. Follow Checklist steps 16 and 17 of the General Procedure (record as required by your facility and add to care plan if appropriate).				

Turning a patient: Logrolling

☐ *Assessment*

1. Follow Checklist steps 1–3 of the General Procedure for Moving a Patient in Bed (assess patient's need to

	Unsatisfactory	Needs More Practice	Satisfactory	Comments
move and ability to move unaided, and check on available assistive devices).				
☐ *Planning*				
2. Follow Checklist steps 4–6 of the General Procedure (plan moving technique, wash your hands, and obtain assistive devices or assistance).				
☐ *Implementation*				
3. Follow Checklist steps 7–9 of the General Procedure (identify patient, raise bed, and put bed in flat position).				
4. With help, move patient to side of bed in one unit.				
5. Raise side rail on that side of bed.				
6. All assistants move to other side of bed.				
7. Place pillows correctly.				
8. Assistants reach across and grasp patient's body.				
9. At count, all turn patient in one unit.				
10. Follow Checklist steps 11–13 of the General Procedure (correctly position patient, have safety devices in place, and wash your hands).				
☐ *Evaluation*				
11. Follow Checklist steps 14 and 15 of the General Procedure (assess for correct alignment and ask patient about comfort).				
☐ *Documentation*				
12. Follow Checklist steps 16 and 17 of the General Procedure (record as required by your facility and add to care plan if appropriate).				
Note: All the movements described can be facilitated by using a turn sheet or pull sheet. See page 139.				

Supine position

	Unsatisfactory	Needs More Practice	Satisfactory	Comments
1. Place patient on back, with spine in straight alignment.				
2. Place low pillow under head.				

	Unsatisfactory	Needs More Practice	Satisfactory	Comments
3. Place arms at side or elevated on pillow, with hands prone.				
4. Place handrolls if needed.				
5. Keep legs straight.				
6. Place trochanter or ankle roll on one or both sides.				
7. Position feet with toes pointed up, and support with footboard, sandbags, or carton.				

Side-lying position

1. Turn patient on side.				
2. Place low pillow under head.				
3. Undertuck pillow along back.				
4. Place lower arm forward of body.				
5. Flex and support lower arm on pillow used for head.				
6. Flex top arm and rest on pillow in front of body.				
7. Place handrolls if needed.				
8. Flex top leg and bring slightly forward.				
9. Place pillow lengthwise between legs.				
10. Support feet with positioning aids to prevent plantar flexion.				

Prone position

1. Place patient on abdomen.				
2. Turn patient's head to one side.				
3. Straighten spine.				
4. Place folded towel under each shoulder.				
5. Place arms flat at side or flexed at elbow near patient's head.				
6. Place handrolls if needed.				
7. Position patient's feet in space between mattress and footboard or use roll under ankles.				

	Unsatisfactory	Needs More Practice	Satisfactory	Comments
Positioning a patient in a chair				
1. Place feet flat against floor.				
2. Position knees and hips at right angle.				
3. Straighten spine.				
4. Support elbows on armrests.				
5. Place handrolls if needed.				
Fowler's position				
1. Place patient in supine position.				
2. Elevate head of bed 18 to 20 inches (approximately 45 degrees).				
High-Fowler's position				
1. Place patient in supine position.				
2. Elevate head of bed to angle of over 45°.				
Semi-Fowler's position				
1. Place patient in supine position.				
2. Elevate head of bed to angle of less than 45° (usually 20–30 degrees).				
Orthopneic position				
1. Have patient sit up in bed with overbed table across lap.				
2. Pad table with pillows and elevate to comfortable height.				
3. Have patient lean forward with head and arms resting on table.				
Dorsal recumbent position				
1. Position patient on back.				
2. Raise knees and separate legs.				
3. Feet remain in position on bed.				
Lithotomy position				
1. Position patient on back.				
2. Raise knees and separate legs.				

	Unsatisfactory	Needs More Practice	Satisfactory	Comments
3. If on table, place feet in stirrups.				

Sims's position

1. Use side-lying position, with single pillow only under head.				
2. Turn far enough onto abdomen so lower arm extends behind patient's back.				

Knee-chest position

1. Have patient kneel on bed or table with hips in air and chest on bed or table.				
2. If special table is available, have patient kneel on platform with head and chest on table.				

Trendelenburg position

1. Position patient on back with head lowered at 45-degree angle.				

| QUIZ |

Short-Answer Questions

1. What is the primary reason for having the bed in the flat position when moving a patient? _____

2. What two important functions are fulfilled by having the patient assist you whenever possible?

    a. _____

    b. _____

3. If the nurse attempts to move a patient by grasping him or her under the axillae, a(n) _____ may occur.

4. A turn sheet should be placed under which part of a patient's body?

    _____

5. List two reasons why patients should be checked after moving.

    a. _____

    b. _____

6. List three reasons for proper and frequent positioning of a patient in bed.

    a. _____

    b. _____

    c. _____

7. To prevent external rotation of the leg when a patient is in the supine position, you might use _____

8. When a patient is in a side-lying position, the top leg is _____ over the lower leg.

9. When a patient is in the prone position, two methods can be used to keep the feet from plantar flexion and possible development of footdrop. What are these two methods?

    a. _____

    b. _____

Multiple-Choice Questions

_____ 10. In all positions the spine should be

    a. slightly flexed.
    b. straight.
    c. slightly extended.
    d. curved.

_____ **11.** A patient's position should usually be changed

      a. every hour.
      b. every two hours.
      c. every four hours.
      d. once per shift.

MODULE 9

Feeding Adult Patients

MODULE CONTENTS

Rationale for the Use of This Skill
General Considerations
    Psychological Overtones
    Influences on Eating Habits
Procedure for Feeding Adult Patients
    Assessment
    Planning
    Implementation
    Evaluation
    Documentation

PREREQUISITES

1. Successful completion of the following modules:

   VOLUME 1
   Module 1 / An Approach to Nursing Skills
   Module 2 / Medical Asepsis
   Module 3 / Safety
   Module 5 / Assessment
   Module 6 / Documentation
   Module 15 / Intake and Output
2. Familiarity with the basic diets used in most institutions.
3. Knowledge of the five major nutrients.

OVERALL OBJECTIVE

To assist and/or to feed patients who are unable to feed themselves independently.

SPECIFIC LEARNING OBJECTIVES

	Know Facts and Principles	Apply Facts and Principles	Demonstrate Ability	Evaluate Performance
1. *Preparation* a. *Environment* b. *Patient (physical and psychological)*	List factors in environment that might affect appetite. Describe optimum position for comfort and ease of eating, and discuss possible modifications. Discuss emotional needs and responses related to eating.	In a specific patient situation, state what needs to be done to prepare patient and environment for meal	In clinical setting, carry out preparation appropriately	Evaluate with instructor
2. *Adaptations of procedure*	List factors that often make adaptations to procedure necessary	Assess muscular and other physical difficulties, including swallowing problems, and emotional reactions	When feeding patient in the clinical setting, vary the procedure appropriately in light of a particular patient's difficulties	Review performance with instructor and patient
3. *Retention and tolerance*	List untoward reactions toward eating and/or being fed	Know problems most commonly experienced by patients being cared for	In the clinical setting, assess for specific responses unique to patient	Share problems with instructor
4. *Documentation*	State importance of monitoring patient's food intake	Be familiar with portions of food items and terms used. Describe amount of food taken and patient's responses	After feeding an individual patient, properly record amounts taken and pertinent observations	Evaluate with instructor

LEARNING ACTIVITIES

1. Review the Specific Learning Objectives.
2. Read the section on nutrition (in the chapter on nutrition) in Ellis and Nowlis, *Nursing: A Human Needs Approach,* or comparable material in another textbook.
3. Look up the module vocabulary terms in the Glossary.
4. Read through the module.
5. Review the steps of the procedure in the Performance Checklist.
6. In the practice setting:
   a. Have a classmate feed you lunch. Try eating half in a recumbent position (lying down) and half in a sitting position in bed. Close your eyes for three minutes while being fed. At this point, have your classmate describe the food to you. Now answer the following questions:
      (1) What was pleasant about the experience?
      (2) What was unpleasant?
   b. Repeat a, only this time you feed your classmate. Discuss the questions from the point of view of the one administering the feeding.
   c. Examine the pictures of feeding aids on page 165. These aids can be purchased commercially or made by members of the patient's family or by the physical therapy department.
7. In the clinical setting:
   a. Observe a patient being fed. What was done that was helpful to the patient? What improvements could have been made?
   b. Feed a patient an entire meal. Note the time when you begin and end the procedure. Answer the following questions for your own learning or discuss them with your instructor.
      (1) How long did the feeding procedure take?
      (2) What conclusions can you draw from the timing?
      (3) What were some of the blocks to effective feeding that you encountered?
      (4) What went well?
      (5) Were you uncomfortable at any point?
      (6) Did the patient appear to be uncomfortable at any point?
      (7) Did you use all the steps of the procedure?
      (8) Did you have to make adaptations? If so, in what way?
      (9) Why were adaptations made?
   c. Record, on a piece of paper, observations you would make on the amount of food taken and the patient's response. Share your notes with your instructor.

VOCABULARY

agility
antiemetic
aspiration
anorexia
body language
condiments
digestion
dysphagia
ethnic
ingestion
NPO
regurgitate
stereotype
tremor

PROVIDING NUTRITION

Rationale for the Use of This Skill

D*uring illness, trauma, or wound healing, the body needs more nutrients than usual. However, many patients, because of weakness, immobility, and/or inability to use one or both of the upper extremities, are unable to feed themselves all or part of a meal. To be sure the patient receives adequate nutrition, the nurse must be knowledgeable, sensitive, and skillful in carrying out the feeding procedure. To promote the patient's well-being, the nurse must also consider the patient's psychological response to being fed.*

Feeding patients has been considered a less than professional skill and has often been relegated to aides or volunteers. This is a shortsighted attitude. You should welcome this extended interaction with patients.[1]

Nursing Diagnoses

Examples of some nursing diagnoses related to nutrition include:

Nutrition, Alteration in: Less than Body Requirements related to, for example, nausea and vomiting.

Nutrition, Alteration in: More than Body Requirements related to, for example, excessive intake of carbohydrates.

Self-Care Deficit: Inability to feed self related to, for example, right upper extremity paralysis.

Knowledge Deficit related to, for example, normal nutrition or "special" diet.

General Considerations

Psychological Overtones

To human beings, eating is ultimately more than taking in food to maintain vital bodily function and metabolism. Meals can be a ritual, a celebration, a habit, and, importantly, a social event.

The psychological aspects of feeding an adult patient are formidable. Supplying food for someone is a satisfying experience for most peo-ple. Many mothers and fathers enjoy providing healthful, attractive diets for their young children. And preparing a festive meal for guests or for a special family occasion is a delight to most homemakers. In the same way, helping a patient eat a meal can be equally challenging and satisfying for you.

To the institutionalized person, the meal takes on new meaning. It may well be the high point of the day, often punctuating an otherwise long, weary day of immobilization. The patient may have the nurse at the bedside for a longer time then than at any other period in the nursing day. However, it is crucial to remember that being fed can be degrading to some patients and may give them a feeling that they are now dependent, unable to carry out for themselves such a simple task as spooning their own food into their mouths.

As with all skills and procedures, whether performed by the professional or the paraprofessional, time and caring are essential components.

Influences on Eating Habits

What affects the manner in which a person eats? At first glance, this seems to be a simple question; however, watching people eat in a restaurant proves otherwise. We can observe in a restaurant that people select very different foods, use condiments in various ways, and show different kinds of "body language" while eating.

Many factors influence eating. For example, eating habits have been affected by escalating food prices during the last few years. Although you must recognize individual differences and not contrive stereotypes, ethnic background also must be considered. More often than not, people enjoy the foods that are prevalent in their family and ethnic group. However, not all blacks like "soul food," nor do all Germans relish sauerbraten.

Age is another important factor. Watching a teenager wolf down two large hamburgers, fries, and a large shake and then rush off to other activities is a totally different experience from joining an elderly couple who linger before a TV set with prepackaged dinners on trays.

Within the institution, a variety of factors may influence how well the patient eats. The portions of servings may be unduly large for a light eater. (Some hospitals request patients to

---

[1]You will note that rationale for action is emphasized throughout the module by the use of italics.

select in advance the size of a serving, usually small, medium, or large.) Unfamiliar mealtimes or food items may also lead to anorexia or lack of appetite. Neuromuscular disturbances can make eating difficult.

The nature of the patient's illness is also important. Remember that illness interferes with both body and mind, and every *illness produces a degree of anxiety within the individual* that may cause decreased eating, increased eating, or erratic eating. An understanding attitude on your part, taking into account all these factors, *will promote a more satisfying outcome to the eating-feeding experience.* Being with the patient during a meal and participating in this significant activity also gives you time for several of your most basic and important functions: assessing, planning, implementing, and evaluating.

Procedure for Feeding Adult Patients

Assessment

1. Identify the type of diet ordered *to determine whether the diet is appropriate for the patient in his or her present condition and to determine whether any special feeding utensils will be needed.* If a patient has just developed a high fever and nausea or is in pain, you may wish to change to a lighter meal *that the patient can digest more easily,* or to delay the meal *until medications can be given to allay the patient's problem.* If you are aware that there is potential for nausea, vomiting, or pain with a particular patient, it is wise to see that the ordered medication is given 20–30 minutes prior to the meal *to enhance the potential for adequate food intake.*

2. Check to see whether there is any reason why the patient's meal should be delayed or omitted. *Scheduled laboratory tests, radiological examinations, and surgery may mean that the patient must be kept "NPO" (nothing by mouth) for a period of time.*

3. Check in the nursing care plan, nursing history, or nursing record for the patient's previous need for assistance. At the same time, note information about cultural or religious limitations, allergies, and specific likes and dislikes. Do your own assessment as well, *because the patient's*

condition may have changed or the previous assessment may have been incomplete.

4. Note any nursing diagnoses related to eating or feeding. *Knowledge of these, along with the related plans of care, can do a lot to make feeding easier and more pleasant for both you and the patient.*

Planning

5. When planning care, take into account the time food trays arrive on the unit *so that tasks and procedures may be scheduled away from mealtime and so that you and/or the patient aren't in the middle of a task or treatment at that time.*

6. Allot enough time for feeding so that you are free of other tasks and can spend uninterrupted time with the patient. This is important *to prevent food from getting cold and the patient from feeling unattended.*

7. Set a tentative goal for how much of the diet the patient will consume, based on physiological status and past performance.

8. Wash your hands *for asepsis.* As the food handler, your hands must be meticulously clean.

Implementation

9. Identify the patient *to be sure you are carrying out the procedure for the correct patient.*

10. Explain what you are going to do. Communication is a skill that is basic to all interaction with patients, and feeding is no exception. Telling patients that they *must* eat in order to get well is, in reality, not helpful and seldom elicits cooperation. It is better to approach the meal as an enjoyable experience both for yourself, as a sharer of time and conversation, and for the patient, for whom it should be a respite from painful experiences that may take place during the day. Approach the patient with the expectation that he or she will join in the procedure willingly and benefit from it.

11. Offer the bedpan or urinal *for patient comfort and so that the meal will not have to be interrupted for reasons of elimination.*

12. Assist in washing the patient's hands and face *to add to comfort and cleanliness.*

13. Prepare the patient's room by removing

163

all unsightly equipment, replacing soiled linens, and arranging the bedside table to receive the tray. Unpleasant odors can be controlled by using an air freshener or opening a window. *A restful, neat, and odor-free environment makes eating more pleasant and aids digestion.*

14. Position the patient comfortably in mid- or high-Fowler's, if possible. *The higher position makes swallowing easier and lessens the risk of choking and aspiration.*

15. If the patient wears eyeglasses or dentures, be sure they are in place *so that the patient can see and chew properly.*

16. Protect the bed linen by using a suitable protective cover. Avoid using the word "bib," *which may be a humiliating term to the patient.* Place a colorful napkin, if available, over the protecting linen for attractiveness.

17. Obtain any special utensils that you have planned to use. Utensils are not always selected for convenience. For example, the fluid "bottle" feeders are fast, convenient facilitators of the feeding process, but they often convey to the patient, "We are treating you like a baby." It is far better to have a few spots of spilled food on the bedding than to diminish, even unintentionally, a patient's dignity. Other utensils, such as those shown in Figure 9.1, *foster self-esteem by allowing patients who are partially disabled to feed themselves.*

18. Check to be sure that the name on the tray corresponds with the name on the patient's identification bracelet and that the food choices marked on the menu correspond with the food on the tray.

19. Assist the patient to prepare the food on the tray as needed. For example, cut food into bite-sized pieces, open milk cartons and cereal boxes, and butter toast. Encourage independence appropriately. Discard all wrappings and clutter before the patient begins to eat.

20. Position yourself at the patient's eye level by sitting, if at all possible. *This establishes an unhurried atmosphere.* (See Figure 9.2.)

21. Involve the patient as much as possible. This can be done best if you work from the unaffected side (the side of the patient least affected by the disease process). *In this way, the patient gains a sense of participation.* Place the tray in such a way that the patient can see the food that is being offered. If the patient is sightless, describing what is on the meal tray is both necessary and helpful. Many such patients can manage with very little assistance if they know where food items are located. Often a clock format is used to assist the sightless patient, e.g., "The milk is at 2 o'clock and the potatoes are at 6 o'clock."

Many disabled patients can hold and enjoy feeding themselves pieces of bread or toast during the meal. Managing their own napkins also *offers them some degree of independence.*

22. Allow choices. Patients have few choices available when they are in the hospital. If a patient is able to specify particular preferences (likes and dislikes) in the menu, communicate this information to the dietician. To someone who is in good health, this may appear unimportant; but to the incapacitated person, it says, "I am still a person," "This nurse cares what I think," "I still have some control."

When possible, find out from the patient what food sequence is preferred. If this is not possible, feed the items in the order in which you would choose to eat them. This is good practice *because it affords the patient a variety of tastes,* which is usually the most pleasant way to eat a meal. If the patient does not respond to being given a choice, feed the more nutritious items of the diet first, *in case the patient's intake capacity is limited.* For example, if the choice is between broth and tea, broth, which is high in protein, would be preferable.

The elderly patient who has difficulty eating because of poorly fitting dentures often prefers to mix eggs, fruit, cereal, and toast together. Although this may strike you as unappetizing, affably feeding this mixture to the patient *serves to develop a good nurse-patient relationship.* Do not feel compelled to change long-standing eating habits, although you may adopt as a long-term goal, for example, arranging for the patient to be fit with comfortable dentures.

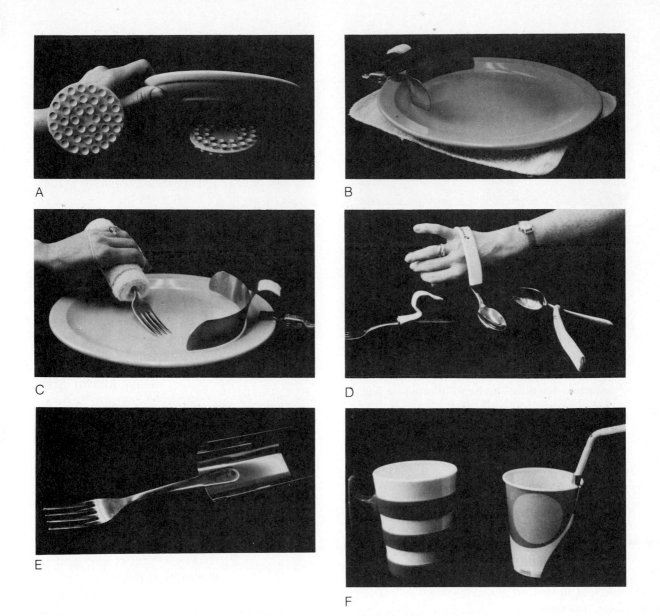

FIGURE 9.1 FEEDING UTENSILS *A:* "Octopus" suction cups for securing plates; *B:* plate secured by wet washcloth, with metal food guard attached to keep food on plate; *C:* washcloth in handroll for easy grip; *D and E:* modified handles; *F:* cup handle and straw secured with pen clip.
Courtesy Florence E. Smith

23. Continue assessment as you feed the patient. Some patients have dysphagia, or difficulty in swallowing. You can easily and accurately assess the patient's muscular agility, mental status, and feelings at this time. Signs such as skin color, respiratory rate, and the presence or absence of tremor can also be assessed.

24. Do not discuss stressful events at mealtime. *It has been shown that digestion is better when a patient is not emotionally upset.*

Try to create a sharing, lighthearted atmosphere.

25. Never hurry a patient's eating. *This can make the patient uncomfortable and fearful of taking up your time.* Feeding, if performed properly, is a time-consuming task, but it can give satisfaction both to you and to the patient.

26. Allow the patient to determine when enough has been eaten *as a way of providing choices.*

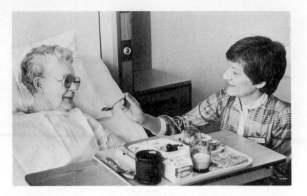

FIGURE 9.2 FEEDING THE OLDER PATIENT
Courtesy Ivan Ellis

27. Remove the tray, offer the bedpan or assist to the bathroom as indicated, and provide hygiene as needed.
28. Reposition the patient. If there have been problems with digestion or vomiting, keep the patient in the high position *so that gravity can help the retention of food in the stomach.* Turning the head to one side *can prevent aspiration if vomiting does occur.*
29. Provide quiet *so that the patient may relax after the meal, which also promotes good digestion.*
30. Wash your hands *for asepsis.*

☐ *Evaluation*

31. Evaluate using the following criteria:
    a. The patient is satisfied and comfortable.
    b. The amount of food and fluid consumed has been observed, as well as measured and recorded if necessary.
    c. Any problems have been noted for later documentation.

☐ *Documentation*

32. Recording the success of the meal, including the patient's response and ability to ingest, is one of your essential duties. Record the food that was taken, either by using the checklist the

institution provides or by charting in more detail on the progress notes, depending on the situation. If food intake has previously presented problems, charting the individual food items and the amounts taken is more accurate.

Add to the nursing care plan any new information related to the patient's likes and dislikes or methods of assisting that you have noted *to enhance continuity of care.*

Examples of Charting   Narrative Charting

11/12/88	
1800	Ate 75% chopped diet with some difficulty swallowing solid food. Feeding facilitated by providing small bites followed by sips of liquids. Left in high-Fowler's position. No emesis.
	Dave Martin, S.N.

POMR Charting

11/12/88		
1800	4.	Dysphagia
	S	"The meat seems to stick in my throat."
	O	Appears to swallow solid foods with difficulty. Fluids taken without difficulty.
	A	Dysphagia with solid food.
	P	Give small bites of solid food alternated with fluids.
		Dave Martin, S.N.

REFERENCES

Carpenito, Lynda. *Handbook of Nursing Diagnosis.* Philadelphia: J. B. Lippincott Company, 1984, pp. 46–48.

PERFORMANCE CHECKLIST

Procedure for feeding the adult patient

	Unsatisfactory	Needs More Practice	Satisfactory	Comments
Assessment				
1. Identify type of diet ordered.				
2. Check to see whether there is any reason why patient's meal should be delayed or omitted.				
3. Check on patient's previous need for assistance.				
4. Note any nursing diagnoses related to eating or feeding.				
Planning				
5. When planning care, take into account the time food trays arrive on the unit.				
6. Plan time for feeding.				
7. Set tentative goal.				
8. Wash your hands.				
Implementation				
9. Identify patient.				
10. Greet patient and explain what you are going to do.				
11. Offer bedpan or urinal.				
12. Assist in washing patient's hands and face.				
13. Prepare patient's room.				
14. Position patient comfortably, preferably in mid- to high-Fowler's.				
15. Provide eyeglasses or dentures if worn.				
16. Protect bed linen.				
17. Obtain any special utensils needed.				
18. Check to be sure that name on tray matches that of patient and that food on tray is consistent with ordered diet.				
19. Assist patient to prepare food on tray.				
20. Position yourself at patient's eye level.				
21. Involve patient as much as possible.				
22. Allow choices.				

	Unsatisfactory	Needs More Practice	Satisfactory	Comments
23. Continually assess patient.				
24. Do not discuss stressful events.				
25. Never hurry the patient's eating.				
26. Allow the patient to determine when enough has been consumed.				
27. Remove tray, offer opportunity for elimination, and provide hygiene.				
28. Reposition the patient.				
29. Provide a quiet atmosphere.				
30. Wash your hands.				
☐ *Evaluation*				
31. Evaluate using the following criteria: a. Patient is satisfied and comfortable.				
b. Amount taken was observed and measured or recorded, if necessary.				
c. Problems encountered noted.				
☐ *Documentation*				
32. Record the following data: a. Type and amount of food taken.				
b. Patient response.				
c. Add new information to the nursing care plan.				

| QUIZ |

Short-Answer Question

1. List four factors that can influence a patient's eating abilities.

    a. _____

    b. _____

    c. _____

    d. _____

Multiple-Choice Questions

_____ 2. Every feeding situation presents which of the following opportunities for the nurse?

   a. Time for health teaching
   b. Determination of the medical diagnosis
   c. Time for nursing assessments to be made
   d. Repositioning of the patient

   Situation: Mr. Swenson, a 63-year-old Scandinavian with a right-sided hemiplegia (paralysis on the right side of the body), has been in the hospital for ten days. The patient's chart states that a soft diet has been ordered and that he is allowed up in a chair q.d. (once daily).

   Lunch trays will be arriving in 20 minutes, and you have been assigned to feed Mr. Swenson. As you enter his room, you see a denture cup on the bedside table and glasses on the overbed table. A urinal is on the floor. Questions 3–10 refer to Mr. Swenson.

_____ 3. From the data given, you determine that Mr. Swenson's feeding problem is

   a. lack of ability to swallow food.
   b. not evident from the information available.
   c. lack of ability to use small-muscle groups to feed himself.
   d. depression brought on by dependency.

_____ 4. Your *first* action in the above situation should be to

   a. introduce yourself and give the reason for your presence.
   b. empty and put away the urinal.
   c. encourage Mr. Swenson to discuss his feelings about being dependent.
   d. reposition Mr. Swenson in a high-Fowler's position for lunch.

_____ 5. If Mr. Swenson must be fed his meal, you should stand on

    a. his left side.
    b. his right side.
    c. either side.

_____ 6. Mr. Swenson's speech is unclear and difficult to understand. Which action should you take?

    a. Don't speak so that he won't feel embarrassed knowing he has to reply.
    b. Carry on a one-sided conversation so that mealtime isn't silent.
    c. Encourage him to speak and take time to try to understand him.
    d. Only make brief comments that require yes or no answers, so that he can devote his energy to eating.

True-False Questions

_____ 7. Mr. Swenson should be encouraged to talk about his anxieties while you are at his bedside feeding him.

_____ 8. Because Mr. Swenson is Scandinavian, he will certainly enjoy the fish on the lunch menu.

_____ 9. The goal for Mr. Swenson in regard to self-feeding this meal should be established only after you check to see what his previous ability has been.

_____ 10. Mr. Swenson ate only half of his meal. This means your feeding plan was unsuccessful.

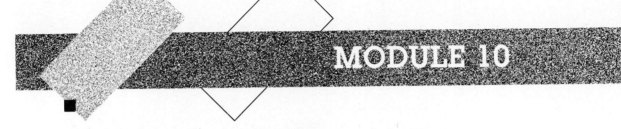

MODULE 10

Assisting with Elimination and Perineal Care

PREREQUISITES

Successful completion of the following modules:

VOLUME 1

Module 1 / An Approach to Nursing Skills
Module 2 / Medical Asepsis
Module 3 / Safety
Module 5 / Assessment
Module 6 / Documentation

OVERALL OBJECTIVE

To assist patients with the use of bedpans or urinals in a hygienic manner, taking into account psychological factors and to provide perineal care according to individual needs.

SPECIFIC LEARNING OBJECTIVES

	Know Facts and Principles	Apply Facts and Principles	Demonstrate Ability	Evaluate Performance
Assisting with Elimination				
1. *Equipment*	Describe equipment needed	Given a patient situation, list appropriate equipment	When caring for patient, select correct equipment	Evaluate own performance with instructor
2. *Assisting with bedpan or urinal*	State three principles for carrying out procedures	Given a patient situation, explain and discuss medical asepsis, psychological needs, and normal conditions of elimination	In the clinical setting, carry out medical asepsis, provide psychological comfort, and approximate normal conditions of elimination	Evaluate own performance with instructor
3. *Procedure*				
a. *Positioning*	Describe positions used for individual patients	Given a patient situation, plan particular procedure correctly	In the clinical setting, individualize procedure to particular patient and carry out plan	Evaluate with instructor using Performance Checklist
b. *Privacy*	State measures to ensure privacy	Given a patient situation, plan privacy measures	In the clinical setting, provide privacy for patient	Evaluate own performance with instructor
c. *Providing bedpan or urinal*	Describe several techniques employed in giving bedpan or urinal	Given a patient situation, plan appropriate technique for giving bedpan or urinal	In the clinical setting, individualize technique for giving bedpan or urinal	Evaluate own performance with instructor

172

d. Cleaning patient	Recognize need for cleanliness	Demonstrate correct cleaning of patient	In the clinical setting, provide cleanliness for patient after use of bedpan or urinal	
4. Documentation	State what should be recorded	Given a hypothetical situation, record as if on chart	Record complete observations in correct format	Evaluate recording with instructor

Giving Perineal Care

1. Equipment	Describe various pieces of equipment	Given a patient situation, simulate correct method for postpartum patient and for patient with a catheter	In the clinical setting, give perineal care to postpartum patient, nonsurgical patient, and catheterized patient, adapting equipment and procedure correctly	Evaluate with instructor using Performance Checklist
2. Psychological comfort	Explain why giving psychological support is important	Given a patient situation, discern possible causes of psychological discomfort	In the clinical setting, provide psychological support to patient	
3. Procedure a. Postpartum patient b. Nonsurgical patient c. Patient with catheter	Describe appropriate adaptations in procedure related to particular patient condition	Given a patient situation, adapt procedure appropriately for a particular patient	In the clinical setting, carry out procedure for postpartum patient, nonsurgical patient, and catheterized patient safely and correctly	Evaluate own performance with instructor
4. Documentation	List what should be recorded	Given a patient situation, record as if on chart	Record observations correctly	Evaluate documentation with instructor

LEARNING ACTIVITIES	VOCABULARY

LEARNING ACTIVITIES

1. Review the Specific Learning Objectives.
2. Read the chapter on elimination in Ellis and Nowlis, *Nursing: A Human Needs Approach,* or a comparable chapter in another textbook.
3. Look up the module vocabulary terms in the Glossary.
4. Read through the module.
5. In the practice setting:
   a. Become familiar with the various pieces of available equipment (different types of bedpans, urinals, perineal packs).
   b. Select a partner and perform the following:
      (1) Pretend you are a patient. Have your partner place you on a bedpan.
      (2) Remain on the bedpan for three minutes in a flat position, then for another three minutes in a sitting position.
      (3) Have your partner remove the bedpan as though you were incapacitated.
      (4) Describe any discomfort you experienced.
      (5) Reverse the roles, repeating (1), (2), (3), and (4).
   c. Using a mannequin, go through the specific procedure for giving perineal care to each of the following:
      (1) A postpartum or perineal surgical patient
      (2) A nonsurgical patient
      (3) A patient with a catheter
6. In the clinical area, with your instructor's supervision:
   a. Place a patient on a bedpan using both methods.
   b. Give a urinal to a male patient.
   c. Administer perineal care to a postpartum patient, a nonsurgical patient, and a catheterized patient.
7. Using the Performance Checklist, evaluate yourself with the help of your instructor.

VOCABULARY

ADLs
bedpan
catheter
defecation
foreskin
fracture pan
genital area
labia
lumbosacral
penis
perineum
renal calculi
smegma
sutures
urethral meatus
urinal
urination
void
vulva

ASSISTING WITH ELIMINATION AND PERINEAL CARE

Rationale for the Use of This Skill

Many patients are unable to use the bathroom for purposes of elimination. They may have an order for complete bed rest or for appliances (traction, casts) that impose immobility. Certain patients who have had recent surgery may be unable to use the bathroom for a day or so. Others who are generally weak may not be able to ambulate to the bathroom part or all of the time. Also, because of their condition, some patients cannot clean themselves properly after eliminating and need the nurse's assistance.

It is one of the nurse's fundamental tasks to help patients with either a bedpan or a urinal and to give perineal care skillfully, being aware of the psychological implications of this care.

Using a bedpan or urinal becomes necessary when the patient is immobilized and has a self care deficit. Helping a patient with this task and assisting with hygiene afterward are basic tasks that you should perform with a minimum of embarrassment and a maximum of skill.[1]

Principles

Keep several principles in mind. First, observe medical asepsis throughout *for your own protection as well as the patient's. When performing these procedures, your hands may come in contact with mucous membrane, which is receptive to infection. It is even more important to protect the patient from the dangers of cross-contamination (contamination from other patients). For practical as well as aesthetic reasons, you must use good aseptic technique.* The CDC recommends the use of clean gloves whenever body substances may be contacted. Wearing gloves during perineal care and when cleaning bedpans is a prudent practice.

Second, the procedure can be embarrassing to you and to the patient. It is important to recognize these feelings in yourself and to know that with experience, assisting with intimate procedures will become less personal and more routine to you. *To lessen a patient's embarrassment or discomfort,* maintain a straightforward attitude and respect the patient's privacy, keeping exposure to a minimum.

Lastly, when you help a patient with any substitution or adaptation of the usual activities of daily living (ADLs), it is important—in terms of efficiency and patient comfort—that you approximate the normal as closely as possible. For a female patient the normal position for urination or defecation is a sitting one; a male commonly stands to urinate and sits to defecate. Therefore, *having a patient assume these positions* when using a bedpan or urinal is very helpful and *may, in some cases, be a strong factor in whether the patient will be able to eliminate.* A male patient, for example, will usually be more successful if he is allowed to stand to urinate. If the patient is unable to stand alone, have him lean on the edge of the bed *for stability* with his feet on the floor. Let the patient have as much control as possible, for example, by giving the patient privacy, allowing the patient to use tissue by himself or herself, and allowing the patient to wash his or her hands afterward. If the patient is unable to perform these activities, you should perform them for the patient.

Types of Bedpans

Bedpans are made of either metal (see Figure 10.1) or plastic and come in two sizes, the smaller being for pediatric patients. *For reasons of asepsis,* each patient has a personal bedpan that is kept in a storage unit in the patient's room. Generally, it is stored with a bedpan cover over it. The cover, which is made of heavy fabric or paper, may be in the form of a loose square or large envelope that slips easily over the bedpan. The paper cover is disposable. A cover should be used *for aesthetic reasons, to conceal the sight of the contents and to decrease odor after the patient has used the bedpan.*

A *fracture pan* is a type of bedpan that was originally designed to be used by patients in casts, who could not use a pan with a high lip. It is smaller and easier to get onto than a standard bedpan. There is a handle toward the front to facilitate handling. Fracture pans also come in two sizes, in plastic or metal, and with a handle for easier placement (see Figure 10.2).

An *emesis basin* (see Figure 10.3) can be used for the rare female patient who, *because of extreme pain or for a medical reason,* should not be raised

---

[1]You will note that rationale for action is emphasized throughout the module by the use of italics.

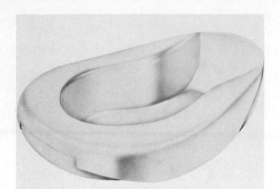

FIGURE 10.1 BEDPAN
Courtesy Vollrath Company

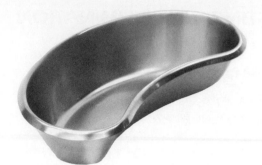

FIGURE 10.3 EMESIS BASIN FOR USE WITH
IMMOBILE FEMALE PATIENT
Courtesy American Hospital Supply Corp., McGaw Park, Illinois

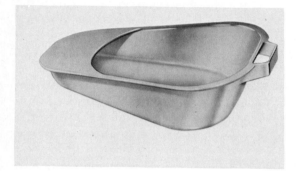

FIGURE 10.2 FRACTURE PAN
Courtesy American Hospital Supply Corp., McGaw Park, Illinois

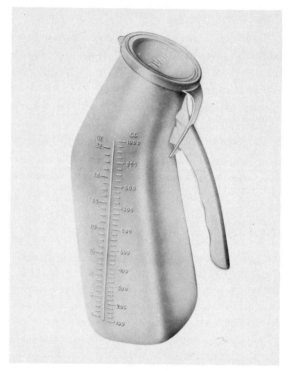

FIGURE 10.4 URINAL FOR MALE USE
Courtesy Vollrath Company

to bedpan height except for defecation. After placing a pad or Chux under the patient *to protect the linen,* hold the emesis basin lengthwise between the legs and firmly against the perineum. Instruct the patient to void. At first a patient may be hesitant, *fearing that she will soil the bed.* Encourage the patient to void freely. Usually the urine flows into the pan with only a drop or so on the pad, and the patient will be very grateful for this easy, more comfortable way to urinate.

A *urinal* is used by the male patient for urination. It is made of plastic or metal with a bottlelike configuration. A flat side allows it to rest without tipping. Urinals are available with or without attached tops or lids (see Figure 10.4). Female urinals are also available.

Comfort Considerations

Although often unavoidable, using a bedpan or urinal is not a pleasant experience. A thin, frag-

ile patient may even feel pain from the pressure of the hard surfaces. Fold a soft pad or small towel over the edges of the pan *to lessen this discomfort.* With metal pans, another source of discomfort is cold. Warm metal pans by holding them under running warm water and then drying them. These simple measures can make the experience less disagreeable.

176

Procedure for Assisting with a Bedpan

☐ *Assessment*

1. Check the patient's activity order and physical status *to ascertain whether a bedpan is necessary.*
2. Review the patient's past use of such equipment and note any problems encountered.

☐ *Planning*

3. Decide how much assistance the patient currently needs and get the help needed.
4. Plan for the specific procedure or technique to be used (see step 10 for options).
5. Wash your hands. Use the principles of medical asepsis throughout. (Washing your hands before you undertake any procedure should become automatic, *to protect both patients and yourself.*)

☐ *Implementation*

6. Explain in general how you plan to proceed. (Of course, if a patient verbalizes the need to eliminate, do not go into detail.)
7. Close the door and curtains *to provide privacy.*
8. Raise the bed to the high position *(for your convenience). For the patient's safety,* put up the side rail on the opposite side of the bed from where you are standing.
9. Take the bedpan, cover, and toilet tissue out of the bedside storage unit. Set the cover and tissue aside. A fracture pan, as previously mentioned, can be used in the same way as a conventional bedpan.
10. There are several ways to put a patient on a bedpan, depending on the patient's condition and his or her ability to help you.
    a. With the patient in a recumbent position and your hand under the small (lumbosacral area) of the back *for support,* ask the patient to raise the buttocks by pushing up with the feet as you push the pan into position under the patient.
    b. A patient in the sitting position who is able to will prefer to simply lift the body by pushing down with the hands and feet as you place the pan in position.
    c. A more immobilized patient must be rolled onto the pan. For this maneuver, again elicit the patient's cooperation. Ask the patient to grasp the side rail on the opposite side of the bed (across from where you are standing) *for stability* as you roll the patient away from you in one plane. Place the pan against the patient, in position. (You may want to pad the pan with a towel *to relieve pressure on the patient's buttocks.*) Now, hold the pan firmly in place as you roll the patient back. Finally, check the position of the pan. If the patient must remain flat, you may want to place a small pillow above the bedpan under the patient's back *for support. Note:* If the patient's bed has a trapeze, make use of this device for placing and removing the bedpan. Have the patient use the trapeze to lift the hips.
11. Raise the side rail nearest you *for safety.*
12. Elevate the head of the bed to mid- or high-Fowler's position, if not contraindicated, as the patient grasps the rails. *This provides a position that approximates what is normal for elimination.* (See Figures 10.5 and 10.6.)
13. Place the toilet tissue and the call bell within the patient's reach.
14. Leave the patient. *Because our culture emphasizes privacy during elimination,* it is very difficult for some patients to eliminate with a nurse in attendance. If possible, it is best to leave the patient for a period of time; if this is not possible, you might step just outside the bed curtains *to be within calling distance if the patient suddenly needs assistance.*
15. When the patient signals, return promptly. *It can be very irritating and uncomfortable for a patient to sit for unnecessarily extended periods of time on a bedpan because a nurse is inattentive. If a patient does not signal you within a reasonable amount of time, return to the patient to ensure safety and comfort.*
16. Put on clean gloves *for asepsis.*
17. If necessary, clean the genital area with

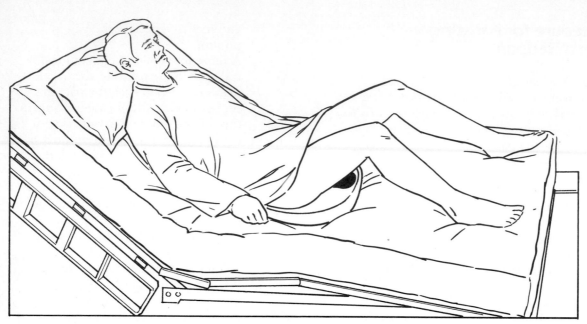

FIGURE 10.5 THE BEDPAN IS PLACED UNDER THE PATIENT WITH THE FLAT SIDE UNDER THE BUTTOCKS

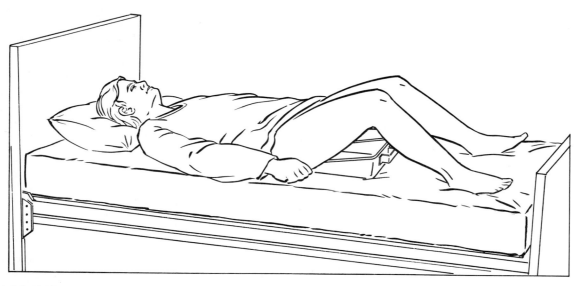

FIGURE 10.6 THE FRACTURE PAN IS PLACED UNDER THE PATIENT WITH THE HANDLE TOWARD THE LEGS AND THE LOW, FLAT SIDE UNDER THE BUTTOCKS

toilet tissue. Most alert patients will be able to clean themselves adequately. Some who are incapacitated may need further assistance. Always clean with fresh tissue from the anterior (urinary) region to the posterior (rectal) region. *Cleaning in this direction minimizes the chance of contaminating the urinary tract with fecal microorganisms.*

18. Remove the bedpan, reversing the method that you used when you placed the patient on the bedpan. If you used the rolling technique, hold onto the pan firmly or get help, *so that the contents do not spill.*
19. Place a cover on the pan.
20. Carry the pan to the bathroom and, if ordered, measure the urine. If a patient is

178

on intake and output, a measuring container is usually kept in the bathroom. You must estimate as accurately as possible, taking into account the amount of toilet tissue used *because the tissue can displace the urine and make measurement inaccurate* (see Module 15, Intake and Output).

21. Collect a specimen of urine or feces, if ordered (see Module 18, Collecting Specimens).

Even when precise measurements or specimens are not ordered, note the amount, color, consistency, and odor, as well as the presence of blood, mucus, or foreign material. *These are important data to convey to the physician and may affect the diagnosis.* A patient who is being observed for renal calculi (kidney stones) may have an order to have all urine strained *so that the small stones or particles can be retained and examined.* If you even suspect that a patient's urine or feces contain blood, in most facilities you can test a specimen on your own *to verify your suspicion* (see Module 20, Performing Common Laboratory Tests).

22. Empty the contents into the toilet and flush.

23. Thoroughly clean the pan with cold water, *which subdues odors and combines with the contents more effectively than hot.* Health regulations require that a container of disinfectant solution and a long-handled brush be kept in the bathroom *for cleaning bedpans.* Wash and rinse the pan thoroughly. Use paper towels for drying. Then return the pan to the patient's storage unit.

24. Remove and dispose of gloves.

25. Give the patient a basin of warm water, a washcloth, soap, and a towel, or a packaged moist towelette so that hygiene can be carried out. Allow the patient to wash the hands and perineal area, if desired. Nurses usually remember to wash their own hands after assisting a patient with a bedpan but sometimes forget that the patient would also like to wash.

26. Place the bed back in the low position *for safety* and lower the rail on the stand side if appropriate. Make the patient comfortable.

27. Dispose of the equipment.
28. Wash your hands *for asepsis.*

Evaluation
29. Note the efficiency of the technique used and how suitable it was for that patient.
30. Identify any specific problems and possible improvements and note them on the nursing care plan.

Documentation
31. Record any problems or unusual observations. Routine elimination is usually recorded on a check list or output sheet.

Procedure for Assisting with a Urinal

The steps used to assist a male patient in using the urinal are essentially the same as those used to assist with a bedpan (see the Performance Checklist), except for a few adaptations.

Never place a urinal between a patient's legs for long periods of time in an effort to control incontinence. *This can irritate and erode the skin of the penis.* If a patient is unable to use the urinal himself, protect the linen with a pad or Chux, place the head of the penis into the opening and tell the patient he can now urinate without soiling the bed linen.

Giving Perineal Care

In the clinical setting, this procedure is sometimes called *pericare.* Perineal care is usually given at the discretion of the nurse upon assessment of the patient. An order is not needed.

Assessment
1. Determine the extent of soiling of the perineal area.
2. Identify the patient's capabilities.

Planning
3. Plan the equipment that will be needed (see step 7, page 180, for options).
4. Decide whether you will need assistance.
5. Wash your hands *for asepsis.* You should wear clean gloves when giving perineal care. *It has been shown that infections can be transmitted through minor breaks in the skin.*

Implementation

6. Explain what you are about to do. Use words the patient understands: "washing your genital area" or "washing between your legs." Again, *the patient may be embarrassed,* so proceed in a professional manner.

7. The selection of equipment will vary with the type of patient to whom you are administering care. Gloves are used for all patients.

   a. *Postpartum or surgical patient*
      (1) Bedpan
      (2) Chux
      (3) Pitcher
      (4) Tap water or antiseptic
      (5) Cotton balls, gauze squares, or "wipes"
      (6) Clean pad or dressing

   b. *Nonsurgical patient*
      (1) Chux
      (2) Washcloth and towel
      (3) Basin of warm water
      (4) Mild soap or cleansing agent

   c. *Patient with a catheter* Research has shown that washing around the catheter insertion site and rinsing thoroughly is sufficient care. The Centers for Disease Control have recommended that special cleaning procedures not be done because they are not associated with decreased incidence of infection.

8. *Provide privacy* by shutting the door and closing the bed curtains.

9. *For purposes of convenience and privacy,* place the patient in the dorsal recumbent position and drape with a bath blanket as you would to catheterize a patient (see Module 39, Catheterization).

10. Proceed as follows:

    a. *Postpartum or surgical patient* Put on gloves. Remove dressing or pads. After placing a Chux under the patient, position the bedpan following step 10 of the Procedure for Assisting with a Bedpan, page 177. Pour tepid tap water or the solution used in your facility over the perineum. Do not spread the labia; *this may allow solution to enter the vagina and might cause infection.* Rinse with clear water. Using cotton balls or gauze, wipe from anterior to posterior *because wiping in this direction lessens the possibility of contamination of the urinary tract from the anal area.* Always clean gently, *to prevent pain and avoid pressure on sutures (stitches).* Use extra gauze squares or cotton balls, if needed, but use each only one time and then discard into waste bag (not bedpan) *to prevent contamination.* Replace any pads or dressings, using sterile materials *for asepsis.* Remove the bedpan, make any necessary observations, and discard the contents. This procedure can also be done with the patient sitting on a toilet.

    b. *Nonsurgical patient* After placing a Chux or pad under the patient, put on gloves and wash the perineum, using warm water and mild soap. Gentle separate the labia of the female patient as you clean, *in order to remove secretions and smegma (an odorous collection of desquamated epithelial cells and mucus).* Clean the male patient beginning with the penile head and moving downward along the shaft. Retract the foreskin of the uncircumcised male gently *to avoid causing irritation or pain, so that the underlying tissue can be cleaned.* All patients should be rinsed, *to remove soap residue,* and dried thoroughly. Replace the foreskin over the head of the penis. Remove the damp pads and make the patient comfortable.

    c. *Patient with a catheter* Put on gloves and wash the perineal area thoroughly with soap and warm water. Clean well around the entire insertion site. Rinse *to remove all soap residue and thus prevent irritation of the mucosa.* The CDC does not recommend any further cleaning procedures or the use of any antiseptic substances around the catheter. These practices do not reduce the rate of urinary tract infection.

11. Replace bed linens and reposition the patient *for comfort.*
12. Dispose of equipment.
13. Wash hands *for asepsis.*

☐ *Evaluation*

14. Check back with patient for feelings of comfort.

☐ *Documentation*

15. Good perineal care is assumed as a part of hygiene. Record any pertinent observations or difficulties with performance.

REFERENCES

Burke, J., et al. "Prevention of Catheter-Associated Infections: Efficacy of Daily Meatal Care Regimens." *American Journal of Medicine* 70, March 1975, 655.

Garner, Julia S., and Martin S. Favero. *Guidelines for Handwashing and Hospital Environmental Control, 1985.* Atlanta: Centers for Disease Control, 1985.

Guidelines for the Prevention of Catheter-Associated Urinary Tract Infections. Atlanta: Centers for Disease Control, 1983.

Examples of Charting   SOAP Note

1/5/88
1630   Impaired skin integrity: Scrotal irritation related to urinary incontinence
S "It hurts between my legs."
O Scrotum reddened and warm to touch.
A Irritation of scrotal area possibly due to intermittent incontinence.
P Offer urinal q.2h. when awake and follow with good perineal care.
             L. Kenny, S.N.

Narrative Style

1/3/88
8 a.m.   Pericare given. Vulva appears reddened. Small am't clear vaginal drainage.
             J. Adams, S.N.

PERFORMANCE CHECKLIST				

Assisting with a bedpan or urinal	Unsatisfactory	Needs More Practice	Satisfactory	Comments
☐ *Assessment*				
1. Check patient's activity order.				
2. Check for past use of bedpan and problems.				
☐ *Planning*				
3. Determine assistance needed.				
4. Plan technique to be used.				
5. Wash your hands.				
☐ *Implementation*				
6. Explain to patient how you plan to proceed.				
7. Provide privacy.				
8. Raise both bed and rail on opposite side.				
9. Obtain pan and other items needed.				
10. Place patient on the bedpan using one of the following: a. Have patient lift up from recumbent position.				
b. Have patient lift up from sitting position.				
c. Roll patient onto the pan.				
11. Raise side rail nearest you.				
12. Elevate patient to sitting position.				
13. Place tissue and call bell within reach.				
14. Leave patient for privacy.				
15. Return when patient signals.				
16. Put on clean gloves.				
17. Clean perineum if necessary.				
18. Remove bedpan.				
19. Place cover on pan.				
20. Carry pan to bathroom; observe and measure any contents as ordered.				
21. Collect any specimens ordered.				
22. Empty contents into bowl and flush.				

182

	Unsatisfactory	Needs More Practice	Satisfactory	Comments
23. Clean pan with cold water.				
24. Remove and dispose of gloves.				
25. Return to patient and offer hygiene items.				
26. Reposition bed and patient for comfort.				
27. Dispose of equipment.				
28. Wash your hands.				
☐ *Evaluation*				
29. Note efficiency of procedure and results.				
30. Identify any problems encountered.				
☐ *Documentation*				
31. Record any unusual observations or problems.				
Giving perineal care				
☐ *Assessment*				
1. Determine the extent of soiling.				
2. Identify patient's capabilities.				
☐ *Planning*				
3. Plan equipment needed.				
4. Decide if you will need assistance.				
5. Wash your hands. Obtain gloves.				
☐ *Implementation*				
6. Explain what you are about to do.				
7. Select appropriate equipment for: a. Postpartum or surgical patient				
b. Nonsurgical patient				
c. Patient with a catheter				
8. Provide privacy.				
9. Drape as appropriate.				
10. Put on gloves and follow appropriate procedure.				
11. Replace bed linens and reposition patient.				

	Unsatisfactory	Needs More Practice	Satisfactory	Comments
12. Dispose of equipment.				
13. Wash your hands.				
☐ *Evaluation*				
14. Check back with patient for comfort.				
☐ *Documentation*				
15. Record any pertinent observations or difficulties.				

QUIZ

Short-Answer Questions

1. List three principles to be followed when assisting a patient with a bedpan or urinal.

    a. _____

    b. _____

    c. _____

2. Name four pieces of equipment that are used to help the bed patient to eliminate.

    a. _____

    b. _____

    c. _____

    d. _____

3. Which two comfort measures should you take for a thin elderly patient who must use a bedpan?

    a. _____

    b. _____

4. Describe two methods for placing a patient on a bedpan.

    a. _____

    b. _____

5. List five of the seven observations that you might make about a patient's urine or feces.

    a. _____

    b. _____

    c. _____

    d. _____

    e. _____

6. Identify three categories of patients who may need special pericare.

    a. _____

    b. _____

    c. _____

7. Describe the procedure for one of the three categories in question 6.

    _____

8. Why is a cover used over a bedpan? _____

    _____

9. Where should specific methods of assisting a patient with using a bedpan be noted? _____

_____

10. Why is all cleansing on the female patient's perineum done from front to back? _____

_____

MODULE 11

Hygiene

MODULE CONTENTS

PREREQUISITES

Successful completion of the following
modules:

VOLUME 1

Module 1 / An Approach to Nursing Skills
Module 2 / Medical Asepsis
Module 3 / Safety
Module 4 / Basic Body Mechanics
Module 5 / Assessment
Module 6 / Documentation
Module 7 / Bedmaking
Module 10 / Assisting with Elimination and
  Perineal Care

OVERALL OBJECTIVE

To provide patients with opportunities for hygiene according to their needs and conditions.

SPECIFIC LEARNING OBJECTIVES

	Know Facts and Principles	Apply Facts and Principles	Demonstrate Ability	Evaluate Performance
1. *Providing hygiene* *a. Baths* *b. Back rubs* *c. Oral care* *d. Hair care* *e. Eye care*	Describe several aspects of hygiene, including baths, back rubs, oral care, hair care, and eye care	Given a patient situation, identify type of bath that should be given and appropriate type of oral and hair care Explain rationale for types of baths, oral care, hair care, and eye care		
2. *Procedures*	Describe procedures	Given a patient situation, state what should be done according to procedures	Demonstrate ability to perform several aspects of hygiene, including baths, back rubs, oral care, and hair care, according to patient's needs. Initiate performance of several aspects of hygiene independently, according to patient's needs.	Evaluate own performance with instructor using Performance Checklist
3. *Recording hygiene measures*	State items to be recorded	Given a patient situation, record appropriate information regarding hygiene	Record hygiene procedures according to facility's procedure	Evaluate own performance with instructor

189

LEARNING ACTIVITIES

1. Review the Specific Learning Objectives.
2. Read the chapter on hygiene in Ellis and Nowlis, *Nursing: A Human Needs Approach,* or a comparable chapter in another textbook.
3. Look up the module vocabulary terms in the Glossary.
4. Read through the module.
5. At home, give yourself a complete sponge bath using the technique for giving bedbaths. This can be done at the bathroom sink, but you should use a basin filled with water (not running water) to simulate the bedside situation. Pay special attention to the following:
   a. The water temperature that feels comfortable to you
   b. Possible chilling due to exposure
   c. The amount of pressure or friction that is comfortable
   d. How easily soap can be rinsed off and how much soap should be used
   e. The effect of "trailing" ends of a washcloth
   f. The need for thorough drying
6. In the practice setting:
   a. Practice giving a complete bedbath, back rub, oral care, hair care, and eye care, using another student as your patient. Have the student comment on his or her comfort. Use the Performance Checklist to evaluate yourself. When you are satisfied with your performance, have your instructor evaluate you.
   b. Describe to your instructor what you would do differently to provide a partial bedbath or a self-bedbath with assistance.
   c. Describe the necessary safety measures for the patient receiving a shower or a tub bath.
   d. Practice denture care if dentures are provided in the practice setting. Use the Performance Checklist to evaluate yourself. When you are satisfied with your performance, have your instructor evaluate you.
   e. Practice care of glasses, hearing aids, and contact lenses if they are provided in the practice setting. Use the Performance Checklist to evaluate yourself. When you are satisfied with your performance, have your instructor evaluate you.
7. In the clinical setting:
   a. Assist a patient with a tub bath or shower and morning care.
   b. Give a complete bedbath and morning care to a patient.

VOCABULARY

asepto syringe
aspirate
axilla
canthus
cariogenic
expectorate
Fowler's position
genital
semi-Fowler's position
sordes
supine
umbilicus

HYGIENE[1]

Rationale for the Use of This Skill

Hospitalized patients have at least as many needs for hygiene measures in their daily lives as you do in yours. Indeed, they may have considerably more. Often, however, they cannot attend to those needs themselves without at least some help. It is the nurse's responsibility to provide patients with the opportunity for hygiene, assisting them as needed, taking into consideration their personal preferences and physical disabilities.[2]

General Procedure for Hygiene

There is a general approach you can use to help patients with the various aspects of hygiene. This can be modified according to the particular aspect of hygiene involved and the degree to which the patient is able to participate.

Assessment

1. Check the chart for any information related to the patient's ability to participate in the procedure being planned—for example, diagnoses, activity orders, or any orders specific to hygiene.
2. Assess the patient for specific symptoms related to diagnosis, for fatigue and level of sedation, and for hygiene preferences.
3. Check to see whether needed special supplies or equipment are already in the room.

Planning

4. Determine whether or not you will need any assistance.
5. Determine what supplies and equipment are needed.
6. Wash your hands *for asepsis*.
7. Obtain the needed supplies.

   Whenever you are doing a procedure that has the potential for bringing you into contact with body secretions, you should put on clean gloves *for asepsis*. You may wish to carry a pair of clean gloves with you at all times. Gloves should be disposed of by turning them inside out as they are removed, leaving the soiled surface enclosed inside the glove. *This provides added protection for housekeeping personnel.*

Implementation

8. Identify the patient *to be sure you are carrying out the procedure for the correct patient.*
9. Explain to the patient what you plan to do and how he or she can participate.
10. Provide for the patient's privacy.
11. Raise the bed to the appropriate working level.
12. Carry out the hygiene procedure planned.
13. Watch the patient carefully for signs of fatigue or other adverse responses.
14. Care appropriately for all equipment and supplies used.
15. Wash your hands *for asepsis*.

Evaluation

16. Evaluate in terms of the following criteria:
    a. Fatigue
    b. Feelings about comfort and cleanliness
    c. Objective signs of cleanliness

Documentation

17. Record the hygiene measure as appropriate for your facility. In many facilities, hygiene measures are recorded on a flow sheet. Information about the patient's preferences and ability to participate is recorded on the nursing care plan. Any information about physical signs and symptoms identified during the procedure can be recorded either on a flow sheet or on the progress notes. See Figure 11.1 for an example of flow sheet entries.

Modifications of General Procedure

For each procedure discussed, *only* the steps in the general procedure that must be modified are presented. You are expected to follow the complete General Procedure for Hygiene when performing any procedure, although we have not repeated all the steps each time. The detailed

---

[1]For infant bathing procedure, see Module 12, Basic Infant Care. For perineal care procedure, see Module 10, Assisting with Elimination and Perineal Care.
[2]You will note that rationale for action is emphasized throughout the module by the use of italics.

SHIFT	23-07	07-15	15-23	23-07	07-15	15-23	23-07	07-15	15-23	23-07	07-15	15-23
PERSONAL HYGIENE: BATH: (Complete Bed Bath, Shower c̄/s̄ help, Sit Shower, Bath c̄ help)		CBB c̄ assist										
ORAL:		self										
BACK CARE:		lotion rub										
PERI-CARE:		Self										
CATH CARE:		N/A										
ACTIVITY: (Bedrest, Amb c̄ help, Dangle, Chair c̄/s̄ help, Up Ad Lib, BR c̄ BRP)		Chair x2 15"										
TURNED & POSITIONED		q 2h when in bed										
DEEP BREATHE & COUGH		q 2h										
ELIMINATION: BM (Number & Description)		1 formed										
SLEEP PATTERNS: (Naps, 1 hour intervals,etc)		naps at intervals										
DIET:	Breakfast	Lunch	Dinner	Breakfast	Lunch	Dinner	Breakfast	Lunch	Dinner	Breakfast	Lunch	Dinner
Type	2 Gm Na											
Amount taken(All, none, fraction)	All	3/4										
Calorie Count												
SIGNATURES 23-07 / 07-15 / 15-23		B. Kucinski,R.N.										
DATE		2-22-88			2-23			2-24			2-25	

ADDRESSOGRAPH:

THE SWEDISH HOSPITAL MEDICAL CENTER
SEATTLE, WASHINGTON

N-1546 Nursing Rev. 6/80 FC/TSHMC

ACTIVITIES OF DAILY LIVING AND TREATMENT

FIGURE 11.1 FLOW SHEET ENTRIES FOR HYGIENE PROCEDURES

procedures, which include all the steps of the General Procedure as well as those steps that need modification, are given in the Performance Checklist.

Bathing Procedures

Apply the principles of asepsis and body mechanics given in Module 7, Bedmaking, to giving various types of bedbaths. *Because a patient receiving a bedbath is very likely to stay in bed while his or her bed is being made,* you may need to refer again to the procedure for making an occupied bed.

Complete Bedbath

☐ *Planning*

7. Gather the necessary equipment:
   a. Basin for water
   b. Soap (patient may have his or her own)
   c. Laundry hamper or bag
   d. Clean linen in the order of use (if you plan to make the bed as well)
   e. Bath blanket, towels, and washcloths as needed. (Remember, you will want to leave a fresh towel and washcloth at the bedside for use at other times during the day.)
   f. Clean gown or pajamas
   g. Supplements to patient's personal toilet articles. (Most patients will bring their own toothbrush and paste or powder, deodorant, comb, and the like; but in some situations this may not be true.)

☐ *Implementation*

12. Give the bath as follows:
    a. Remove the top linen, placing a bath blanket over the patient before removing the top sheet. (See Module 7, Bedmaking, Occupied Beds, step 12, page 117.)
    b. Give oral care at this point if you have not done so already. (See Oral Care, pages 199–202.)
    c. Obtain water for the bath. This may be done when you are rinsing the oral hygiene articles.
    d. Position the patient for the bath. Usually the supine position is used unless the patient cannot tolerate it. In some cases it may be necessary to use a semi-Fowler's or even Fowler's position *for the patient's comfort or safety.* Move the patient to your side of the bed *to decrease the need for reaching.*
    e. Bathe the patient in the following order.
       (1) Spread a towel across the patient's chest, tucking it under the chin.
       (2) Make a mitt out of the washcloth. Tucking one edge of the washcloth under your thumb, wrap it in thirds around your hand, tucking the final edge under your thumb as well (see Figure 11.2).

           Bring the far edge of the washcloth up and tuck it under the near edge. *Using a mitt prevents loose, cool ends of the cloth from dragging across the patient.* As long as the mitt does not come apart, it may be left on the hand.
       (3) Wash the patient's face. This is generally done *without* soap, but be certain to ask the patient for his or her preference. Many patients are able to do this portion of the bath themselves. Wash the eyes from the inner canthus to the outer canthus; rinse the cloth after washing each eye.

           Use gentle but firm strokes when you wash the face, *so that the patient feels clean.*

           Be sure to wash *behind* the ears as well as on the upper surfaces, using soap.

           You may want to use soap on the neck even if you didn't on the face. Wash just the front and the sides of the neck. *The back part can be washed when the back is done.* Rinse and dry the neck after washing.
       (4) Remove the patient's gown.
       (5) Place the towel lengthwise under the far arm. If you have moved the patient toward the side of the bed on which you are working, it should not be too far to reach,

193

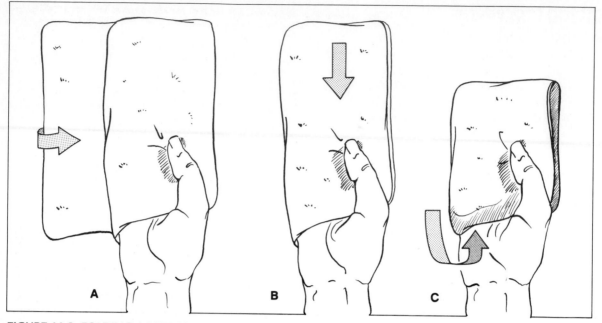

FIGURE 11.2 FOLDING A MITT FOR BATHING *A:* Fold washcloth lengthwise in thirds around your hand; *B and C:* fold top end of cloth down and tuck under bottom end.

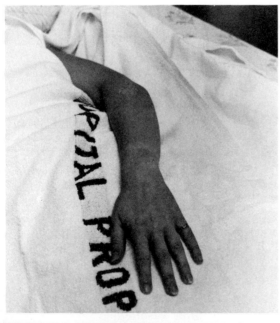

FIGURE 11.3 DRAPING FOR WASHING PATIENT'S ARM Position patient's arm across body, with towel lengthwise underneath.
Courtesy Ivan Ellis

especially if you place a towel across the patient's chest and have him or her place the arm on top of it (see Figure 11.3). Do the far arm first *to avoid leaning over or dripping dirty water on the part that is already washed.* Using long, firm strokes toward the center of the body (*to increase venous return*), wash the far hand, arm, and axilla in that order. Rinse and dry thoroughly.

Often the hands have been washed before the bath or are not very dirty. Some patients, however, really enjoy the opportunity to soak their hands in a basin. In any case, wash the hands thoroughly, being certain to dry well between the fingers. Use an orangewood stick to clean under the nails if needed.

(6) Next place the towel under the near arm and wash the near hand, arm, and axilla in the same way.

(7) Fold the bath blanket down to

the waist. Place the towel over the bath blanket, *so that it is nearby and easy to reach for drying the patient. It may also be used for warmth between washing and rinsing.*

Wash the chest, being certain to wash, rinse, and dry thoroughly under the breasts of a female patient. Leave the chest covered with the towel while rinsing the mitt. Rinse and dry the chest.

(8) Fold the bath blanket down to the pubic bone, leaving the towel over the chest. Wash, rinse, and dry the lower abdomen, paying particular attention to the umbilicus. Remove the towel and replace the bath blanket over the chest and arms.

(9) Remove the bath blanket from the far leg only, tucking it under the near leg and up around the hip *to avoid exposure and drafts.* Place the towel lengthwise under the far leg (see Figure 11.4).

(10) Bending the leg at the knee, slide the basin onto the bed and place the patient's foot in it. Place the foot carefully in the basin, *so as not to spill the water.* In some facilities the basins used for bathing may be too small to carry out this procedure for patients with large feet.

(11) Wash the leg, using long, firm strokes toward the center of the body *to increase venous return.* Rinse and dry.

(12) Wash and rinse the foot, being careful to do each toe separately. Remove the basin from the bed. Dry the foot, giving special attention to the areas between the toes *to prevent irritation and injury to the skin.*

(13) Wash the near leg and foot in the same way (steps 9–12).

(14) Change the bath water.

(15) Turn the patient on the side,

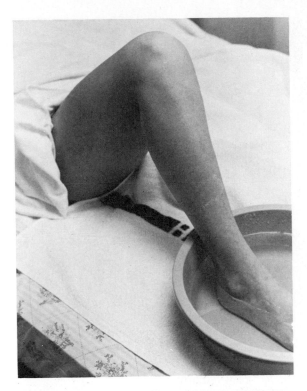

FIGURE 11.4 DRAPING FOR WASHING PATIENT'S LEG   Uncover only one leg at a time, keeping rest of patient's body covered.
Courtesy Ivan Ellis

facing away from you. Very few patients will be comfortable lying on the abdomen, although this may be done. Drape the patient as shown in Figure 11.5, with the bath blanket drawn down to the hips and a towel tucked lengthwise behind and beside the back.

(16) Wash, rinse, and dry the back, using long, firm strokes. Remember to include the back of the neck.

(17) Wash, rinse, and dry the buttocks. If the patient is incapacitated, it may be necessary to wash the peri-anal area at this time. If this area is soiled with stool, put on gloves before bathing it.

(18) A back rub may be given at this point if the purpose is to stimulate or invigorate the

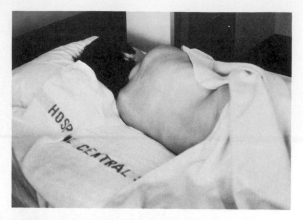

FIGURE 11.5 DRAPING FOR WASHING PATIENT'S
BACK
Courtesy Ivan Ellis

patient. If, however, you wish to
make the back rub a more
relaxing experience for the
patient, you can wait until after
the bath is completed.

(19) Change the bath water.

(20) Wash the genital area.
In many cases, a patient will be
able to wash himself or herself.
In this case, your responsibility is
to see to it that everything
needed is within reach. You may
want to stay within hearing
distance or instruct the patient
to call you with the call light. Be
sure the patient understands
what you expect to be done.

If a patient is not able to
wash his or her own genital area,
you should do so. Put on clean
gloves *for asepsis*. Wash, moving
gently from front to back (clean
to dirty), making certain to wash
and dry carefully between
opposing skin surfaces (See
Module 10, Assisting with
Elimination and Perineal Care.)
Remove and dispose of gloves.

f. Help the patient put on a clean gown
or pajamas.

g. Comb or brush and arrange the
patient's hair. (See Hair Care, pages
202–203.)

h. File or cut the patient's fingernails
and toenails. Since some facilities do

not permit nail cutting, especially of
diabetic patients, be sure you know
the policy and follow it.

i. The male patient may shave at this
point if he wants to. You may have to
assemble his shaving equipment,
which will vary depending on the type
of razor he prefers. If he is unable to
shave himself, this task is also your
responsibility. Most facilities have an
electric razor you can use if the
patient needs help. If your facility
requires you to use a safety razor and
you do not know how, ask for
assistance.

j. Make the occupied bed. (See Module
7, Bedmaking, Occupied Beds, pages
117–118.) Be sure to return the bed
to the low position at the completion
of this procedure *for safety*.

k. Set the patient's room in order; wash
and return the bath basin to the
patient's storage unit; and put away
the patient's personal articles, leaving
a washcloth and towel for use during
the day. Be sure the patient has
everything he or she will need
throughout the day within reach.

Partial Bedbath

A partial bedbath is given for several reasons, *including a patient's inability to tolerate a full bath and
a lack of need or desire for a full daily bath.* A partial
bedbath usually includes the face, neck, hands,
axillae, and perineum. The back may also be included if the patient can tolerate it. Perform a
back rub for any patient on bed rest.

Self-Bedbath

This type of bath is given *when a patient is, for
some reason, unable to take a shower or a tub bath but
is able to move about freely in bed.* The self-bedbath
is usually a complete bath. Your responsibility is
to provide the basin of water, bath blanket, and
other necessary articles and to be ready to assist
at the call of the patient. Your assistance may be
needed for the feet and legs, and is necessary for
the back and buttocks. Do not omit the back rub
simply because a patient is able to bathe
unaided.

Tub Bath

Tub baths are generally used *for cleaning purposes only, although at times therapeutic agents can be added.* If your facility requires a physician's order for a tub bath, be sure you have the order before you offer the patient a bath.

⬜ *Planning*

5. Prepare the tub area. *It is frustrating for everyone involved to arrive at the tub room only to find it already in use.*

9. After checking to make sure the tub is clean, fill the tub about half full with warm water (100–115°F).

⬜ *Implementation*

10. Assist the patient to the tub room. Be certain to check which method of ambulation is appropriate. Bring all needed items (towel, deodorant, pajamas, and the like).

11. Hang a sign on the door indicating that the room is occupied *to protect the privacy of the patient.*

12. a. Help the patient into the tub.
    b. Assist the patient as needed. If the patient is quite helpless, you may need a second person to assist while you wash. Some patients may be able to support themselves but will need your help with the bath. If there are no safety strips on the bottom of the tub, place an extra bath towel on the bottom of the tub *to prevent slipping.* If the patient is quite independent, you may leave for a few minutes while the bath is being taken. The bed may be made at this time. Be certain, however, to tell the patient how to use the emergency call signal before you leave. If the patient seems weak, do *not* leave. Be sure to wash the patient's back.
    c. Assist the patient out of the tub. Get help if you think you might need it. *Both you and the patient are too valuable to injure.*
    d. Assist the patient with drying.
    e. Help the patient to put on a clean gown or pajamas.
    f. Assist the patient back to his or her room.

14. Return to the tub room.
    a. Clean the tub in the manner prescribed by your facility.
    b. Discard the used linen.
    c. Put the "unoccupied" sign on the door and/or notify the staff person next in line that the tub is ready for use.

Shower

A patient may take a standing shower independently, or a shower may be given in a shower chair. In any case, patients usually prefer showers to bedbaths. If your facility requires a physician's order for a patient to have a shower, be sure you have the order before offering the patient a shower.

⬜ *Planning*

7. Prepare the shower area.

⬜ *Implementation*

10. Assist the patient to the shower room or stall. If a chair shower is to be given, you can transport the patient in the shower chair. The safest way to do this is to pull the chair backward down the hall, with at least one hand grasping the patient's shoulder.

11. Hang a sign on the door indicating that the room is occupied *to protect the privacy of the patient.*

12. a. Assist the patient as necessary. Run the shower until the water is warm (100–115°F); then adjust it to the patient's preference. Place a paper shower mat or bath towel on the floor *to prevent slipping.*

    At this point, a patient who can take a shower independently may be left (with a call bell within reach), but leave for no more than ten minutes. A patient having a chair shower may need assistance throughout or only at the end of the shower. In any case, check frequently to be certain that the patient is all right.
    b. Assist the patient with drying if necessary. Help the patient put on a clean gown or pajamas.
    c. Assist the patient back to his or her room.

14. Return to the shower room.
    a. Clean the stall and shower chair in the manner prescribed by your facility.
    b. Discard used linen.
    c. Put the "unoccupied" sign on the door.

Back Rub Procedure

Perhaps one of the most talked-about and least-performed aspects of nursing care is the back rub. A daub of lotion smeared over a patient's back in 30 seconds or less is *not* a back rub, but frequently that is all a patient gets.

All patients deserve a back rub at least twice a day (tradition dictates a back rub during or after the bath and at bedtime), but it is of particular importance for those confined to bed *because it stimulates circulation* and generally relaxes them. However, back rubs may certainly be done more frequently if a patient needs or desires them.

Use the lotion generally provided in the "hospitality kit" for rubbing the back. It is a nice touch to warm it slightly before use by placing it under warm running water for a few moments. Once you begin a back rub, *it is more pleasant and relaxing for the patient* if at least one hand remains in contact with his or her back until you have finished (see Figure 11.6). This is not difficult to do if the lotion is within easy reach.

Be aware of the patient's response to your touch and question the patient about areas that are especially tight or tense. Ask which areas he or she would like special attention to be given to. Also give special attention to any reddened areas.

There are many acceptable ways to perform a back rub. We prefer the following method.

☐ *Planning*

5. Secure lotion or another rubbing agent of the patient's preference.

☐ *Implementation*

12. Give the back rub:
    a. Move the patient close to your side of the bed *to decrease the distance you need to reach.* Position the patient on his or her abdomen if possible. If this is not possible because of the patient's condition or the presence of tubes, a side-lying position with the patient

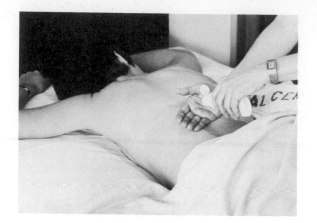

FIGURE 11.6 RETAINING TOUCH DURING BACK RUB   At least one hand should remain in contact with patient's back at all times, even when you are pouring lotion. (Let the back of your hand rest on the patient's back.)
Courtesy Ivan Ellis

facing away from you is adequate, also. Pull the top covers down below the buttocks.
    b. Pour a small amount of lotion into your hand and rub your palms together, *to get the lotion on both hands.*
    c. With your feet apart (the outside one ahead of the inside one *so that you can rock back and forth while maintaining good posture and body mechanics*), place your hands at the sacral area, one on either side of the spinal column.
    d. Rub toward the neckline, using long, firm, smooth strokes.
    e. Pause at the neckline and, using your thumbs, rub up into the hairline, while using your fingers to massage the sides of the neck.
    f. With a kneading motion, rub out along the shoulders. Continue the kneading motion and move down one side of the trunk with both hands until you are again at the sacral area.
    g. Then, placing your hands side by side with the palms down, rub in a figure-8 pattern over the buttocks and sacral area (see Figure 11.7). Move the figure 8 back and forth to include the entire buttocks area, an area that is often neglected.
    h. Next, again using the kneading

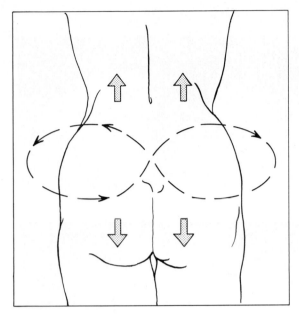

FIGURE 11.7 *FIGURE-8 TECHNIQUE IN BACK RUB*

motion, move up the opposite side toward the shoulder.
  i. Ask the patient if there are any areas that he or she would especially like rubbed.
  j. Complete the back rub using long, firm strokes up and down the back (shoulders to sacrum and back to shoulders).
  k. Replace the top covers, reposition the patient, and lower the bed.
14. Return the lotion to the bedside stand.

Oral Care

Oral care is a too often neglected or inadequately done part of hygiene. Ideally the patient should be offered the opportunity for oral care before breakfast, after all meals, and at bedtime. Not all patients will want oral care this frequently, but it should still be offered. Oral care is especially important for patients who are receiving oxygen and for patients who have nasogastric tubes in place, as well as for those on NPO (nothing by mouth). Many will be able to take care of this aspect of their hygiene independently, provided the equipment is conveniently placed.

If a patient can perform his or her own oral care but is confined to bed, you should provide the necessary articles: toothbrush, toothpaste or

powder (usually brought to the facility by the patient), cup of water, emesis basin, and face towel. Some patients also use dental floss.

Toothbrushing

Brushing is correctly done using a small, soft brush. Many dentists recommend a four-row, level, straight-handled brush. Holding the brush at a 45° angle, use a small, vibrating, circular motion with the bristles at the junction of the teeth and gums. Use the same action on the front and the back of the teeth.

Use a back-and-forth brushing motion over the biting surfaces of the teeth. Brush the tongue last and then rinse the mouth. It is wise to rinse after eating if brushing cannot be done. Mouthwashes can be used if desired, but remember that their antiseptic value is questionable.

⬜ *Planning*
  7. Assemble the equipment as listed above.

⬜ *Implementation*
  12. Give oral care.
    a. Place a towel under the patient's chin, tucking it behind the shoulders.
    b. Put on clean gloves *for asepsis.*
    c. Moisten the toothbrush with water from a glass and spread a small amount of toothpaste on it. If no cleansing agent is available, plain water is adequate. Baking soda is a substitute that also freshens the breath.
    d. Brush the teeth according to the procedure above, allowing the patient to expectorate into the emesis basin.
    e. Allow the patient to rinse his or her mouth with water, followed by a mouthwash if desired.
    f. Wipe the patient's mouth.
  14. a. Rinse equipment and return it to its appropriate place.
    b. Remove and dispose of gloves.
    c. Return bed to low position.

Flossing

Flossing should be done once daily *to remove plaque (organisms trapped in a mucous base), which if not removed causes tooth and gum disease.* Plaque forms in 24 hours, after which it can be removed

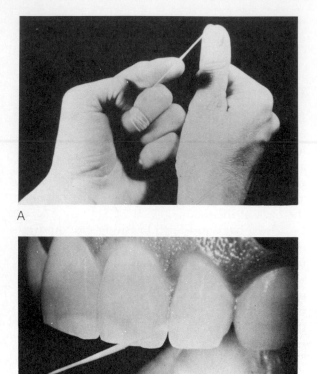
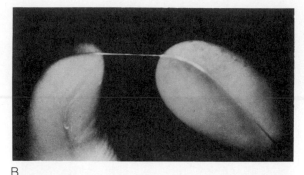
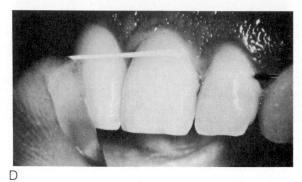

FIGURE 11.8 FLOSSING THE TEETH
Courtesy Ivan Ellis

only by a visit to the dentist's office. Floss is correctly held as demonstrated in Figure 11.8. Remember, however, that control of the floss is more important than how it is held.

Carry out flossing both between the teeth and between the gums and each individual tooth, taking care not to injure the delicate mucous membranes. The mouth should be rinsed after flossing *to remove debris.*

Patients who can sit in Fowler's or even semi-Fowler's position can often do most of their oral care independently. If they cannot, use the following procedure.

Oral Care for Unconscious Patients

Unconscious patients are completely dependent on you for their oral care. *Because these persons may be "mouth breathers" and are not taking food or fluids by mouth,* sordes (foul matter that collects on the lips and mouth) accumulates rapidly. A suitable procedure for the oral care of unconscious patients is as follows.

Planning

7. Assemble the equipment. Many facilities have prepared mouth care kits that include tongue blades, applicators, mouthwash, and the like. Suction should be available. Raise the bed to a comfortable working height.

Implementation

12. Give oral care.
    a. Place the patient in semi-Fowler's position, if possible, with the head turned toward you. If the patient's head cannot be raised, leave him or her flat and turn the head toward you.
    b. Place a towel under the patient's chin, tucking it in beneath the shoulders.
    c. Put on clean gloves *for asepsis.*
    d. Place a padded tongue blade (made by wrapping 4 × 4s around a tongue blade and taping them securely) in the patient's mouth. Use this to hold the mouth open and prevent the patient from biting down on your hands or utensils.

e. Moisten toothbrush very lightly and avoid highly foaming cleansing agents.

f. Brush all tooth surfaces as previously discussed.

g. Using oversized cotton-tipped applicators, or gauze or a washcloth wrapped around your index finger, clean all surfaces of the mouth, including the palate, inner cheeks, and tongue. A variety of cleansing agents can be used. A mixture of hydrogen peroxide and water, half and half, is probably as good as anything, and it is not cariogenic, as buttermilk and milk of magnesia are. *Commercial agents often contain lemon, which can etch the teeth, and glycerin, which actually absorbs moisture from the tissue.* Therefore the use of such agents is not wise, particularly for unconscious patients or patients who are receiving nothing by mouth. If a large accumulation of sordes is present, it may be necessary to remove it in stages, so as not to damage the tissue.

h. Rinse the patient's mouth with small amounts of water, either allowing it to drain into the emesis basin by gravity or using an asepto syringe to aspirate it.

i. Wipe the patient's mouth.

j. Lubricate the lips as needed. Use a water-soluble agent to prevent the aspiration of any oils.

k. Return the bed to the low position.

14. Rinse and replace the equipment, then remove and dispose of gloves.

Procedure for Care of Dentures

Patients often want to care for their dentures themselves. If so, your responsibility, once again, will be to provide them with the necessary articles. A patient may have brought a denture brush and cleansing agent to the hospital, but if not, a regular toothbrush and paste or powder will suffice. Provide the patient with a partially filled bath basin over which to wash the dentures, *so that if they fall they will not break.* The patient will also need a glass of water *for rinsing.*

If you care for the dentures yourself, keep the following facts in mind.

Planning

7. A special denture brush and denture cleaner may be available. If not, use a regular toothbrush and cleansing agent.

Implementation

12. Clean the dentures.
    a. Put on clean gloves *for asepsis.*
    b. To assist a patient with removal, apply downward pressure with the index fingers from above the dentures. It may help if the patient inflates his or her cheeks *to break the suction.* If no assistance is needed, it works well to have the patient remove his or her own dentures and place them in a denture cup for you.
    c. Handle dentures with care. *If dropped, they often break.* For this reason they are usually cleaned over a sink that is partially filled with water, *to break the fall in case they are dropped.*
    d. Take the dentures to the sink in the denture cup. Use a denture brush if the patient has one. Note that the longer side of the brush is used for the tooth surface and the smaller part for brushing the inner surface. Be certain to do the brushing over a basin of water. Some people like to pad the basin with a towel instead of putting water in it. Both measures are taken *to prevent breakage in case the dentures are dropped.*
    e. Have the patient rinse out his or her mouth before reinserting the dentures. Some like to use a soft toothbrush to brush the gums and tongue.
    f. Then rinse the dentures and return them to the patient, fitting the upper dentures in first. If dentures are to be stored (for an unconscious patient or at night if necessary), they should be stored in a covered container, carefully labeled, and preferably placed in a drawer or other area *where they are not likely to be brushed off onto the floor.* Whether or not they should be stored in water depends on the material of which they are made.

Check with the patient or the patient's family.

g. Dry the patient's mouth.

Hair Care

Brushing and Combing

A patient's hair should be combed and brushed daily. Generally this is done along with other hygiene activities and at other times throughout the day as necessary. Hair care is especially important to the patient, *since morale is often directly related to appearance.*

Hair care is usually done after the bath. Whenever it is done, these are some important points to remember.

☐ *Planning*

7. Assemble the equipment. The patient will probably have brought his or her own comb, brush, and other hair care items to the facility. A mirror may be available as a part of the overbed table.

☐ *Implementation*

12. Provide hair care.

a. Place a face or bath towel over the pillow *to keep it clean.*

b. The patient who is able to comb and brush his or her own hair should be placed in Fowler's position with the hair care items on the overbed table. Assist the patient as necessary.

The helpless or unconscious patient may be flat or in a semi-Fowler's position.

c. Turn the patient's head away from you and bring the hair back toward you. Brush hair with few tangles in two or three large sections. Matted hair may have to be separated into small sections and treated with a cream rinse or alcohol *to remove the snarls.*

d. Hold a section of hair 2 to 3 inches from the end. Comb the end until it is free of tangles. Gradually move toward the scalp, combing 2 to 3 inches at a time until the hair is tangle-free. You should be very gentle *to avoid causing pain.*

e. Turn the patient's head in the opposite direction and repeat steps 5 and 6.

f. Arrange the hair as neatly and simply as possible. Braiding may be the most appropriate style for long hair. (The family can bring in barrettes and ribbons to make your job easier.) Use cream or spray if it is needed or if the patient wants it.

g. Remove towel.

14. Place towel in a laundry hamper or bag. Clean the comb and brush and return them, along with the other toilet articles, to the bedside stand.

Shampooing

Many patients whose illnesses keep them in the hospital for only a few days do not want or need shampoos during that time. Other patients, however, may *need* shampoos, not only *to remove oil and dirt and to increase circulation to the scalp, but to improve appearance and morale as well.* Before giving a shampoo, check to see whether a physician's order is needed.

Generally, a shampoo is not given at the same time as the bath *because it is a tiring procedure.* The obvious exception is when a patient can shower. The equipment and general procedure you will use for those patients who need a shampoo and cannot shower will vary with the facility. In some places, the patient is taken on a stretcher to an area away from his or her room where there is a sink at the right height with room for the stretcher, too. In most facilities, however, the patient remains in bed and the shampoo is given using pitchers of warm water and a trough arrangement *to guide the water into a receptacle on the floor or chair beside the bed.*

Use this general procedure for giving a shampoo.

☐ *Planning*

7. Assemble the equipment, including bath blanket, two towels, shampoo, commercial rinse or vinegar, plastic square to protect the bed, pitcher, trough (if not available in the facility, you can make one from a plastic or rubber sheet with rolled towels under the edges), and basin to collect water (see Figure 11.9).

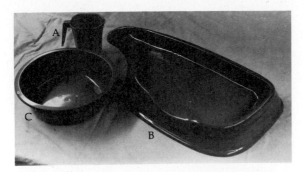

FIGURE 11.9 EQUIPMENT FOR SHAMPOOING PATIENT'S HAIR IN BED   Water is poured from the pitcher (A) over the patient's hair, drains down through the trough (B) beneath the patient's head, and falls into the basin (C) below.
Courtesy Ivan Ellis

 Implementation

12. Shampoo hair.

   a. Remove the top linens and position a bath blanket. (See Module 7, Bedmaking, Occupied Beds, step 12, page 117.)

   b. Place the plastic square under the patient's head and shoulders.

   c. Place a towel around the patient's shoulders and neck, with the ends of the towel coming together in front.

   d. Place or arrange a trough under the patient's head with one end extending to the receptacle for water.

   e. Wet the hair, taking care to keep water out of the patient's eyes. Some patients like to hold a folded washcloth over their eyes *to protect them.*

   f. Shampoo and rinse twice, using only a small amount of shampoo and rinsing thoroughly. Use cream rinse or half-and-half vinegar and water rinse as desired by the patient. Rinse again.

   g. Dry the patient's hair, ears, and neck with a towel. If an electric hair dryer is available, you may find it helpful, particularly if a patient has long hair.

   h. Comb or brush and arrange the hair, allowing the patient to assist if able. If hair-setting materials are available, a female patient may wish to set, or

have you set, her hair, in which case you would comb it at a later time.

   i. Remove the plastic square, towels, trough, pitcher, and basin.

   j. Replace the top bed linen, removing the bath blanket after the top sheet is in place.

   k. Allow the patient to rest.

14. Return equipment to be cleaned.

Eye Care

The eyes of the healthy individual need no special care other than that given during the usual bathing procedure. However, if there is a neurologic deficit that prevents the blink reflex from operating or if the person is comatose, the eyes need special care to prevent drying of the surface, which can lead to ulceration and permanent vision impairment.

The physician may order a product known as "artificial tears" to keep the eye surface moist or may order that the eyes be patched for protection.

Assessment

1. Check the chart to determine whether there is a physician's order relative to eye care.

2. Assess the patient's ability to blink.

3. Check to see whether there are eye care supplies in the patient's room. You will need a clean eye pad and tape. Commercially prepared eye pads are oval in shape and *do not have lint that could get in the eye.* If these are not available, clean gauze squares can be substituted. Many hospitals use sterile pads *for extra safety from microorganisms. However, the eye will be closed, and the pad will contact only the exterior of the eyelid; therefore, sterile pads are not essential.* Follow the policy of your facility.

Planning

4. Wash your hands *for asepsis.*

5. Obtain the needed supplies.

Implementation

6. If the eyelids are not clean, clean them at this time. Use a clean washcloth and clear warm water. Wipe the exterior of each

eye from the medial aspect to the lateral aspect. Dry the eyes in the same way.

7. If artificial tears are ordered, instill them into the eyes at this time. (See Module 50 for directions on administering eye drops.)

8. Observe the surface of the eyes closely *to detect any irritation or inflammation.*

9. Gently close each eyelid and hold it closed while the eyepad is placed over it.

10. Secure the eyepad with tape so that it holds the eye closed. *The eyelid will protect the surface of the eye from foreign bodies and allow tears to keep the surface moist.*

11. Repeat steps 9 and 10 for the second eye.

12. Put away or dispose of equipment.

13. Wash your hands *for asepsis.*

▢ *Evaluation*

14. Evaluate whether the pad is holding the eye closed.

15. Check skin around eye for irritation resulting from tape.

▢ *Documentation*

16. Routine care for eyes may be recorded on a flow sheet or on the narrative progress notes. If eye medication was instilled, follow directions for recording medications (see Module 50).

Contact Lens Care, Removal, and Insertion

When a patient wears contact lenses, self-care is the best way to ensure that the care is done properly. However, an individual who enters a hospital in an emergency may have contact lenses in place that must be removed *to prevent complications associated with excessive wear.* During a stay, an incapacitated patient may need assistance with routine care and placement of contact lenses.

▢ *Assessment*

1. Ascertain that the patient has contact lenses in place.

2. Determine what type of lenses are being worn (i.e., soft lenses or hard lenses).

▢ *Planning*

3. Wash your hands *for asepsis.*

4. Obtain a clean container in which to store the contact lenses. If a regular contact lens container is not available, use sterile specimen jars that have been carefully marked with the patient's name and the information that these are contact lenses. The left and right lenses should be separated and marked as left or right. Hard lenses may be stored dry; however, both hard and soft lenses may be stored in sterile saline or special soaking solution.

▢ *Implementation*

5. Use a flashlight to examine the eye and determine where the contact lens is resting. *The lens will reflect light and be visible.* Without this, it is often difficult to see the lens.

6. Care for the lenses in the following way:
   a. Hard lenses
   (1) *Removing the lens*
   Place a drop of saline or lens solution in the eye *to moisten the surface and facilitate removal.*
   Place one forefinger on the upper lid and one on the lower lid.
   Raise the upper lid and gently push in on the lower lid at the lower margin of the lens. *This should raise the lower edge of the lens and allow it to pop out.*
   (2) *Cleaning the lens*
   Clean the lens with lens cleaning solution by moistening the lens and rubbing it gently between your fingers. Be sure to hold the lens over a basin or sink with water in it in case you drop the lens. Rinse the cleaning solution off with sterile saline or wetting solution.
   (3) *Replacing the lens*
   Place the lens on the tip of the index finger with the concave surface up.
   Wet with wetting solution or sterile saline *to avoid drying the eye surface.*
   Hold the eye open with the thumb and index finger of the other hand.

Tip the lens onto the surface of the eye.

Have the patient blink *to position the lens.*

b. Soft lenses
   (1) *Removing the soft lens*
   Place a drop of saline or lens wetting solution in the eye *to moisten the surface and facilitate removal.*

   Place the forefinger on the upper lid and the thumb on the lower lid and open the eye wide.

   Using the other forefinger and thumb, gently pinch up on the lens. *It is flexible and will fold and lift out.*

   (2) *Cleaning the soft lens*
   Place the lens in the palm of one hand.

   Apply a few drops of cleaning solution and rub both surfaces of the lens thoroughly *to remove accumulated sediment.*

   Rinse with rinsing solution or sterile saline *to remove cleansing agent.*

   Store in saline or replace in eye.

   (3) *Inserting the soft lens*
   Hold the lens carefully pinched between thumb and forefinger.

   Open eye with other thumb and forefinger.

   Place lens onto eye surface and release.

   Have patient blink *to position the lens.*

Evaluation

7. Evaluate in terms of patient comfort and whether the patient can see adequately.

Documentation

8. Record that the patient wears contact lenses on the nursing care plan.

9. Note in the chart the disposition of contact lenses (whether they were sent home with a relative or stored in the bedside stand) in order *to prevent concern over their possible loss and to prevent liability of the hospital for loss of the lenses.*

Example of Charting   POR Style

4/10/88
1600   Interim note: Contact lenses Contact lenses removed from both eyes, placed in labeled sterile specimen bottles, and sent home with Mrs. Evans (mother of patient).

J. Johnson, N.S.

Care of Glasses

It is probable that most nursing students have worn some type of eyeglasses, either regular glasses or sunglasses, at some time. Therefore, it seems somewhat unnecessary to describe the care of glasses. However, in the busy care environment, it is easy to forget certain essentials.

Cleaning Glasses   Whenever you clean glasses, use water and soap to clean them before polishing them dry. *This prevents the fine scratches on the surface of glasses that dust particles can cause.* Many glasses are now made of plastic, *which is much more susceptible to scratching than traditional glass;* therefore, extra care is needed.

Glasses should be washed at the beginning of the day. *A soiled surface that is tolerable when it accumulates gradually during the day is very disturbing when the glasses are put on at the beginning of the day.*

Protecting Glasses   When glasses are removed, place them in a glasses case *for protection* if at all possible. If a case is not available, place the glasses in a bedside drawer, *where they are more protected.* Always place them with the glass surface up *to avoid scratches on the glass.* Be careful where glasses are placed *so that they do not get accidentally knocked on the floor.*

Care of Hearing Aids

Currently available hearing aids are finely adjusted electronic devices. They can be damaged by rough handling. The ear piece can be lifted out of the ear. A notation should be made on the nursing care plan or patient record of the need for a hearing aid and the ear in which it should be placed *to facilitate appropriate care by other care givers.*

Cleaning the Hearing Aid

To clean the earpiece, gently wipe it off with a dry tissue. If ear wax has become embedded in the small opening in the earpiece, it can be cleaned out with a special cleaning instrument that comes with the hearing aid. The patient may have this at home.

Protecting the Hearing Aid

If the hearing aid is not going to be used for a period of days, the battery should be removed for storage. This prolongs the life of the battery and protects the hearing aid. The hearing aid must be kept dry because any moisture can interfere with its functioning. Place the hearing aid in a bedside drawer or other safe place to prevent its being knocked to the floor.

Example of Charting   **Narrative Style**

4/10/88
4:00 pm   Hearing: Wears hearing aid in left
             ear. Pt. able to insert aid and
             adjust volume independently.
                    K. Robertson, N.S.

PERFORMANCE CHECKLIST				

General procedure for hygiene	Unsatisfactory	Needs More Practice	Satisfactory	Comments
Assessment				
1. Check chart for information related to patient's ability to participate in the procedure being planned.				
2. Assess patient for specific symptoms.				
3. Check to see what supplies are in room.				
Planning				
4. Determine assistance needed.				
5. Determine what supplies and equipment are needed.				
6. Wash your hands.				
7. Obtain needed supplies.				
Implementation				
8. Identify patient.				
9. Explain procedure to patient.				
10. Provide for patient's privacy.				
11. Raise bed to appropriate working level.				
12. Carry out hygiene procedure planned.				
13. Watch patient for adverse responses.				
14. Care for equipment and supplies.				
15. Wash your hands.				
Evaluation				
16. Evaluate in terms of the following criteria: a. Fatigue				
b. Feelings about comfort and cleanliness				
c. Objective signs of cleanliness				
Documentation				
17. Record as appropriate for your facility.				

Complete bedbath

	Unsatisfactory	Needs More Practice	Satisfactory	Comments
☐ *Assessment*				
1. Follow Checklist steps 1–3 of the General Procedure for Hygiene (check chart, assess patient, check supplies).				
☐ *Planning*				
2. Follow Checklist steps 4–6 of the General Procedure (determine assistance, determine needed supplies, wash hands).				
3. Obtain supplies: basin, soap, hamper, clean linen, bath blanket, clean garment, toilet articles).				
☐ *Implementation*				
4. Follow Checklist steps 8 and 9 of the General Procedure (identify patient and explain procedure).				
5. Follow Checklist steps 10 and 11 of the General Procedure (provide privacy and raise bed).				
6. Proceed with the bedbath.				
a. Remove top linen and place bath blanket.				
b. Give oral care if not already done.				
c. Obtain water.				
d. Position patient (see Complete Bedbath, step 12d, page 193).				
e. Bathe the patient in the following order: (1) Spread towel across patient's chest.				
(2) Make mitt out of washcloth.				
(3) Wash patient's face.				
(4) Remove patient's gown.				
(5) Place towel under far arm and bathe, rinse, and dry far hand, arm, and axilla.				
(6) Place towel under near arm and bathe, rinse, and dry near hand, arm, and axilla.				
(7) Spread towel across patient's chest and wash, rinse, and dry chest to waist.				
(8) Wash, rinse, and dry abdomen.				
(9) Place towel under far leg.				

	Unsatisfactory	Needs More Practice	Satisfactory	Comments
(10) Place patient's foot in bath basin.				
(11) Wash, rinse, and dry far leg.				
(12) Wash, rinse, and dry far foot.				
(13) Wash near leg and foot.				
(14) Change water.				
(15) Assist patient to turn and drape.				
(16) Wash, rinse, and dry back.				
(17) Wash, rinse, and dry buttocks.				
(18) Give back rub if desired.				
(19) Change water.				
(20) Wash genital area or give patient an opportunity to do so.				
f. Help patient put on clean gown.				
g. Assist patient with hair care.				
h. Assist patient with nail care.				
i. Assist male patient with shaving.				
j. Make occupied bed and return to low position.				
k. Tidy up area.				
7. Follow Checklist steps 13–15 of the General Procedure (watch patient response, care for equipment, wash your hands).				
☐ *Evaluation*				
8. Evaluate as in step 16 of the General Procedure (fatigue, subjective comfort, and cleanliness).				
☐ *Documentation*				
9. Record as in step 17 of the General Procedure.				

Tub bath

☐ *Assessment*				
1. Follow Checklist steps 1–3 of the General Procedure for Hygiene (check patient record, assess patient, check for supplies in room).				

	Unsatisfactory	Needs More Practice	Satisfactory	Comments
Planning				
2. Follow Checklist steps 4–7 of the General Procedure (determine assistance, determine needed supplies, wash your hands, obtain supplies and prepare tub room).				
Implementation				
3. Follow Checklist steps 8 and 9 of the General Procedure (identify patient and explain procedure).				
4. Assist patient to tub room.				
5. Hang occupied sign.				
6. In tub room: a. Help patient into tub.				
b. Assist with bathing as needed.				
c. Assist patient out of tub.				
d. Assist with drying.				
e. Help with donning garments.				
f. Assist patient to return to room.				
7. Watch for adverse response as in step 13 of the General Procedure.				
8. Return to tub room and clean area.				
9. Wash hands.				
Evaluation				
10. Evaluate as in step 16 of the General Procedure (fatigue, subjective comfort, cleanliness).				
Documentation				
11. Record as in step 17 of the General Procedure.				

Shower

	Unsatisfactory	Needs More Practice	Satisfactory	Comments
Assessment				
1. Follow Checklist steps 1–3 of the General Procedure for Hygiene (check patient record, assess patient, check for supplies in room).				

	Unsatisfactory	Needs More Practice	Satisfactory	Comments
☐ *Planning*				
2. Follow Checklist steps 4–7 of the General Procedure (determine assistance, determine needed supplies, wash your hands, obtain supplies and prepare shower room).				
☐ *Implementation*				
3. Follow Checklist steps 8 and 9 of the General Procedure (identify patient and explain procedure).				
4. Assist the patient to the shower room.				
5. Hang privacy sign on door.				
6. Give shower.				
a. Assist patient as necessary.				
b. Assist patient to return to room.				
7. Watch patient for adverse responses as in step 13 of the General Procedure.				
8. Return to the shower room and clean area.				
9. Wash your hands.				
☐ *Evaluation*				
10. Evaluate as in step 16 of the General Procedure (fatigue, subjective comfort, cleanliness).				
☐ *Documentation*				
11. Record as in step 17 of the General Procedure.				

Back rub

	Unsatisfactory	Needs More Practice	Satisfactory	Comments
☐ *Assessment*				
1. Follow Checklist steps 1–3 of the General Procedure for Hygiene (check patient record, assess patient, check for supplies in room).				
☐ *Planning*				
2. Follow Checklist steps 4–7 of the General Procedure (determine assistance, determine needed supplies, wash your hands, obtain lotion).				

211

	Unsatisfactory	Needs More Practice	Satisfactory	Comments
Implementation				
3. Follow Checklist steps 8–11 of the General Procedure (identify patient, explain procedure, provide privacy, and raise bed).				
4. Give back rub.				
a. Move patient to your side of bed and position.				
b. Pour small amount of lotion into hand and rub hands together.				
c. Place hands on sacral area, one on either side.				
d. Rub toward neckline.				
e. Massage into hairline.				
f. Knead along shoulders and down one side of trunk.				
g. Rub in figure-8 pattern over buttocks and sacral area.				
h. Knead up opposite side toward shoulders.				
i. Seek response from patient.				
j. Complete back rub by moving from shoulders to sacrum and back to shoulders.				
k. Replace covers, reposition patient, and lower bed.				
5. Watch for adverse responses as in step 13 of the General Procedure.				
6. Return lotion to storage.				
7. Wash your hands.				
Evaluation				
8. Evaluate as in step 16 of the General Procedure (fatigue, subjective feelings, objective appearance of comfort).				
Documentation				
9. Record as in step 17 of the General Procedure.				

Oral care procedure

	Unsatisfactory	Needs More Practice	Satisfactory	Comments
(The student serving as patient should provide his or her own toothbrush and cleansing agent.)				
☐ **Assessment**				
1. Follow Checklist steps 1–3 of the General Procedure for Hygiene (check patient record, assess patient, check for supplies in room).				
☐ **Planning**				
2. Follow Checklist steps 4–7 of the General Procedure (determine assistance, determine needed supplies, wash hands, obtain supplies).				
☐ **Implementation**				
3. Follow Checklist steps 8–11 of the General Procedure (identify patient, explain procedure, provide privacy, and raise bed).				
4. Provide oral care. a. Place towel under patient's chin.				
b. Put on clean gloves.				
c. Moisten toothbrush and apply cleansing agent.				
d. Brush teeth (see Toothbrushing, page 199).				
e. Allow patient to rinse with water.				
f. Wipe patient's mouth.				
g. Return bed to low position.				
5. Follow Checklist steps 13–15 of the General Procedure (watch patient for adverse response, care for equipment and supplies, and wash hands).				
☐ **Evaluation**				
6. Evaluate as in step 16 of the General Procedure (fatigue, subjective feelings, objective appearance of cleanliness).				
☐ **Documentation**				
7. Record as in step 17 of the General Procedure.				

Oral care for unconscious patients

	Unsatisfactory	Needs More Practice	Satisfactory	Comments
☐ *Assessment*				
1. Follow Checklist steps 1–3 of the General Procedure for Hygiene (check patient record, assess patient, check for supplies in room).				
☐ *Planning*				
2. Follow Checklist steps 4–7 of the General Procedure (determine assistance, determine needed supplies, wash hands, obtain supplies).				
☐ *Implementation*				
3. Follow Checklist steps 8–11 of the General Procedure (identify patient, explain procedure, provide privacy, and raise bed).				
4. Provide oral care. a. Position patient.				
b. Place towel under patient's chin.				
c. Put on clean gloves.				
d. Place padded tongue blade in patient's mouth.				
e. Moisten toothbrush.				
f. Brush teeth (see Toothbrushing, page 199).				
g. Use swabs or gauze to cleanse all surfaces of the mouth.				
h. Rinse patient's mouth.				
i. Wipe patient's mouth.				
j. Lubricate lips as needed.				
k. Return bed to low position.				
5. Follow Checklist steps 13–15 of the General Procedure (watch patient for adverse response, care for equipment and supplies, and wash hands).				
☐ *Evaluation*				
6. Evaluate as in step 16 of the General Procedure (fatigue, subjective feelings, objective cleanliness of mouth).				

	Unsatisfactory	Needs More Practice	Satisfactory	Comments
Documentation				
7. Document as in step 17 of the General Procedure.				
Care of dentures				
Assessment				
1. Follow Checklist steps 1–3 of the General Procedure for Hygiene (check patient record, assess patient, check for supplies in room).				
Planning				
2. Follow Checklist steps 4–7 of the General Procedure (determine assistance, determine needed supplies, wash hands, obtain supplies).				
Implementation				
3. Follow Checklist steps 8–11 of the General Procedure (identify patient, explain procedure, provide privacy, and raise bed).				
4. Clean dentures. a. Put on clean gloves.				
b. Assist patient with removal of dentures.				
c. Handle dentures with care.				
d. Take to sink in denture cup and clean.				
e. Have patient rinse mouth and clean gums if desired.				
f. Replace moist dentures, upper first, or store dentures in denture cup.				
g. Dry the patient's mouth.				
5. Follow Checklist steps 13–15 of the General Procedure (watch patient for adverse response, care for equipment and supplies, and wash hands).				
Evaluation				
6. Evaluate as in step 16 of the General Procedure (fatigue, subjective feelings, objective cleanliness of mouth).				
Documentation				
7. Document as in step 17 of the General Procedure.				

Hair care

	Unsatisfactory	Needs More Practice	Satisfactory	Comments
☐ *Assessment*				
1. Follow Checklist steps 1–3 of the General Procedure for Hygiene (check patient record, assess patient, check for supplies in room).				
☐ *Planning*				
2. Follow Checklist steps 4–7 of the General Procedure (determine assistance, determine needed supplies, wash hands, obtain supplies).				
☐ *Implementation*				
3. Follow Checklist steps 8–11 of the General Procedure (identify patient, explain procedure, provide privacy, and raise bed).				
4. Provide hair care. a. Place a towel over the pillow.				
b. Position patient.				
c. Turn head away and arrange hair toward you.				
d. Brush gently in two or three sections.				
e. Turn head toward you, rearrange hair.				
f. Repeat step d on the other side of the head.				
g. Arrange hair neatly and simply.				
h. Remove towel.				
5. Follow Checklist steps 13–15 of the General Procedure (watch patient for adverse response, care for equipment and supplies, and wash hands).				
☐ *Evaluation*				
6. Evaluate as in step 16 of the General Procedure (fatigue, subjective feelings, objective cleanliness).				
☐ *Documentation*				
7. Document as in step 17 of the General Procedure.				

Shampooing

	Unsatisfactory	Needs More Practice	Satisfactory	Comments
☐ *Assessment*				
1. Follow Checklist steps 1–3 of the General Procedure for Hygiene (check patient record, assess patient, check for supplies in room).				
☐ *Planning*				
2. Follow Checklist steps 4–7 of the General Procedure [determine assistance, determine needed supplies, wash hands, obtain supplies (trough, pitcher, basin, plastic sheet, shampoo, rinse agent, and towels)].				
☐ *Implementation*				
3. Follow Checklist steps 8–11 of the General Procedure (identify patient, explain procedure, provide privacy, and raise bed).				
4. Give the shampoo. a. Remove top linens and place bath blanket.				
b. Place plastic square under patient's head and shoulders.				
c. Place towel around patient's shoulders and neck.				
d. Arrange trough under patient's head.				
e. Wet the hair.				
f. Shampoo and rinse twice, rinsing thoroughly.				
g. Dry hair, ears, and neck.				
h. Assist the patient to comb and arrange hair.				
i. Remove equipment.				
j. Replace top linen and remove bath blanket.				
k. Allow patient to rest.				
5. Follow Checklist steps 13–15 of the General Procedure (watch patient for adverse response, care for equipment and supplies, and wash hands).				
☐ *Evaluation*				
6. Evaluate as in step 16 of the General Procedure (fatigue, subjective feelings, objective cleanliness).				

	Unsatisfactory	Needs More Practice	Satisfactory	Comments
☐ *Documentation*				
7. Document as in step 17 of the General Procedure.				
Eye care				
☐ *Assessment*				
1. Check for physician's orders.				
2. Assess patient's ability to blink.				
3. Check to see whether supplies are in room.				
☐ *Planning*				
4. Wash your hands.				
5. Obtain needed supplies.				
☐ *Implementation*				
6. Clean eyelids if necessary.				
7. Instill artificial tears if necessary.				
8. Observe surface of eye for irritation or inflammation.				
9. Close eyelid and place eyepad over it.				
10. Tape eyepad in place.				
11. Repeat steps 6–10 for second eye.				
12. Care for equipment.				
13. Wash your hands.				
☐ *Evaluation*				
14. Evaluate whether eyepad is holding eye closed.				
15. Check skin around eye for tape irritation.				
☐ *Documentation*				
16. Record eye care on flow sheet or progress notes.				
Contact lens care, removal, and insertion				
☐ *Assessment*				
1. Ascertain presence of contact lenses.				
2. Determine type of lenses being worn.				

	Unsatisfactory	Needs More Practice	Satisfactory	Comments
☐ *Planning*				
3. Wash your hands.				
4. Obtain container for contact storage.				
☐ *Implementation*				
5. Use flashlight to check for lens position.				
6(a). Care for hard lenses: a. Remove the lenses.				
(1) Place drop of saline or lens solution in the eye.				
(2) Place forefingers on upper and lower lid.				
(3) Raise upper lid and push in on lower lid at lens margin.				
b. Clean the lenses.				
(1) Work over a basin or sink with water in it.				
(2) Use cleaning solution.				
(3) Rub gently between fingers.				
c. Replace the lenses.				
(1) Place lens on tip of finger, concave surface up.				
(2) Wet with wetting solution or sterile saline.				
(3) Hold eye open with thumb and forefinger of opposite hand.				
(4) Tip lens onto surface of eye.				
(5) Have patient blink.				
6(b). Care for soft lenses: a. Remove the lenses.				
(1) Place a drop of saline or lens wetting solution in the eye.				
(2) Place forefinger on upper lid and thumb on lower lid.				
(3) Gently pinch lens up with opposite thumb and forefinger.				

	Unsatisfactory	Needs More Practice	Satisfactory	Comments
b. Clean the soft lenses.				
(1) Place lens in palm of one hand.				
(2) Apply cleaning solution and rub both surfaces.				
(3) Rinse lens.				
c. Insert the soft lenses.				
(1) Hold lens pinched between thumb and forefinger.				
(2) Open eye with other thumb and forefinger.				
(3) Place lens onto eye surface and release.				
(4) Have patient blink.				
☐ *Evaluation*				
7. Evaluate in terms of patient comfort and patient vision.				
☐ *Documentation*				
8. Record that patient wears contact lenses on the nursing care plan.				
9. Note on the chart the disposition of contact lenses that were removed.				

Care of glasses

1. Clean the glasses.				
a. Use soap and water.				
b. Polish dry.				
c. Clean at the beginning of the day.				
2. Protect the glasses.				
a. Place in glasses case.				
b. Place in bedside drawer or where they won't get knocked to the floor.				
c. Place with glass surface up.				

Care of hearing aids

1. Clean the hearing aid.				
a. Use a dry tissue.				

	Unsatisfactory	Needs More Practice	Satisfactory	Comments
b. Use special instrument to remove ear wax from opening.				
2. Protect the hearing aid.				
a. Remove battery if hearing aid will be out for several days.				
b. Keep dry.				

QUIZ

Multiple-Choice Questions

_____ 1. The temperature of the water for bathing and shampooing has been described as "warm." This means

    a. 75–90°F.
    b. 90–105°F.
    c. 100–115°F.
    d. 110–125°F.

_____ 2. The preferred position for bathing the patient in bed is

    a. prone.
    b. supine.
    c. semi-Fowler's.
    d. Fowler's.

_____ 3. The partial bedbath usually includes which of the following areas of the body? (1) face and neck; (2) hands; (3) axillae; (4) perineum

    a. 1 and 2
    b. 1 and 2
    c. 2, 3, and 4
    d. All of these

Short-Answer Questions

4. How are soft contact lenses stored? _____

_____

5. How are hard contact lenses removed? _____

_____

6. Why are glasses cleaned with soap and water instead of simply being polished while dry? _____

_____

7. What should be done to store a hearing aid for several days?

_____

_____

True-False Questions

_____ 8. A patient's face should be washed with soap and water.

_____ 9. When washing the arms, long, firm strokes toward the center of the body are used to decrease venous return.

_____ **10.** The back of the neck is washed separately from the front of the neck.

_____ **11.** You should always cut and file the patient's toenails and fingernails.

_____ **12.** A patient should be offered the opportunity for oral care before breakfast, after all meals, and at bedtime.

_____ **13.** The unconscious patient does not need oral care.

_____ **14.** Toothbrushing is correctly done using a small, soft brush.

_____ **15.** Dentures should be brushed over a basin of water.

_____ **16.** The hair of the hospitalized patient should be washed and combed or brushed daily.

MODULE 12

Basic Infant Care

MODULE CONTENTS

PREREQUISITES

Successful completion of the following
modules:

VOLUME 1

Module 1 / An Approach to Nursing Skills
Module 2 / Medical Asepsis
Module 3 / Safety
Module 4 / Basic Body Mechanics
Module 5 / Assessment
Module 6 / Documentation
Module 11 / Hygiene
Module 21 / Applying Restraints

OVERALL OBJECTIVE

To provide basic daily care for infants and to implement safety measures in all aspects of care.

SPECIFIC LEARNING OBJECTIVES

	Know Facts and Principles	Apply Facts and Principles	Demonstrate Ability	Evaluate Performance
1. Diapering a. Types	Identify types of diapers in common use			
b. Folding cloth diapers	Know methods of folding cloth diapers and advantages of each method	Determine appropriate way to fold diaper for particular situation	Fold diaper in both triangle-fold and rectangle-fold shapes.	Evaluate own performance using Performance Checklist
c. Cleaning	State rationale for frequent diaper changes. Know purpose of cleaning perineal area and buttocks with each diaper change.	Decide when to change infant's diaper based on rationale. Given a situation, select appropriate materials for cleaning infant during diapering.		
d. Fastening diapers	List two ways diapers are fastened	Given a situation, determine appropriate way to fasten diaper	Fasten diaper, handling safety pins correctly	
e. Skin problems	Describe symptoms of diaper rash and scald	Given a description of infant, identify whether diaper rash or scald is present	In the clinical setting, identify diaper rash and scald	
f. Diapering procedure	List steps of procedure		Change infant's diaper correctly and safely, using appropriate materials and methods for cleaning	Evaluate diapering by checking for fit and comfort. Evaluate own performance using Performance Checklist.

	Know Facts and Principles	Apply Facts and Principles	Demonstrate Ability	Evaluate Performance
2. Bathing	Discuss special considerations for bathing infant	Given a situation, describe correct procedure for bathing infant	Bathe infant correctly and safely	Evaluate own performance with instructor
3. Bottle feeding	Describe two positions for bottle feeding	Plan appropriate feeding position for particular infant	Bottle-feed infant	Evaluate by measuring infant's intake
a. Temperature	State usual temperature for bottle. State method for testing temperature.	Given a situation, decide whether to warm formula	Correctly distinguish safe temperature for bottle feeding	Evaluate own performance with instructor
b. Burping	Describe two positions for burping		Burp infant after feeding	Evaluate by checking whether infant has burped
4. Feeding solids	Describe two positions for feeding solids to infants	Plan appropriate position for particular infant	Feed solids to infant correctly	Evaluate by recording infant intake
a. Temperature	State proper temperature for solid foods	Identify safe method for warming infant's food	Demonstrate method to determine temperature of food	Evaluate own performance with instructor
5. Safety measures a. Tying a clove hitch	State purpose of clove-hitch restraint	Identify situation in which clove-hitch restraint is needed	Correctly and safely tie clove-hitch restraint	Evaluate own performance using Performance Checklist
b. Using crib restraints	State purpose of crib restraints	Identify situations in which crib restraints are needed	Correctly and safely apply crib restraints	Evaluate own performance using Performance Checklist
c. Elbow restraints	State purpose of elbow restraints	Identify situations in which elbow restraints are needed	Correctly and safely apply elbow restraints	Evaluate own performance using Performance Checklist

d. *Mummying*

State purpose of mummying

Identify situations in which mummying is needed

Given a situation, identify correct type of restraint to be used

Correctly and safely apply mummy restraint to infant

Evaluate own performance using Performance Checklist

Evaluate choice with instructor

LEARNING ACTIVITIES

1. Review the Specific Learning Objectives.
2. Look up the module vocabulary terms in the Glossary.
3. Read through the module.
4. In the practice setting:
   a. Diapering
      (1) Inspect both cloth and disposable diapers.
      (2) Practice folding diapers using both the rectangle-folded and triangle-folded methods. Fold them to provide extra thickness in the front (used for males and for females lying on the abdomen). Then refold to provide extra thickness in the back (used for females lying on the back).
      (3) Diaper an infant mannequin, using the Performance Checklist as a guide. Practice opening and closing safety pins with one hand while keeping the other hand on the "infant."
      (4) Arrange for your instructor to check you when you feel competent.
   b. Bathing
      (1) Bathe an infant mannequin using the procedures described.
   c. Bottle feeding
      (1) Practice holding an infant mannequin for bottle feeding.
      (2) Practice both methods of holding an infant mannequin for burping.
      (3) Have your instructor check your performance.
   d. Feeding solids
      (1) Practice feeding an infant mannequin solids while holding it on your lap.
   e. Safety measures
      (1) Practice tying a clove-hitch knot. Have your instructor check the knot.
      (2) Improvise an arm or use a mannequin's arm and tie it to a stationary object (the bed frame or an armboard) using a clove-hitch knot.
      (3) Inspect elbow restraints if they are available.
      (4) Practice mummying an infant mannequin using the two methods outlined in the module.
      (5) Have your instructor check your performance.

VOCABULARY

burp
cardiac sphincter
circumcise
clove hitch
colic
cradle cap
fontanel
foreskin
gastro-colic reflex
macerate
macular
smegma

BASIC INFANT CARE

Rationale for the Use of This Skill

*I*ncluded in the care of hospitalized infants are feeding, bathing, and diapering. Special efforts are needed to maintain safety for infants, both in general care and throughout all procedures. To provide this safety, the nurse must carry out special measures and use equipment, such as restraints, correctly.[1]

Diapering

Types of Diapers

Many hospitals use disposable diapers (see Figure 12.1). These have the advantage of decreasing laundry and ensuring that no cross-contamination occurs. Most have a waterproof cover that protects the linen from urine and stool. Disposable diapers come in a variety of sizes based on the weight of the infant, making proper fit possible. Some infants do develop skin sensitivity to paper products, however.

Cloth diapers can be softer and less irritating for some infants. Plastic pants are optional, and should be omitted for some infants—for example, a newborn, whose skin is sensitive to urine accumulation. Cloth diapers generally come in one size but can be folded to accommodate different-size infants. Also, several diapers can be folded together *to provide an absorbent diaper for overnight use on older infants or toddlers.* Some cloth diapers are available in prefolded shapes.

Folding Cloth Diapers

There are a variety of methods for folding diapers. We explain two common ones in this module. *The purpose of any type of fold is to provide a diaper that:*

1. *is the correct size for the infant.*
2. *fastens safely and securely.*
3. *is thickest where greatest absorbency is needed.*
4. *is comfortable for the infant to wear.*
5. *retains both urine and stool in the diaper.*

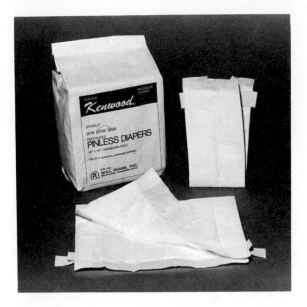

FIGURE 12.1 DISPOSABLE DIAPER
Courtesy Searle Medical Products USA, Inc.

No one folding method is ideal, and you may devise your own adaptations for specific situations.

Triangle folding provides the greatest mobility for an infant's legs. A diaper can be folded with its maximum thickness in the front for boys or for girls who sleep on the abdomen, and with maximum thickness in the back for girls who sleep on the back. Alter the size by changing the size of the initial square into which the diaper is folded and by changing the width to which the triangle is folded.

To fold, follow the diagrams in Figure 12.2.

1. Fold the diaper into a square (A). The size may be altered at this point.
2. Holding one corner of the square firmly in place, fold the two adjacent corners toward the middle of the diaper, forming an elongated diamond shape (B). The final width of the diaper can be altered by changing the amount the two corners overlap.
3. Fold the corner you have been holding down over the other two, creating a long triangle.
4. Now, fold the last corner, which is the smallest angle of the triangle, toward the center (C). The length of the diaper may be altered by changing the amount that is folded up.

---

[1]You will note that rationale for action is emphasized throughout the module by the use of italics.

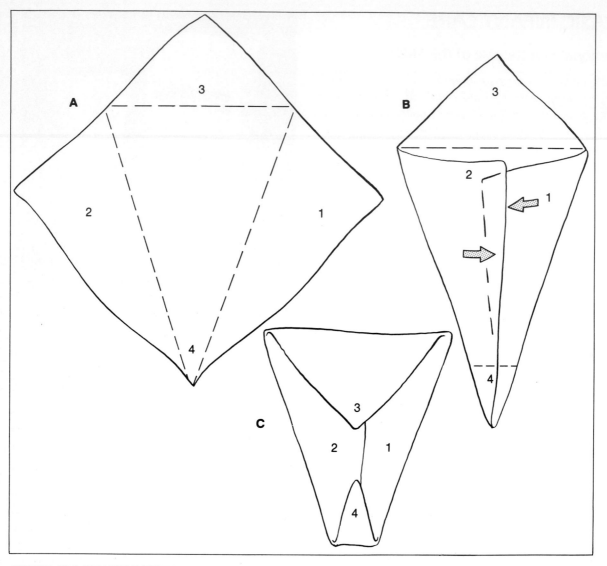

FIGURE 12.2 TRIANGLE-FOLDING A DIAPER

Rectangular folding provides the greatest width between the legs and is often better at containing loose stools than is a triangle-folded diaper. The size can be changed very simply. Alter the width by changing the width of the initial fold. Alter the length by simply folding over the front or the back until the diaper is the desired length.

To fold, follow the diagrams in Figure 12.3.

1. Use a square diaper and fold the two outer edges in to form a long rectangle (A).
2. Divide the rectangle into thirds by either (B) folding the top third down to put the added thickness in the back or (C) folding the bottom third up to put the added thickness in the front.

Cleansing at Diaper Changes

Cleansing is needed any time a diaper is changed *because stool and urine left on the skin will cause skin irritation.* Facilities usually establish a routine for this procedure. Several methods are presented here.

1. The simplest method is to wash with a mild soap and water, then rinse thoroughly. Keep a washcloth and towel at the side of the crib for this purpose.
2. Use cotton balls saturated in baby oil or baby lotion. This method does not require rinsing because the baby oil does not irritate the skin.

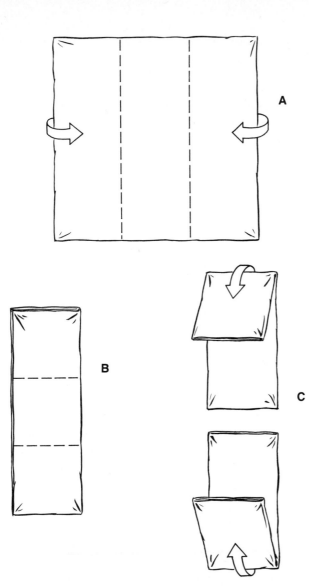

FIGURE 12.3 RECTANGLE-FOLDING A DIAPER

3. Use disposable wipes that contain baby oil or lotion for cleansing. Again, rinsing is not needed because there is no irritating substance present.

Fastening Diapers

Disposable diapers come with attached tapes for fastening. These are both convenient and safe. Use safety pins to fasten all other diapers. Remember that open safety pins are *always* a hazard. Close pins as soon as they are removed and place them out of reach. *Then, even if you have misjudged the infant's reach, he or she will pick up a closed, not an open, pin.*

When you are ready to fasten a diaper, place the pin horizontally, with the point toward the infant's side. *If the pin later opens, it will be less likely to cause injury* because it is pointed away from vital tissue. Also, always place your hand between the infant and the diaper you are pinning. *Then, if you push the pin completely through the diaper, you will stick your own hand and not the infant.* If a safety pin does not slide easily into the diaper, stick the point into a bar of soap to lubricate it *so that it enters easily.*

Skin Problems

Diaper rash is a skin reaction that appears as a macular to solid redness in the perineal area. It may be caused by:

1. prolonged contact with urine.
2. irritation from ammonia formed as the urine decomposes.
3. maceration from wetness.
4. irritation from residual detergents or cleansing agents in a diaper.
5. irritation from the harsh surface of a diaper.

Scald occurs rapidly and appears as a totally reddened area much like a burn. It happens when the stool or urine contains harsh ingredients that cause a chemical-type burn of the skin.

The best way to prevent diaper rash or scald is *to change diapers frequently, clean the skin with each change to remove residual urine or feces, and wash diapers correctly (with mild soap and thorough rinsing).* If diaper rash persists, consult a physician. *Infants are prone to* candida *(a fungal infection), which can have an appearance similar to that of diaper rash.*

If an infant is having frequent, loose, or diarrheal stools, a heavy, non–water soluble ointment (petroleum jelly, A & D ointment) may be applied at the time of the diaper change *to protect the skin from contact with the stool.* You must check your facility's policy regarding the use of ointments.

Powders can also be used to help the skin remain dry. Do not let powder get into the air, where the infant might inhale it, because *it acts as an irritant to the respiratory tract.* Place a small amount on your hand and smooth it over the infant's skin. Use only a thin coating; *large amounts tend to gather in clumps that can irritate the skin. Some infants are sensitive to the perfume in baby powder, and this can cause skin irritation also.* Because of the problems associated with its use, some facilities do not use baby powder at all. Cornstarch is an inexpensive substitute that does not tend to cause irritation.

Diapering Procedure

Although gloves are not generally worn for routine diaper changes, if your hospital has a policy that clean gloves are to be worn whenever you have actual or potential contact with body substances, you should wear them. Otherwise, practice conscientious handwashing after changing diapers.

Assessment

1. Check the infant to see whether the diaper is dry.
2. Determine the infant's physical development, with emphasis on its ability to roll over and grasp.

Planning

3. Select the type of diaper fold to be used or the size of disposable diaper needed.
4. Plan the method of securing the diaper (pins or tapes).
5. Wash your hands *so that you do not introduce microorganisms to the infant.*
6. Obtain a clean diaper and cleansing equipment.

Implementation

7. Fold the diaper if necessary.
8. Place the infant on his or her back in the crib or on a clean surface. Make sure the infant is safe from falling. *Never* leave an infant out of the crib or with side rails down.
9. Unfasten the soiled diaper. Close the safety pins as you remove them, and set them aside out of the infant's reach.
10. Remove the soiled diaper, using the clean portion of the diaper to wipe away stool. Wipe from front to back *to avoid spreading microbes from the anal area to the vagina or urethra.*
11. Clean the diaper area thoroughly. Take extra care to clean in all folds, around the scrotum on a boy and between the labia on a girl. For a girl, be sure you clean from the anterior region to the posterior region *so that you do not contaminate the*

urinary meatus with bacteria from the rectal area. If there was a large amount of stool or urine, the infant may need more extensive bathing. Change all wet or soiled clothing. Be careful about leaning over a male infant—urine can be sprayed a long distance.

12. Lift the infant's buttocks by grasping both ankles with one hand and place a clean diaper under the infant (see Figure 12.4).
13. Pull the front of the diaper up between the infant's legs, *so that it fits snugly around the abdomen.* Fasten with pins or tapes (see Figure 12.5). Always put the pins into the diaper so that the point is toward the outside. *That way, if the pin comes open, it will be less likely to jab the infant.*
14. Be sure that the infant is secure and protected from falling.

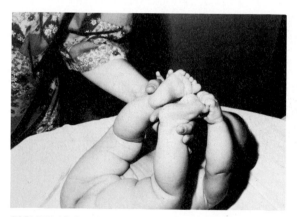

FIGURE 12.4 LIFTING AN INFANT BY THE ANKLES TO PLACE A DIAPER
Courtesy Ivan Ellis

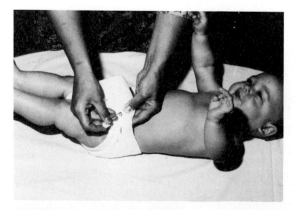

FIGURE 12.5 DIAPER IN PLACE
Courtesy Ivan Ellis

15. Dispose of the soiled diaper.
16. Wash your hands.

Evaluation

17. Check the diaper for secure fit and comfort.

Documentation

18. Record the number of diaper changes and the appearance and any unusual odor of the urine and stool. In situations in which the amount of output is critical, you may be required to weigh the soiled diapers.

Bathing

General Information

An infant is given a bedbath in much the same manner as an adult. Keeping the infant warm and safe are of primary importance. Among the special considerations for bathing an infant are the following:

Safety Everything must be within reach before beginning; one hand must remain in contact with the infant at all times.

Holding the Infant Any method of holding an infant must *provide support for the head and neck and keep the infant close to your body to lessen the chance of injury or dropping.* The *football hold* does all of these things. In the football hold, the infant is held with the head in the palm of the hand, the back on the forearm, and the feet between the arm and your side (see Figure 12.6). If the infant can sit in a basin with support, keep one of your arms behind the infant, holding onto the infant's far arm. *This leaves your other arm free, yet keeps the infant secure.* Even with an older infant who can sit unaided, you should still keep one hand on the infant at all times. Remember, a tub is slippery and infants move very quickly. Do not immerse an infant whose umbilicus is not completely healed *because an infection might result.*

Shampooing This is usually done each time an infant is bathed to *prevent a scale accumulation called cradle cap.* Hold the infant football-style, with the head over the basin, so that the scalp can be gently scrubbed and thoroughly rinsed with strokes going away from the infant's face.

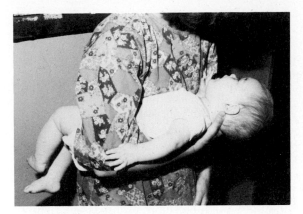

FIGURE 12.6 THE FOOTBALL HOLD
Courtesy Ivan Ellis

Eye Care Without soap, clean each eye from inner to outer canthus, using a clean area of the washcloth for each eye *so that microorganisms are not transferred from one eye to the other.*

Folds Infants have many creases and folds. Take care to wash and dry carefully in all of them. *Moisture left in creases causes skin breakdown.*

Perineal Care For the female infant, be sure to clean between the labia and in all folds from front to back. For the uncircumcised male infant *gently* retract the foreskin only as far as it will go easily, and return it to its normal position after cleansing the exposed surfaces. *Secretions left under the foreskin may cause irritation and be a focus for infection, with resulting adhesions.*

Bathing Procedure

Assessment

1. Determine the physical development and size of the infant.
2. Check for clothing, linen, and supplies needed.

Planning

3. Wash your hands *for asepsis*.
4. Gather the necessary equipment. You will need a basin, mild soap, a washcloth, a towel, clean clothing for the infant, and possibly clean linen.

Implementation

5. Identify infant *to be sure you are carrying out the procedure for the correct infant.*
6. Fill the basin with warm water. Check the temperature by using a sensitive part of

235

your arm, such as the elbow. It should be comfortably warm, never hot, *to prevent burns*. If a bath thermometer is available, use water at 100°F to 105°F.

7. Place the basin on a firm surface. On a towel in the crib may be the safest place.
8. Wash and dry the infant's face. Be very careful with the soap.
9. Hold the infant securely in a football hold, with the head over the basin (see Figure 12.6).
10. Shampoo the scalp. Use your fingertips, not your fingernails, and massage firmly. If any scales are present, remove them from the hair with a fine comb. Do not hesitate to wash over the fontanels (soft spots). In some facilities, the scalp (including the area behind the ears) is wiped with a small amount of baby oil on a cotton ball *to help prevent scales*.
11. Rub the head dry with a towel.
12. Undress the infant. Keep the infant dressed during the shampoo *to prevent chilling*.
13. Hold the infant securely as you place him or her in the water. Use a towel in the basin *to decrease slipping*.
14. Keep one hand securely on the infant while bathing with the other *to prevent injury* (see Figure 12.7).
15. Wash and rinse the shoulders, arms, and chest, then move on down the body.
16. Lift the infant out of the water and lay him or her on the towel.
17. Wrap the infant while you dry *to prevent chilling*.
18. Diaper and redress the infant.
19. If the crib must be made, place the infant at one end while you make up the other.
20. Put side rails up before you leave the infant. Refasten the crib net if necessary *for safety*.
21. Empty and clean the basin.
22. Dispose of soiled linen.
23. Wash your hands *for asepsis*.

☐ *Evaluation*
24. Check the infant for comfort and safety.

☐ *Documentation*
25. Chart observations made during the bath.
26. Enter the bath on the checklist or flow sheet for daily care.

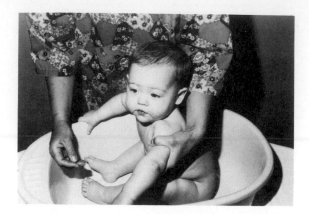

FIGURE 12.7 *BATHING AN INFANT IN A BASIN*
Courtesy Ivan Ellis

Feeding

Bottle Feeding Procedure

☐ *Assessment*
1. Assess the physical development of the infant.
2. Check the order for formula.
3. Check whether a specialized nipple or feeding device is needed.

☐ *Planning*
4. Correctly identify the formula *for safety*.
5. Identify whether the formula is to be warmed. Although warming the formula is optional, *an infant with decreased energy levels will have to use energy to restore body heat if given cold formula*. Also, *chilled food takes longer to digest*. Therefore, the feeding should be at room temperature or slightly warmer. If the feeding is warmer than room temperature, use it as soon as it is warmed, *so that it is not a source of bacterial growth*. Most hospitals routinely use formula at room temperature.
6. Wash your hands *for asepsis*.
7. Obtain and warm formula, if necessary.
8. Test for temperature. This is commonly done by shaking a few drops of formula onto the inner aspect of the wrist. The formula should feel only lukewarm—not hot.

☐ *Implementation*
9. Check the infant's identification *to be sure*

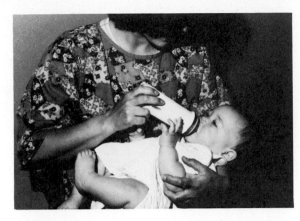

FIGURE 12.8 BOTTLE-FEEDING AN INFANT
Courtesy Ivan Ellis

you are carrying out the procedure for the correct infant.

10. Try to sit in a comfortable position, in a pleasant area, while you feed an infant. *Atmosphere is transmitted to infants and affects their feeding and digestion.*

11. Ideally, hold the infant in your arms while you bottle-feed. When an infant cannot be removed from the crib or isolette (because of equipment, traction, need for oxygen), substitute hand touch and support for whole-body contact. Tuck a bib or clean cloth under the infant's chin *to wipe up dribbles and spills.* Hold the infant with the head slightly elevated *to facilitate swallowing.* Hold the bottle so that the nipple is filled with fluid, not air (see Figure 12.8). Although sucking infants usually swallow some air, you should try to keep the amount to a minimum. *Excessive swallowed air causes distention, discomfort, and sometimes regurgitation.*

12. If the infant feeds quickly, remove the bottle *for an occasional rest.*

13. After the feeding is completed, burp the infant *to help expel swallowed air.* The two positions most commonly used are the *over-the-shoulder* and the *on-the-lap* positions (see Figures 12.9 and 12.10). A small infant should be burped after each ounce as well as at the end of the feeding. Place the bottle on a clean, safe surface while you burp the infant; do not place it on the floor. By *gently* patting or rubbing the infant's back you *encourage the*

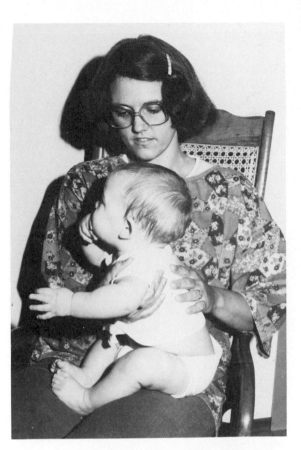

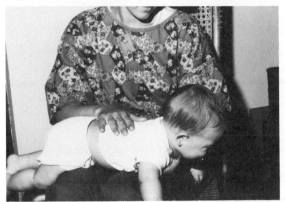

FIGURE 12.9 HOLDING AN INFANT ON THE LAP FOR BURPING—TWO POSITIONS
Courtesy Ivan Ellis

relaxation of the cardiac sphincter and the release of retained air. Place the bib or cloth where it will protect your clothing while you burp the baby.

14. Change the infant's diaper if necessary. *Small infants commonly defecate while eating because of the gastro-colic reflex.*

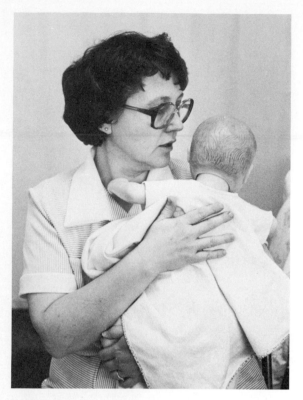

FIGURE 12.10 HOLDING AN INFANT OVER THE SHOULDER FOR BURPING
Courtesy Ivan Ellis

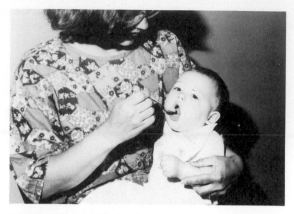

FIGURE 12.11 FEEDING AN INFANT ON THE LAP
Courtesy Ivan Ellis

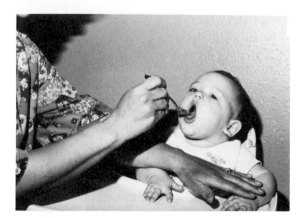

FIGURE 12.12 FEEDING AN INFANT IN A HIGHCHAIR
Courtesy Ivan Ellis

15. Return the infant to the crib. Position the infant on the abdomen, with the head to the side, or on the side, *so that if the infant spits up, aspiration will not occur.* An infant positioned on the right side is more likely to burp out air without bringing formula with it *because the sphincter is on the left side of the stomach.*
16. Wash your hands *for asepsis.*

☐ *Evaluation*
17. Compare the infant's intake with his or her usual intake and with the usual intake for an infant of this age and size.
18. Check the infant for comfort and safety.

☐ *Documentation*
19. Record the kind and amount of formula taken.

Feeding Solids to an Infant

☐ *Assessment*
1. Assess the infant's physical development.
2. Identify the type of food ordered *in order*

to determine appropriateness for the infant in his or her present condition.
3. Check to see whether any special feeding device is necessary.

☐ *Planning*
4. Wash your hands *for asepsis.*
5. Obtain the proper food and a small spoon.

☐ *Implementation*
6. Identify the infant *to be sure you are carrying out the procedure for the correct infant.*
7. Position the infant comfortably, either on your lap (Figure 12.11) or in a highchair (Figure 12.12).
8. Use a bib *to protect the infant's clothing.*
9. Check the food *to be sure it is a comfortable temperature. Hot food can burn an infant's*

238

tender mouth and chilled food takes longer to digest, so slightly warm or room temperature food is usually used. Remember that infants have not established the strong likes and dislikes of adults and will usually eat what they are fed. They do, however, respond to nonverbal cues of aversion from the person who is feeding them. Also, feeding plainer foods (cereals, vegetables) before feeding fruits usually results in better acceptance of the plainer foods. *This is because once infants have tasted the naturally sweet fruit, they will prefer to continue eating it.*

10. Give small bites and place them well into the infant's mouth.
11. Scrape the food that is pushed back out of the mouth into the spoon and refeed. Hungry infants will often eat rapidly and complain loudly if food appears too slowly.

    Infants frequently put their hands into their mouths, smearing the food. You can minimize this by providing something for the infant to hold, by fending off the hands with your free hand, or by actually holding the arms (see Figures 12.11 and 12.12).
12. When you have finished, wash the infant.
13. Diapering also may be needed *because the stimulus of food often causes defecation.*
14. Wash your hands *for asepsis.*

Evaluation
15. Compare the infant's intake with his or her usual intake and with the usual intake for an infant of this age and size.
16. Check the infant for comfort and safety.

Documentation
17. Record the amount of food taken. In some facilities and/or situations you may be required to record the *kinds* of foods taken as well.

Restraints and Safety Devices

Maintaining safety for the infant is a major concern. Since it is impossible for an adult to be with the infant or young child at all times, special restraints and safety devices are used *to prevent falls, to prevent interruption of therapy,* and *to prevent the young child from behaving in ways that will cause harm* (such as scratching lesions or pulling off dressings). *There are many procedures in which the infant must be kept very still and must be prevented from kicking or hitting at the person performing the procedure.* Restraints are useful in many of these situations. It will be your responsibility to determine when restraints or safety devices are needed and which type to use.

General Procedure for Applying Restraints and Safety Devices

Assessment
1. Check the age and developmental level of the infant.
2. Identify hazards in the environment related to the infant's age and developmental level.
3. Identify the purpose for which the safety device is needed.

Planning
4. Plan the type of safety device to be used for the infant.
5. Plan for intervals at which to recheck the infant.
6. Wash your hands *for asepsis.*
7. Obtain the appropriate safety device.

Implementation
8. Identify the infant *to be sure you are carrying out the procedure for the correct infant.*
9. Put the appropriate safety device in place, following either the instructions for use or the specific directions given below.

Evaluation
10. Check the circulation in the extremities distal to any restraint, *to determine whether the device is restricting circulation.*
11. Check the skin under any restraint for skin damage.
12. Check the infant for safety and comfort.
13. Wash your hands *for asepsis.*

Documentation
14. Note the type of safety device used, the reason for it, and the time applied.
15. Record all evaluative checks done.

Specific Safety Precautions

Many different kinds of restraints are available for infants. *Crib nets* are used to keep an active

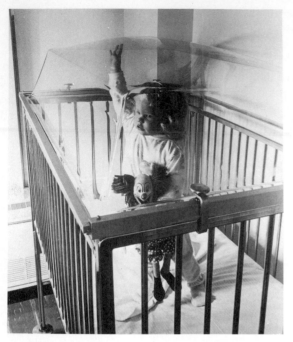

FIGURE 12.13 PLEXIGLAS CRIB DOME
Courtesy American Hospital Supply Corp. and Bafti-Dom Crib Top

infant or toddler in the crib while still allowing some freedom of movement. Clear Plexiglas *domes* (see Figure 12.13) are also used for the same purpose.

Chest restraints can be used to secure an in-fant to a highchair. On occasion, they may be used to keep an infant restrained in a crib. (See Module 21, Applying Restraints.)

Sandbags provide a useful way to immobilize an infant. A sandbag is heavy enough so that an infant cannot push it out of the way. Make sure that the sandbag does not cause pressure on the infant's tender skin.

A soft *fabric tie* can be used to immobilize an extremity. Use a clove-hitch tie (see Figure 12.14), *which ensures that the loop will not tighten and restrict circulation if the infant struggles.* Whenever you use a tie for a restraint, watch the infant closely to make sure that he or she does not become entangled in it. Always attach the end of a tie to a stable part of the crib (bed), like the frame, and not to a movable part, like the side rail. *This prevents injury when the position of the movable part is changed.*

Elbow restraints are used to immobilize the elbow joint and *to prevent an infant or young child from touching his or her own face and head.* To be effective, elbow restraints must be incorporated in a jacket or applied over a long-sleeved shirt and pinned at the wrist. *This prevents the infant from pulling the arms up and out of the restraint.* (See Module 21, Applying Restraints.) Commercial elbow restraints are widely available, but substitutes can be constructed from tongue blades, tape, and cardboard.

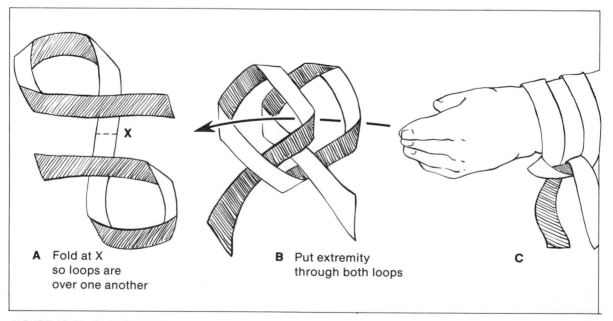

A Fold at X so loops are over one another

B Put extremity through both loops

C

FIGURE 12.14 CLOVE HITCH

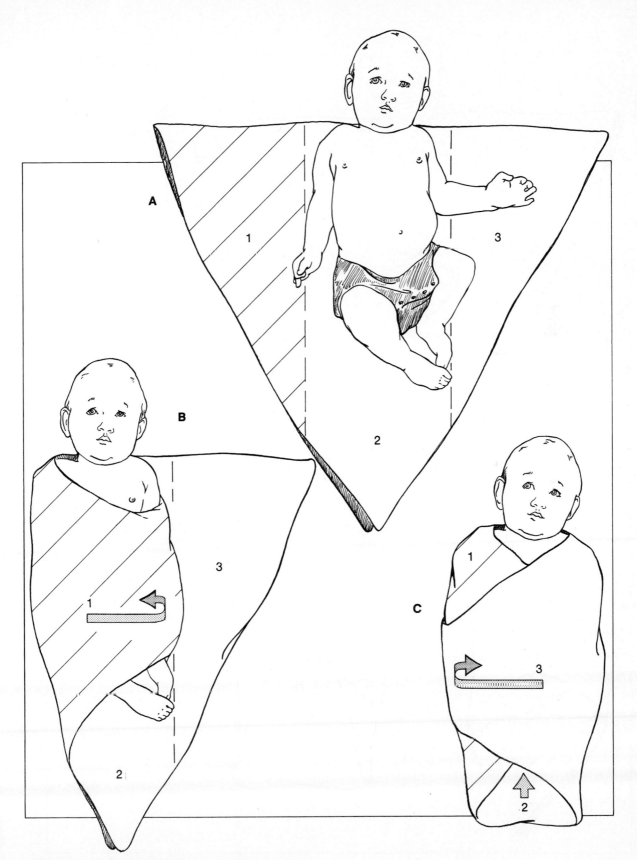

FIGURE 12.15 MUMMY RESTRAINT: CHEST COVERED

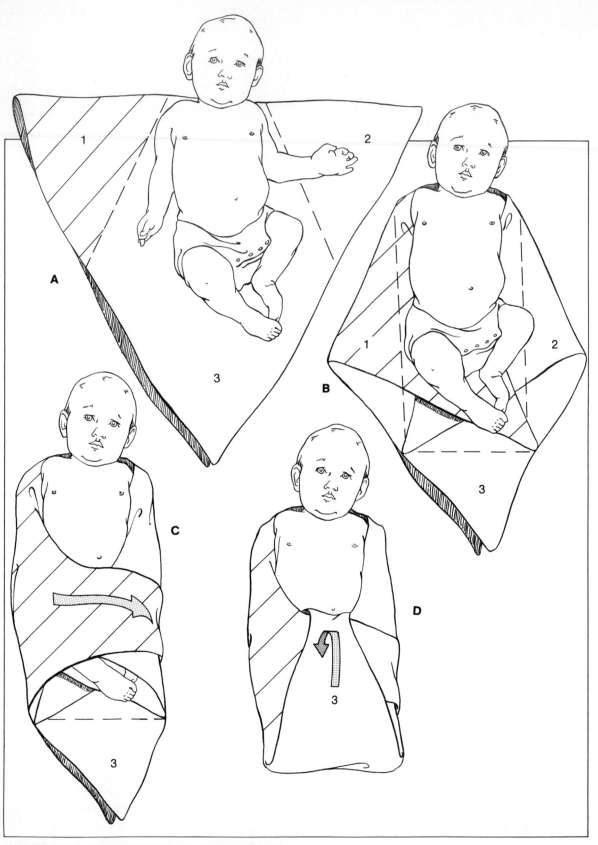

FIGURE 12.16 MUMMY RESTRAINT: CHEST EXPOSED

Mummying

One way to immobilize an infant safely during a procedure such as venipuncture is to wrap the infant tightly in a manner called *mummying* or *swaddling. A secure restraint allows the procedure to be done more quickly and protects the infant from the harm that might occur if he or she were to move during the procedure.* You can alter the swaddling to provide access to whatever part of the body is needed. To expose only the neck and head, follow the diagrams in Figure 12.15.

For the two types of mummying described, the steps in the general procedure that are modified are presented. The detailed procedures, which include all the steps of the general procedure as well as the modified steps, are given in the Performance Checklist.

Head and Neck Exposed

⬜ *Implementation*

8. Identify the infant.
9. **a.** Obtain a clean small sheet and fold it into a triangle.
   b. Place the sheet under the infant with the long, straight edge lying across under the shoulders and the opposite point under the feet (A).
   c. Fold one side corner over the infant's arm, across the chest, and around the other arm. Tuck this side under the infant's back (B). This securely anchors both arms.
   d. Fold the bottom point up over the feet.
   e. Then wrap the other side corner over the top of and around the infant. Note that one person can then hold the infant, yet all extremities are restrained.

f. Pin or simply hold in place.

A mummy wrap can also be done to allow the chest and abdomen to be uncovered, as shown in Figure 12.16.

Chest and Abdomen Exposed

⬜ *Implementation*

8. Identify the infant.
9. **a.** Start with a triangle-folded sheet.
   b. Place the sheet under the infant as before (A).
   c. Wrap one corner over the infant's arm and under the infant's back.
   d. Repeat with the other arm (B). The ends of the sheet will emerge on either side of the infant's legs and hips.
   e. Wrap first one end and then the other tightly around the infant's legs (C).
   f. Fold the bottom point up over the feet.
   g. Pin or tuck the bottom edge over the infant's arms (D).

Wrapping for Circumcision

To immobilize an infant during circumcision, a *circumcision board* is usually used. The infant is wrapped securely, in the correct position, against the board, *which prevents the infant from moving during the procedure.* The exact manner of wrapping, using the board, is determined both by the device itself and by the specific procedure in your hospital. If the facility has no specific procedure, modify the swaddling procedures given above for use with the available device.

PERFORMANCE CHECKLIST	Unsatisfactory	Needs More Practice	Satisfactory	Comments
Diaper folding				
1. Triangle folding a. Fold into square.				
b. Hold one corner and fold adjacent corners into center, forming diamond shape.				
c. Fold corner down, creating long triangle.				
2. Rectangle folding a. Fold two outer edges in to form a long rectangle.				
b. Fold top third of rectangle down or bottom third of rectangle up.				
Diapering procedure				
☐ *Assessment*				
1. Check infant for dry diaper.				
2. Determine physical development of infant.				
☐ *Planning*				
3. Select type of diaper fold or size of disposable diaper.				
4. Plan method for securing diaper.				
5. Wash your hands.				
6. Obtain clean diaper and equipment.				
☐ *Implementation*				
7. Fold diaper if necessary.				
8. Place infant on back in safe, clean location.				
9. Unfasten soiled diaper, fastening pins before setting them down.				
10. Remove soiled diaper, wiping away stool.				
11. Clean diaper area thoroughly.				
12. Lift infant and place clean diaper underneath.				
13. Pull diaper up between infant's legs and fasten securely.				
14. Be sure infant is safe.				
15. Dispose of soiled diaper.				

	Unsatisfactory	Needs More Practice	Satisfactory	Comments
16. Wash your hands.				
☐ *Evaluation*				
17. Check diaper for fit and comfort.				
☐ *Documentation*				
18. Record number of diaper changes, appearance and odor of urine and stool, and weight of soiled diapers if required.				

Bathing procedure

	Unsatisfactory	Needs More Practice	Satisfactory	Comments
☐ *Assessment*				
1. Determine physical development of infant.				
2. Check for supplies needed.				
☐ *Planning*				
3. Wash your hands.				
4. Gather the necessary equipment: basin, mild soap, wash cloth, towel, clean clothing, and clean linen.				
☐ *Implementation*				
5. Identify infant.				
6. Fill basin with warm water (100 to 105° F).				
7. Place basin on safe surface.				
8. Wash and dry infant's face.				
9. Hold infant over basin.				
10. Shampoo scalp.				
11. Rub head dry with towel.				
12. Undress infant.				
13. Hold infant securely and place in basin.				
14. Keep one hand on infant while bathing.				
15. Wash and rinse shoulders, arms, chest, etc.				
16. Lift infant out of water and place on towel.				
17. Wrap infant while you dry to prevent chilling.				
18. Diaper and redress infant.				

	Unsatisfactory	Needs More Practice	Satisfactory	Comments
19. Place infant at one end of crib while making other end.				
20. Put up side rails and refasten crib net.				
21. Empty and clean basin.				
22. Dispose of soiled linen.				
23. Wash your hands.				
☐ *Evaluation*				
24. Check infant for comfort and safety.				
☐ *Documentation*				
25. Record observations made during bath.				
26. Enter bath on checklist or flow sheet.				

Bottle feeding procedure

☐ *Assessment*				
1. Determine physical development of infant.				
2. Check order for type of formula.				
3. Check need for specialized feeding device.				
☐ *Planning*				
4. Identify formula.				
5. Determine whether or not formula is to be warmed.				
6. Wash your hands.				
7. Obtain formula and warm, if necessary.				
8. Test formula for temperature on wrist.				
☐ *Implementation*				
9. Check infant's identification.				
10. Pick up infant and sit in a comfortable position.				
11. Hold infant in your arms. Tuck bib under infant's chin and slightly elevate the head.				
12. Remove bottle for occasional rest.				
13. Burp infant.				

	Unsatisfactory	Needs More Practice	Satisfactory	Comments
14. Change infant's diaper.				
15. Return infant to crib. Position infant on right side or on abdomen with head to side.				
16. Wash your hands.				
☐ *Evaluation*				
17. Compare infant's intake with usual intake for an infant of this age and size and with usual intake for this child.				
18. Check infant for comfort and safety.				
☐ *Documentation*				
19. Record kind and amount of formula taken.				

Feeding solids

	Unsatisfactory	Needs More Practice	Satisfactory	Comments
☐ *Assessment*				
1. Assess physical development of infant.				
2. Check order for type of food.				
3. Check need for specialized feeding device.				
☐ *Planning*				
4. Wash your hands.				
5. Obtain correct food and spoon.				
☐ *Implementation*				
6. Check infant's identification.				
7. Position infant.				
8. Put bib on infant.				
9. Check temperature of food.				
10. Give small bites.				
11. Refeed as needed.				
12. Wash infant as needed.				
13. Diaper if necessary.				
14. Wash your hands.				

	Unsatisfactory	Needs More Practice	Satisfactory	Comments
☐ *Evaluation*				
15. Compare infant's intake with usual intake for an infant of this age and size and with usual intake for this child.				
16. Check infant for comfort and safety.				
☐ *Documentation*				
17. Record amount of food taken and kinds of food, if necessary.				

General procedure for applying restraints and safety devices

	Unsatisfactory	Needs More Practice	Satisfactory	Comments
☐ *Assessment*				
1. Determine age and development of infant.				
2. Identify environmental hazards.				
3. Identify purpose.				
☐ *Planning*				
4. Plan type of device to be used.				
5. Plan intervals for rechecking infant.				
6. Wash your hands.				
7. Obtain device.				
☐ *Implementation*				
8. Identify infant.				
9. Put device in place.				
☐ *Evaluation*				
10. Check circulation in extremities distal to restraint.				
11. Check skin under restraint.				
12. Check infant for comfort and safety.				
13. Wash your hands.				

	Unsatisfactory	Needs More Practice	Satisfactory	Comments
☐ *Documentation*				
14. Note type of device used and time applied.				
15. Record evaluative checks.				

Mummying

	Unsatisfactory	Needs More Practice	Satisfactory	Comments
☐ *Assessment*				
1. Follow Checklist steps 1–3 of the General Procedure for Applying Restraints and Safety Devices (determine age and development of infant, identify environmental hazards, identify purpose).				
☐ *Planning*				
2. Follow Checklist steps 4–7 of the General Procedure (plan type of device to be used, plan intervals for rechecking infant, wash your hands, obtain device).				
☐ *Implementation*				
3. Identify infant.				
4. Head and neck exposed: a. Get and fold clean sheet.				
b. Place sheet under infant.				
c. Fold one corner over arm, across chest, around other arm, and under back.				
d. Fold bottom up.				
e. Fold second corner over top of infant and around body firmly.				
f. Pin or hold in place.				
5. Chest and abdomen exposed: a. Obtain triangle-folded clean sheet.				
b. Place sheet under infant.				
c. Wrap one corner over arm and under back.				
d. Repeat for other side.				
e. Wrap ends securely around legs.				
f. Fold bottom point up over feet.				
g. Pin or tuck bottom edge over arm.				

	Unsatisfactory	Needs More Practice	Satisfactory	Comments
Evaluation				
6. Follow Checklist steps 10–13 of the General Procedure (check circulation, check skin, check infant for comfort and safety, wash your hands).				
Documentation				
7. Follow Checklist steps 14 and 15 of the General Procedure (note type of device used and time applied, record evaluative checks).				

| QUIZ |

Short-Answer Questions

1. What is an advantage of a triangle-folded cloth diaper? _____
   _____

2. Why is the perineal area cleaned at the time of a diaper change? _____
   _____

3. What should be done with safety pins while changing a baby's diaper?
   _____

4. Differentiate between diaper rash and scald. _____
   _____

5. What precaution should be taken when using baby powder, and why?
   _____

6. How would you test a bottle feeding for proper temperature? _____
   _____

7. What is one method of minimizing the amount of air swallowed during
   bottle feeding? _____

8. Why should you feed an infant plain food (such as cereal) before fruits?
   _____

9. Why is a clove hitch used to tie an arm restraint? _____
   _____

10. List three safety measures that must be followed when bathing an infant.
    a. _____
    b. _____
    c. _____

U N I T III

SKILLS TO
EXPAND
ASSESSMENT

MODULE 13

Inspection, Palpation, Auscultation, and Percussion

PREREQUISITES

Successful completion of the following modules:

OVERALL OBJECTIVE

To achieve beginning skills in inspection, palpation, auscultation, and percussion, and thereby to enhance assessment and nursing care.

SPECIFIC LEARNING OBJECTIVES

	Know Facts and Principles	Apply Facts and Principles	Demonstrate Ability	Evaluate Performance
1. Inspection	Define inspection. List six areas to be included in inspection.		Include color, odor, size, shape, symmetry, and movement appropriately when performing inspection	Evaluate own performance with instructor
a. Pupils	List three aspects of pupils to include in inspection. Explain pupillary reaction to light. Explain accommodation. Explain convergence.	Describe patient situations in which inspection of pupils is needed	Inspect pupils of patient for size, shape, and equality. Check pupillary reaction to light and accommodation. Check pupillary convergence.	Evaluate with instructor using Performance Checklist
b. Neck veins	State position in which neck veins are normally collapsed	Place patient in position in which neck veins are normally collapsed.	Identify jugular veins of neck and assess	Evaluate with instructor using Performance Checklist
	Describe how to estimate venous pressure without special equipment. State normal venous pressure values in centimeters.	Given specific values, state whether venous pressure is within normal limits.	Estimate venous pressure of patient with distended neck veins	

2. *Palpation*	Define palpation. List four areas or conditions that can be identified using palpation.	Given patient situations, choose parameters to be measured by palpation	Using palpation, identify softness, rigidity, temperature, position, and size appropriately	Evaluate own performance with instructor
	State two items of information to be included in explanation to patient prior to palpation	Given a patient situation, state what should appropriately be included in explanation to patient	In the clinical setting, give appropriate explanation to patient before palpating	Evaluate with instructor using Performance Checklist
a. *Edema*	State four areas of body where dependent edema might be found	Given a patient situation, state where dependent edema might be found	In the clinical setting, evaluate patient for presence of dependent edema	Evaluate with instructor using Performance Checklist
	Define *periorbital edema* and *pretibial edema*		In the clinical setting, evaluate patient for presence of periorbital edema	
b. *Ascites*	Define *ascites*. State how to differentiate between obesity and ascites.	State one problem patient might have as a result of ascites	In the clinical setting, test for presence of fluid wave	Evaluate own performance with instructor
c. *Breasts*	List five parameters to be observed in inspecting breasts of male or female patients. Describe characteristics of breast tissue in younger female, older female, and menstruating female. Describe how to palpate breast.	Given a patient situation, describe what characteristics of breast tissue might be present	Include size, symmetry, skin color, vascularity, and skin retraction when inspecting breasts of male or female patient. In the clinical setting, palpate breasts of male or female patient.	Evaluate own performance with instructor	Evaluate with instructor using Performance Checklist.

	Know Facts and Principles	Apply Facts and Principles	Demonstrate Ability	Evaluate Performance
d. Abdomen and liver	List four observations to be made when inspecting abdomen. List three parameters that may be demonstrated when palpating abdomen. Describe procedure for palpation of liver.	Describe patient situations in which palpation of abdomen is needed	Include bulges, bruises, scars, and symmetry when inspecting abdomen of patient. Palpate abdomen, moving systematically and gently. In the clinical setting, palpate for liver of patient.	Evaluate own performance with instructor. Evaluate with instructor using Performance Checklist.
e. Digital exam of rectum	List signs and symptoms of fecal impaction. Describe procedure for digital exam of rectum.	Describe patient situations in which digital exam of rectum is needed	In the clinical setting, perform digital exam	Evaluate with instructor using Performance Checklist
3. Auscultation	Define auscultation. State two ways in which nurse can help control environmental noise level.	Given a patient situation, state what might be done to control noise level	Take steps to control noise level before attempting auscultation	Evaluate with instructor using Performance Checklist
a. Heart	List three areas commonly auscultated. List three aspects of heartbeat to be evaluated with use of auscultation. Describe where first and second heart sounds are usually heard most easily.	Describe patient situations in which auscultation of heart is needed	Accurately discern rate, rhythm, and intensity of heartbeat of assigned patient. Listen for first and second heart sounds in correct locations.	Evaluate with instructor using Performance Checklist
b. Bowel sounds	List situations in which bowel sounds may be diminished. List situations in which bowel sounds may be increased.	Given a patient situation, predict whether bowel sounds will be diminished or increased	In the clinical setting, listen for bowel sounds in a systematic fashion	Evaluate with instructor using Performance Checklist

State why auscultation of abdomen should be carried out prior to palpation and percussion.			
c. *Lungs*	List situations in which breath sounds may be absent or decreased. List conditions that might cause breath sounds to be increased. Define *adventitious sounds*.	Given a patient situation, predict whether breath sounds will be decreased or increased	In the clinical setting, identify adventitious sounds on auscultation of lungs	Evaluate with instructor using Performance Checklist
4. *Percussion* a. *Chest* b. *Abdomen*	Define *percussion*. Describe percussion procedure. Define *resonance, tympany, dullness,* and *flatness.* State where and in what situation(s) each sound might be heard.	Given a patient situation, state what sound might be heard on percussion	In the clinical setting, demonstrate percussion of chest and abdomen	Evaluate with instructor using Performance Checklist
5. *Documentation*	State observations that should be included in record with regard to inspection, palpation, auscultation, and percussion	Given a patient situation, record appropriate items accurately	In the clinical setting, chart findings of inspection, palpation, auscultation, and percussion completely and accurately	Evaluate with instructor using Performance Checklist

LEARNING ACTIVITIES

1. Review the Specific Learning Objectives.
2. Read the section on observation (in the chapter on the nursing process) in Ellis and Nowlis, *Nursing: A Human Needs Approach,* or comparable material in another textbook.
3. Look up the module vocabulary terms in the Glossary.
4. Read through the module.
5. In the practice setting, with a partner and under supervision:
   a. Test the reaction of your partner's pupils to light and accommodation, and for convergence, using the Performance Checklist as a guide. Chart your observations.
   b. Identify the jugular veins of your partner bilaterally while he or she is lying supine. Gradually elevate the head of the bed to a 45-degree angle. Note when the jugular veins collapse. Is your partner's venous pressure within normal limits?
   c. Assess your partner for edema of the ankles. If any is present, rate it on a scale of 1+ to 4+. Is periorbital edema present?
   d. Inspect and palpate your partner's breasts. Practice communicating as you would with a patient.
   e. Observe and palpate the four quadrants of the abdomen.
   f. Palpate for the liver.
   g. Practice the digital exam for fecal impaction on a mannequin. Have your partner evaluate your performance, including communication, using the Performance Checklist.
   h. Using the diaphragm of the stethoscope:
      (1) Practice listening to your own cardiac rate and rhythm.
      (2) Identify first and second heart sounds, using the carotid pulse as a guide.
      (3) Repeat steps (1) and (2) using your partner as a patient.
   i. Listen to all four quadrants of your partner's abdomen for bowel sounds.
   j. Systematically listen to your partner's lungs, both anteriorly and posteriorly. Then listen to your partner's lungs in the supine and side-lying positions. If you hear rales, ask your partner to cough, and listen again to see whether they have cleared.
   k. Practice percussion technique on a hard surface, such as a desk or table. Then practice on your thigh to get used to percussing on a body surface. Using the procedure as a guide, practice percussing your partner for resonance, tympany, dullness, and flatness. Do systematic percussion of the chest and abdomen.
   l. Have your partner evaluate your technique using the various checklists. He or she should also evaluate your explanations and your regard for the "patient's" comfort and modesty.
   m. Change roles, and repeat steps a–l.
   n. When you are both satisfied with your performances, have your instructor evaluate you.
6. In the clinical setting:
   a. Practice inspection, palpation, auscultation, and percussion techniques as frequently as possible, with a staff nurse or your instructor to supervise, assist, and evaluate.
   b. Practice the above techniques independently, and compare your findings with those of the staff nurse responsible for the care of the patient.

VOCABULARY

accommodation
adventitious sounds
alveoli
apex
apical pulse
auscultation
base
bell
bronchi
consensual

constriction
convergence
dependent edema
diaphragm
diastole
digital
dullness
edema
flatness
impaction
inspection
objective
palpation
percussion
periorbital edema
pretibial edema

rales
rebound tenderness
resonance
retraction
rhonchi
stethoscope
subjective
symmetry
symphysis pubis
systole
trachea
tympany
umbilicus
venous pressure
wheezes
xiphoid process

INSPECTION, PALPATION, AUSCULTATION, AND PERCUSSION

Rationale for the Use of This Skill

The nurse is expected to perform various aspects of the basic physical exam on a daily basis when caring for hospitalized patients. Observations, augmented by skills in inspection, palpation, auscultation, and percussion, give the nurse a better data base for nursing care and give the physician valuable input into the medical diagnosis and treatment of patients.

The development of the skills presented in this module requires frequent practice. The module is not meant to provide you with the detail and depth necessary to do a complete physical examination; it is meant to give you the beginning skills that will enable you to make a more complete nursing assessment.

The four general processes included in a physical examination are difficult to separate totally from one another. Despite the overlapping of certain areas, we will attempt to discuss each process as a single entity.[1]

General Procedure for Examination

For all of these examinations, you will need to use the following general procedure. You may perform all the specific examinations or only those indicated at the time.

1. Prepare for the examination.
   a. Wash your hands *for asepsis. Washing in warm water also warms the hands. Warm hands are more comfortable for the patient and prevent involuntary tensing of muscles, which could interfere with palpation.*
   b. Obtain needed equipment. The equipment needed for each specific examination is listed in the procedure for that examination.
   c. Explain the examination to the patient *to provide information and relieve anxiety.*

---

[1]You will note that rationale for action is emphasized throughout the module by the use of italics.

   d. Provide privacy *to protect the patient's modesty and self-esteem.*
2. Carry out the specific examination as described.
3. Conclude the examination.
   a. Restore the patient to a position of comfort.
   b. Return the unit to its previous condition.
   c. Remove supplies.
   d. Wash your hands *for asepsis.*
4. Document your findings. Whatever you have learned during your examination should be documented in the patient's record.

Inspection

Inspection is closely related to observation, but it is more involved with physical than with social information. Although it is primarily visual in nature, inspection also includes the sense of smell.

You will want to work out your own system for the inspection process *to avoid missing any area.* You can use the body systems approach, a head-to-toe approach, or a combination of the two, but the emphasis should be on a *systematic* approach.

Whichever system you use, inspection should include observations of color, odor, size, shape, symmetry, and movement (or lack of it). In each instance, you will be comparing what you see with what is "normal" for someone of the patient's age group.

When you observe something significant, you must elicit information about the finding. For example, what were the precipitating factors? How long has the finding existed in this state? Is there pain associated?

Pupils

The nurse is frequently called on to observe the pupils and their reaction to light. Usually performed as a part of "neuro signs," *this is often done when neurological disease is present or suspected.*

1. Prepare for the examination as discussed.
2. Inspect size, shape, and equality of pupils.
3. Inspect the pupillary reaction to light.
   a. Holding the lid open with one hand, shine a light (a common flashlight is

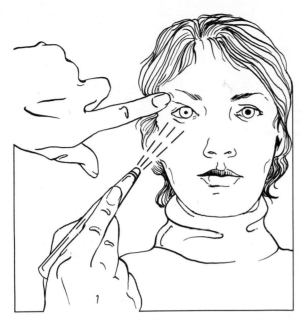

FIGURE 13.1 *TESTING THE PUPILLARY REACTION TO LIGHT   The light source is brought in from the side.*

generally used) on one pupil at a time, bringing the light in from the side (see Figure 13.1).

  b. Observe what happens to the pupil.
    (1) Does it constrict?
    (2) If it does constrict, does it do so rapidly, or is it sluggish?

  c. Observe what happens to the opposite eye when the light is shined into one pupil. The normal pupil has a consensual reaction; that is, it constricts along with the eye that is exposed to light.

  d. Repeat steps a to c on the other eye. Are the reactions the same?

4. Test the pupillary reaction to accommodation. (This is not routinely done in all settings.)

  a. Ask the patient to look at an object in the distance, then at your fingers, which are held 5 to 10 cm from the bridge of the patient's nose.

  b. Note the pupillary constriction (the pupils should constrict as they attempt to accommodate).

  c. Note whether the pupils converge (i.e., stay focused on the finger and thus move toward the nose and toward one another).

5. Conclude the examination as discussed.

6. Document your observations on the patient's record. A variety of forms have been designed for pupillary observations (see Figure 13.2), and one of them may be in use in your clinical facility. The abbreviations PERL (pupils equal and reactive to light), PERLA (pupils equal and reactive to light and accommodation), and PERRLA (pupils equal, round, and reactive to light and accommodation) are commonly used in charting pupillary observations.

Neck Veins

You will often be called on to inspect the distention of the jugular veins for an estimation of venous pressure. When a person is standing, or sitting at an angle greater than 45 degrees to the horizontal, the jugular veins of the neck are normally collapsed. If these veins are distended in a position above 45 degrees, an abnormally high venous pressure is present.

1. Prepare for the examination as discussed.

2. Have the patient lie flat on his or her back. Watch for dyspnea. (Patients with distended neck veins are often unable to lie flat without experiencing dyspnea.)

3. Identify the jugular veins bilaterally.

4. Gradually elevate the head of the bed to a 45-degree angle, watching to see when the jugular veins collapse.

5. If the jugular veins remain distended at 45 degrees, venous pressure may be estimated by measuring the vertical distance (in centimeters) from the right atrium level (midchest) to the upper level of distention. If this procedure is carried out frequently, mark the right atrial level on the patient's chest, *to ensure consistent measurements.* Venous pressure of between 4 and 10 cm is considered normal.

6. Conclude the examination as discussed.

7. Document the estimated venous pressure on the patient's record.

Palpation

Palpation involves the sense of touch and in most cases is used simultaneously with inspection. Using the palms, fingers, and tips of the fingers, the nurse can identify softness, rigidity,

VITAL SIGN RECORD

PUPIL SIZE AND REACTION

0 - - 0	Equal	R	Reacts
. - - 0	Unequal	NR	Does not react

Example: left smaller, no reaction

O	R	.	NR

CONSCIOUSNESS

Normal
Responds verbally
Disoriented
Moves only to pain
Deeply comotose

MISCELLANEOUS

Medicines
Fluids
Treatments
Pain
Paralysis

DATE	HOUR	B.P.	P	R	TEMP	PUPILS RIGHT	PUPILS LEFT	

BALLARD COMMUNITY HOSPITAL

SEATTLE, WASHINGTON

VITAL SIGNS RECORD

FIGURE 13.2 FORM FOR RECORDING PUPILLARY OBSERVATIONS

and temperature and determine position and size. You will also use palpation to measure the rate and quality of the peripheral pulses.

Again, explanation is extremely important in obtaining the cooperation of the patient as you palpate. Explain what is being done, why it is being done (if appropriate), and what the patient can do to make it easier for both of you.

Edema

Edema is the abnormal accumulation of fluid in the intercellular tissues of the body. Edema is often dependent; that is, it occurs in dependent areas of the body (the hands, feet, ankles, and sacrum, where excess fluids pool as a result of gravity).

Periorbital edema (around the soft tissue of the eyes) is also relatively common. It may have diagnostic significance, or, in women, it may simply be related to cyclical hormonal changes. This type of edema is usually soft and resilient, not pitting (which occurs when a depressed area is temporarily created in response to palpation).

To palpate for edema, use the fingertips of the index and middle fingers, pressing firmly over a bony area (see Figure 13.3). When you remove your fingers, observe the area for pitting and continue to watch to see how long it takes for the depressed area to disappear. Edema is generally rated on a scale of 1+ to 4+. 1+ is a slight depression that disappears quickly; 4+ is a deep depression that disappears slowly. *Because the scale is subjective,* daily weights and circumferential measurements of extremities are often used to provide more objective data.

Measuring the number of centimeters the edema extends up the tibia beyond the malleoli is another way of obtaining a more objective measure of edema of the lower extremities.

Ascites

Ascites is a large accumulation of fluid in the peritoneal cavity that can cause respiratory distress because of the pressure of the fluid on the diaphragm. It is sometimes difficult to identify ascites, especially in an obese person. One way to differentiate between obesity and ascites is to test for a fluid wave, which indicates the presence of fluid in the peritoneal cavity. One side

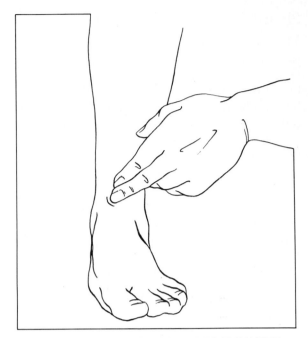

FIGURE 13.3 APPLYING PRESSURE TO EVALUATE PRETIBIAL EDEMA

of the abdomen is tapped. If the impact of the tap is felt by the other hand, you have demonstrated the presence of a fluid wave.

Ongoing assessment of ascites usually includes periodic measurement of abdominal girth. You will need a felt-tip marker and a measuring tape to carry out this procedure.

1. Prepare for the examination as discussed, placing the patient in the supine position.
2. Place the palm of your hand against the lateral abdominal wall.
3. With the other hand, tap the opposite wall of the abdomen and check for fluid wave.
4. Identify the area of greatest girth *in order to measure the extent of the ascites.*
5. Using the felt-tip marker, place marks at the same level on each side of the patient's abdomen *to facilitate consistent measurement.*
6. Place the tape measure around the abdomen at the marks and note the abdominal girth. *Abdominal girth is the circumference of the body at the level of the abdomen.*
7. Conclude the examination as discussed.
8. Document the patient's girth on the record.

Breasts

The most common site of cancer in the female is the breast. The examination of the breasts in male patients is important, too. Cancer of the breast does occur in males, although much less frequently than in females. Again, the procedure is a combination of inspection and palpation.

1. Prepare for the examination as discussed.
2. Ask the patient to disrobe to the waist and to be seated with hands in the lap.
3. Observe the nipples for color, discharge, and retraction ("dimpling").
4. Observe the breasts for size, symmetry, skin color, vascularity, and skin retraction.
5. Ask the patient to raise the hands above the head, and particularly observe for irregularities in skin texture or dimpling.
6. Have the patient lie down.
7. Starting with the upper outer quadrant and moving systematically in one direction or the other, use the palmar aspect of your fingers to palpate each breast in turn. Palpate the breast by gently compressing the breast tissue against the chest wall. The consistency of breast tissue varies among females, primarily according to age: that of younger women is firm and elastic; that of older women is more stringy and nodular. In addition, be aware of the stage of the menstrual cycle of menstruating females because the breasts can be particularly sensitive at the time of menstruation.
8. Conclude the examination as discussed.
9. Document your findings on the patient's record.

Abdomen and Liver

Although the palpation of the abdomen can be a very sophisticated procedure, we describe a fairly simple version here. In a complete examination, first auscultate the abdomen, then palpate and percuss. *Palpation and percussion can change the bowel sounds.*

Palpation of the liver is part of the overall procedure. The normal liver is not palpable. An enlarged nontender liver indicates chronic disease; an enlarged tender liver indicates acute disease.

1. Prepare for the examination as discussed.

2. To make your examination systematic and to clarify your descriptions, mentally divide the abdomen into quadrants. The horizontal line extends across through the umbilicus; the vertical line extends downward from the xiphoid process to the symphysis pubis. The four quadrants are the *right upper quadrant* (RUQ), the *right lower quadrant* (RLQ), the *left lower quadrant* (LLQ), and the *left upper quadrant* (LUQ). (See Figure 13.4.)
3. Ask the patient to breathe through the mouth *to enhance relaxation.*
4. Observe the abdomen. Note the condition of the skin, including any bulges, bruises, or scars, and observe for symmetry.
5. Use the palmar surfaces of your fingers to palpate.
6. Moving systematically, palpate gently for tone (softness versus rigidity), swelling, and tenderness.
7. Also assess for rebound tenderness (pain that is elicited when you release your hand quickly after slow palpation). Rebound tenderness is a symptom of peritonitis.
8. Ask the patient to inhale.
9. Standing to the right of the patient, place your left hand under the rib cage and use the palmar surface of the fingers of your right hand to palpate just below the right costal margin. If the liver edge is palpable, it will descend below the right

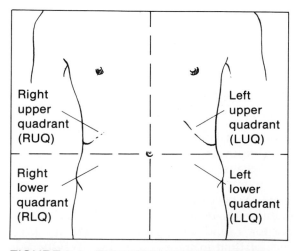

FIGURE 6.4   THE FOUR QUADRANTS OF THE ABDOMEN

costal margin, and the number of centimeters it descends below that margin should be noted.

10. Conclude the examination as discussed.
11. Document your findings on the patient's record.

Digital Examination of the Rectum

A digital examination of the rectum is usually performed when fecal impaction is suspected, usually based on the patient's complaint of long-term or abnormal constipation, or the leakage of watery stool in the absence of actual bowel movements.

1. Prepare for the examination as discussed and gather the following equipment:
   a. Clean rectal gloves
   b. A lubricant
   c. A bedpan
2. Assist the patient to the left lateral position, with the knees drawn up toward the abdomen. Other positions can be used, but this is usually the most comfortable for both patient and nurse.
3. Put on gloves.
4. Lubricate the gloved index finger.
5. Spread the patient's buttocks apart with your other hand.
6. Ask the patient to bear down while you gently insert your index finger into the rectum.
7. Ask the patient to breathe in and out through the mouth *to enhance relaxation.*
8. Move your examining finger in a circle. A hard mass that fills the rectum is probably a fecal impaction. You may be able to break it up and remove it with your gloved finger by bending the finger and gently removing small amounts at a time into the bedpan. (Sometimes oil-retention enemas are given *to help soften the fecal mass and assist in its discharge.*)
9. Remove the glove by turning it inside out over the soiled surface. Dispose of it in the waste receptacle designated for heavily soiled items. This may not be in the patient's room because of the potential for odor.
10. Conclude the examination as discussed.
11. Document your findings on the patient's record.

Auscultation

Auscultation refers to listening (usually with a stethoscope) to sounds produced by the body *in order to differentiate normal from abnormal sounds.* To perform auscultation, you must first be able to recognize the normal variation in sounds. Gradually, through constant practice, you will begin to recognize deviations from normal. Only a sophisticated practitioner can evaluate the significance of the abnormal sounds.

Stethoscopes come equipped with a bell, a diaphragm, or preferably both. With this last type, you can switch from one to the other by turning the chestpiece or by flipping a lever. Low-pitched sounds are better heard with the bell placed lightly against the skin; high-pitched sounds are better heard with the diaphragm pressed firmly against the skin. Many nurses purchase their own stethoscopes *to ensure quality and consistency.*

An important aspect of auscultation is the control of the noise level in the environment. This is extremely important *if you are to detect all sounds.* In addition, instruct the patient not to talk during this aspect of the examination.

Heart

You can begin to recognize heart sounds by listening first to your own heart and then to those of other students. Starting at the fifth left intercostal space near the sternum, listen all the way over to the nipple line and laterally, until you find the position in which you can hear best.

In the clinical setting, if you have difficulty hearing the heart, have the supine patient roll partially over to the left, or have the sitting patient lean slightly forward. In either case, the sounds should be easier to hear *because the heart has moved closer to the chest wall.* Heart sounds that are very difficult to hear are termed *distant,* and those that are easily heard are termed *clear.* Heart sounds are often more difficult to hear in obese or barrel-chested patients.

Evaluate cardiac rate, rhythm, and intensity first. In some facilities, all patients who are receiving a digitalis preparation have an apical pulse taken prior to the administration of the digitalis, *to ensure an accurate heart rate count that is within the parameters for giving that drug.* Note *regular* irregularities (those that occur regularly

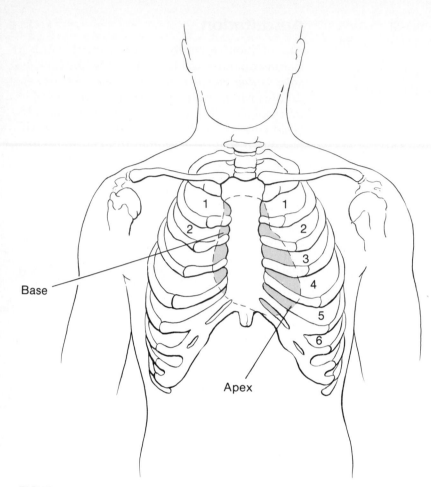

Base

Apex

FIGURE 13.5 *THE APEX AND BASE OF THE HEART*

every third beat, for example), as well as occasional missed or early beats (irregular irregularities). Abrupt changes in rate or rhythm should also be noted.

You should be able to differentiate between the first and second heart sounds (S_1 and S_2). (This is more easily accomplished at normal and slow rates.) Heart sounds are created by the closing of valves in the heart. Systole occurs between the first and second sounds, and diastole between the second and first sounds. The first sound is more easily heard in the area of the fifth left intercostal space near the nipple line (the apex); the second sound is more easily heard in the area of the second intercostal space immediately to the right of the sternum (the base) (see Figure 13.5). The sounds over the apex are usually heard more easily with the bell of the stethoscope; the sounds over the base of the heart are usually heard more easily with the

diaphragm. You should, however, feel free to experiment with both on any given patient to determine which gives you the best sound.

If you have difficulty distinguishing the sounds, identify the carotid pulse while you listen to the heart. The carotid pulse occurs simultaneously with the first heart sound.

Certain sounds (third and fourth) are generally considered abnormal, as are other sounds associated with cardiac pathology. These are beyond the scope of this text.

Lungs

As you did with the heart, you can begin by listening to your own lungs, although it will probably be easier to listen to those of another student, or to a record of lung sounds if available. You should try to discern normal breath sounds

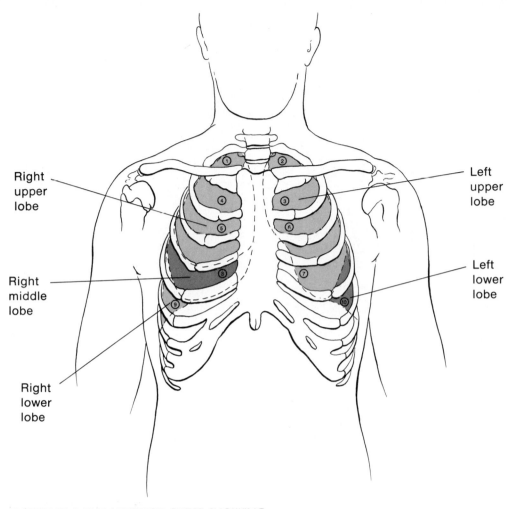

Right
upper
lobe

Left
upper
lobe

Right
middle
lobe

Left
lower
lobe

Right
lower
lobe

FIGURE 13.6 *THE ANTERIOR CHEST, SHOWING PATTERN OF STETHOSCOPE PLACEMENT*

and abnormal, or adventitious, sounds. Again, to attain any degree of skill, you must practice frequently.

Use the diaphragm of the stethoscope, pressed firmly against the skin, to auscultate the lungs. The patient should be in a sitting position, if possible. If not, roll the patient from side to side so that you can listen to all areas. If the patient is able to cooperate, ask him or her to breathe slowly in and out through an open mouth when the stethoscope is placed on the back. Auscultation should be done both anteriorly and posteriorly in a systematic manner, comparing one side to the other. (See Figures 13.6 and 13.7. Note the location of the lobes of the lungs in the figures. The lower lobes are heard only in a very small area on the anterior chest; conversely, the upper lobes are heard only in a small area of the posterior chest.)

Breath sounds are the sounds created by the movement of air in the trachea, bronchi, and alveoli. Normally, the expiratory phase is twice as long as the inspiratory phase. *On auscultation, however, you do not hear all of the expiratory phase,* so that it will seem shorter than the inspiratory phase. In cases of bronchial obstruction, chronic lung disease, or shallow breathing (as might be seen in a patient with incisional pain after abdominal surgery), breath sounds may be absent or decreased. In a condition that causes consolidation of lung tissue, such as pneumonia, the breath sounds may be louder or increased.

You may hear many abnormal sounds superimposed on the breath sounds. Among these are rales, rhonchi, wheezes, and friction rubs. In many facilities the practice is to describe the sounds instead of using terms that might be misunderstood.

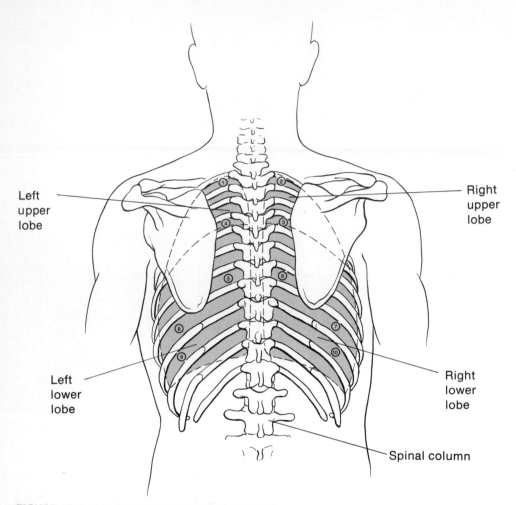

Left
upper
lobe

Right
upper
lobe

Left
lower
lobe

Right
lower
lobe

Spinal column

FIGURE 13.7 *THE POSTERIOR CHEST, SHOWING PATTERN OF STETHOSCOPE PLACEMENT*

Rales   Rales result from air passing through moisture (due to secretions) in the respiratory passages. They are usually heard on inspiration. Fine rales have a crackling sound; coarse rales are similar in quality but louder. If you hear rales, ask the patient to cough and listen again. *Often a patient who has been lying quietly has some rales in the bases that clear when he or she coughs.*

Rhonchi   Rhonchi are caused by air passing through respiratory passages that have narrowed or been partially obstructed by secretions, edema, tumors, and the like. Rhonchi are usually low-pitched and often alter in quality after the patient coughs.

Wheezes   Like rhonchi, wheezes are caused by air passing through partially obstructed respiratory passages, but they are higher-pitched *because they originate in smaller passages.* Wheezes have a whistlelike tone. Although they are more commonly heard during expiration, rhonchi and wheezes can be heard during any phase of respiration.

Pleural Friction Rubs   Pleural friction rubs are caused by the rubbing together of inflamed and roughened pleural surfaces. The sound is rough and scratchy, somewhat like two pieces of sandpaper being rubbed together. Friction rubs are heard on both inspiration and expiration. If this sound correlates with the rate and rhythm of the heartbeat, not the respirations, it is a pericardial friction rub.

Bowel Sounds

Normal bowel sounds, which indicate normal peristaltic activity, are relatively high-pitched and occur every 5 to 15 seconds. The absence of sound or the presence of very soft sounds (commonly called diminished bowel sounds) indicates the inhibition of bowel motility, as would occur in inflammatory processes or in the postoperative state. Increased bowel sounds (or hyperactive bowel sounds) occur with gastroenteritis or after a laxative has been taken. Loud, high-pitched rushing sounds, usually accompanied by pain, may indicate a bowel obstruction.

To listen for bowel sounds, lightly place the diaphragm of the stethoscope on the abdomen. Auscultate all four quadrants in a systematic fashion. Start with the right lower quadrant *because bowel sounds are often most pronounced (and most easily heard) there.*

Procedure for Auscultation

This procedure includes the auscultation of the three areas presented here: heart, lungs, and bowels.

1. Prepare for the examination as discussed. While preparing,
   a. Explain to the patient what you plan to do. Ask the patient not to speak while you are trying to listen.
   b. Control the noise in the environment. For example, turn off the television and close the door.
   c. Screen the patient or pull the curtain around the bed.
2. Fan-fold the patient's gown or pajama top up to the shoulders.
3. To auscultate the heart:
   a. Place the patient in the supine position.
   b. Fan-fold the bed linen down to the patient's waist.
   c. Warm the diaphragm of the stethoscope in your hands.
   d. Place the diaphragm at the fifth left intercostal space near the sternum and listen, moving laterally until you can hear the heart sounds clearly.
   e. Count the cardiac rate.
   f. Evaluate the cardiac rhythm, noting any regular or irregular irregularities.
   g. Listen for the first and second heart sounds, correlating the carotid pulse with the first heart sound.

4. To auscultate the lungs:
   a. Assist the patient to a sitting position, if possible; if not, roll the patient from side to side.
   b. Ask the patient to breathe slowly in and out through an open mouth.
   c. Using the diaphragm of the stethoscope, listen to the anterior chest, beginning with the apex on one side and comparing with the other side.
   d. Then move to the posterior chest and listen, beginning with the upper lobes and moving to the lower.
   e. If any rales or rhonchi are present, ask the patient to cough and listen again to see whether they have cleared.
5. To auscultate the bowels:
   a. Fan-fold the patient's gown or pajama top down to cover the chest.
   b. Fan-fold the bed linen down to the symphysis pubis.
   c. Place the diaphragm of the stethoscope lightly against the skin of the right lower quadrant, moving systematically until you have listened to all four quadrants. If no sounds are heard in a quadrant, continue to listen in that quadrant for a minimum of two to five minutes.
6. Conclude the examination as discussed.
7. Document your findings.

Percussion

Percussion involves striking a body surface to produce sounds that enable an experienced examiner to determine whether the underlying tissues are air-filled, fluid-filled, or solid. The examiner both hears (sounds change with the density of the tissue beneath) and feels the effects of percussion.

Because percussion penetrates only about 5 to 7 centimeters into the chest, it will not detect deep lesions.

Sounds

Resonance   Resonance is the normal sound heard when the lung is percussed. You can elicit this sound by percussing the lung at the right anterior portion of the third interspace. The sound is low in pitch and not loud.

271

Tympany Tympany results from air trapped in an enclosed chamber. It is loud and high in pitch. You can hear this sound if you percuss over the stomach. It is especially marked after a carbonated beverage has been consumed.

Dullness Dullness occurs with consolidation or increased density of lung tissue, as in the case of pneumonia. It is a short, high-pitched sound. You can elicit dullness by percussing over the diaphragm.

Flatness Flatness is a short, high-pitched sound completely without resonance or vibration. Fluid in the chest or abdomen can produce this sound. You can hear the sound by percussing over solid tissue—your thigh, for example.

Method

Although we present the process (the actual procedure appears in the Performance Checklist), along with examples of the kinds of sounds that can be elicited, to be able to detect abnormal sounds, you will first have to practice on normal individuals to become familiar with normal sounds.

1. Prepare for the examination as discussed.
2. Place the middle finger of your nondominant hand firmly against the body surface to be percussed. Keep the palm and other fingers off the skin.
3. With the tip of the middle finger of your dominant hand, strike the base of the distal phalanx of the finger against the body

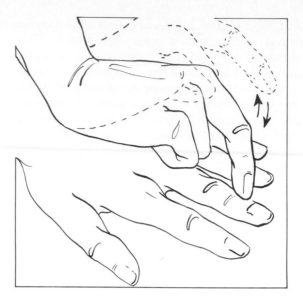

FIGURE 13.8 PERCUSSION

surface, just behind the nail bed (see Figure 13.8). Use a wrist action, and make the blow brief. Remove the striking finger immediately *to avoid attenuating the vibrations.*

4. Systematically percuss the chest, comparing one side to the other.
5. Percuss each quadrant of the abdomen. Dullness may indicate the presence of fluid. Tympany in the left upper quadrant may indicate a gastric air bubble.
6. Conclude the examination as discussed.
7. Document your findings.

PERFORMANCE CHECKLIST

	Unsatisfactory	Needs More Practice	Satisfactory	Comments
General procedure				
1. Prepare for the examination.				
a. Wash your hands.				
b. Obtain equipment needed (if any).				
c. Explain the examination to the patient.				
d. Provide privacy as needed for the type of examination.				
2. Carry out the specific examination.				
3. Conclude the examination.				
a. Restore the patient to a position of comfort.				
b. Restore the unit to appropriate condition.				
c. Care for the equipment.				
d. Wash your hands.				
4. Document your findings.				
Inspecting the pupils				
1. Prepare for examination as in the General Procedure (wash hands, obtain equipment, explain, and provide privacy).				
2. Inspect size, shape, and equality of pupils.				
3. Test reaction of pupils to light.				
a. Constriction and rate				
b. Consensual response				
4. Test reaction of pupils to accommodation.				
a. Constriction				
b. Convergence				
5. Conclude the examination as in the General Procedure (restore patient, restore unit, care for equipment, and wash hands).				
6. Document your findings.				
Inspecting the neck veins				
1. Prepare for examination as in the General Procedure (wash hands, obtain measuring device, explain, and provide privacy).				

	Unsatisfactory	Needs More Practice	Satisfactory	Comments
2. Have patient lie flat on back.				
3. Identify jugular veins bilaterally.				
4. Gradually elevate head of bed to 45-degree angle.				
5. Measure vertical distance in centimeters from right atrium to upper level of distention.				
6. Conclude the examination as in the General Procedure (restore patient, restore unit, return measuring device, and wash hands).				
7. Document your findings.				
Palpating the breasts				
1. Prepare for examination as in the General Procedure (wash hands, explain, and provide privacy).				
2. Have patient disrobe and be seated with hands in lap.				
3. Observe nipples for color, discharge, and dimpling.				
4. Observe breasts for size, symmetry, skin color, vascularity, and skin retraction.				
5. Have patient raise hands above head, and observe for irregularities in skin texture and dimpling.				
6. Have patient lie down.				
7. Palpate each breast systematically.				
8. Conclude the examination as in the General Procedure (restore patient, restore unit, and wash hands).				
9. Document your findings.				
Palpating the abdomen and liver				
1. Prepare for examination as in the General Procedure (wash hands, explain, and provide privacy).				
2. Mentally divide abdomen into quadrants.				
3. Ask patient to mouth-breathe.				
4. Observe abdomen for skin condition and symmetry.				

	Unsatisfactory	Needs More Practice	Satisfactory	Comments
5. Using palmar surfaces of your fingers, palpate patient's abdomen.				
6. Move systematically, palpating for tone, swelling, and tenderness.				
7. Assess for rebound tenderness.				
8. Ask patient to inhale.				
9. Palpate for liver.				
10. Conclude the examination as in the General Procedure (restore patient, restore unit, and wash hands).				
11. Document your findings.				

Examining the rectum

	Unsatisfactory	Needs More Practice	Satisfactory	Comments
1. Prepare for examination as in the General Procedure (wash hands, obtain clean gloves and lubricant, explain, and provide privacy).				
2. Put patient in left lateral position.				
3. Place gloves on hands.				
4. Lubricate gloved index finger.				
5. Spread patient's buttocks.				
6. Gently insert finger into patient's rectum.				
7. Ask patient to mouth-breathe.				
8. Move examining finger in a circle, breaking up and removing any fecal material found.				
9. Conclude the examination as in the General Procedure (dispose of glove, restore patient, restore unit, and wash hands).				
10. Document your findings.				

Auscultating the heart, lungs, and bowels

	Unsatisfactory	Needs More Practice	Satisfactory	Comments
1. Prepare for examination as in the General Procedure (wash hands, obtain stethoscope, explain, and provide privacy).				
2. Control environmental noise.				
3. Raise patient's gown or pajama top to shoulders.				

	Unsatisfactory	Needs More Practice	Satisfactory	Comments
4. Heart:				
a. Place patient in supine position.				
b. Fan-fold bed linen to patient's waist.				
c. Warm diaphragm of stethoscope.				
d. Position diaphragm.				
e. Locate apical pulse and count rate.				
f. Evaluate rhythm.				
g. Listen for first and second heart sounds, correlating carotid pulse with first heart sound.				
5. Lungs:				
a. Assist patient to sitting position, or roll from side to side.				
b. Ask patient to mouth-breathe.				
c. Auscultate anterior chest, comparing right and left sides.				
d. Auscultate posterior chest, comparing right and left sides.				
e. If rales or rhonchi are present, have patient cough and listen again.				
6. Bowels:				
a. Fan-fold patient's gown or pajama top down over chest.				
b. Fan-fold bed linen to patient's symphysis pubis.				
c. Systematically listen to all four quadrants of abdomen, beginning with right lower quadrant.				
7. Conclude the examination as in the General Procedure (restore patient, restore unit, clean and replace stethoscope, and wash hands).				
8. Document your findings.				
Percussing the chest and abdomen				
1. Prepare for examination as in the General Procedure (wash hands, explain, and provide privacy).				
2. Remove patient's gown or pajama top.				
3. Fan-fold bed linen to patient's waist.				

	Unsatisfactory	Needs More Practice	Satisfactory	Comments
4. Place patient in sitting position.				
5. Percuss patient's chest systematically.				
6. Have patient lie down.				
7. Percuss each quadrant of patient's abdomen.				
8. Conclude the examination as in the General Procedure (restore patient, restore unit, and wash hands).				
9. Document your findings.				

QUIZ

Short-Answer Questions

1. List five elements that should be included in inspection.

a. _____

b. _____

c. _____

d. _____

e. _____

2. Before testing the pupillary reaction to light and accommodation, for what three things should the nurse inspect the pupils?

a. _____

b. _____

c. _____

3. In what position are the jugular veins normally collapsed?

_____

4. Between what values is venous pressure considered normal?

_____

5. List three elements that the nurse should include in the explanation to the patient prior to palpation.

a. _____

b. _____

c. _____

6. Where is periorbital edema found? _____

7. Why should the nurse be aware of the patient's stage in the menstrual cycle when palpating the breasts of a female? _____

8. When examining the abdomen, why should auscultation be done before palpation and percussion? _____

9. In what area is the first heart sound usually most easily heard?

_____

10. Name one situation in which breath sounds might be absent or decreased.

_____

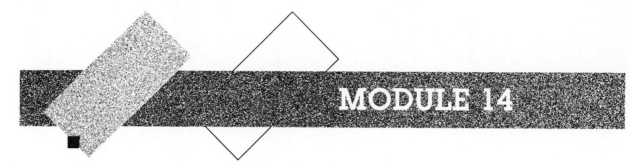

MODULE 14

Admission, Transfer, and Discharge

PREREQUISITES

1. Successful completion of the following modules:

   VOLUME 1

   Module 1 / An Approach to Nursing Skills
   Module 2 / Medical Asepsis
   Module 3 / Safety
   Module 5 / Assessment
   Module 6 / Documentation

2. Modules 22 and 23, Transfer and Ambulation, may be essential for admitting some incapacitated patients.
3. Modules 16, 17, and 18, Temperature, Pulse, and Respiration, Blood Pressure, and Collecting Specimens, may be necessary in a facility that requires the admitting person to collect such data.

OVERALL OBJECTIVE

To admit, transfer, and discharge patients, taking into consideration both general nursing concerns and the needs of individual patients.

SPECIFIC LEARNING OBJECTIVES

	Know Facts and Principles	Apply Facts and Principles	Demonstrate Ability	Evaluate Performance
Admission				
1. *Introduction and orientation* a. *Staff* b. *Environment* c. *Expectations and role*	State rationale for introducing patient to staff and environment. State rationale for orienting patient to expectations and role and discussing patient's expectations.	List information specific patient would need on admission	When admitting a patient, introduce staff present and environment, and discuss expectations for patient's behavior	Elicit patient's evaluation of adequacy of introductions and orientation
2. *Immediate needs* a. *Physical* b. *Emotional*	Discuss various physical needs patient may have on admission. Discuss various emotional needs patient may have on admission.	Given a patient situation, identify physical needs that take priority. Given a patient situation, identify emotional needs that take priority.	When admitting a patient, take action to meet immediate needs, both physical and emotional	Check patient for evidence of comfort and relaxation
3. *Baseline assessment* a. *Observation* b. *Physical examination* c. *Interview and history taking*	List initial observations that must be made. List information that should be obtained.	Given data on a new patient, identify observations needed for patient. Given data on a new patient, outline interview to be done.	When admitting a patient, make appropriate observations. Obtain needed information through interview.	Use the Basic Data Gathering Guide in Module 5, Assessment, to evaluate completeness of assessment
4. *Care of personal property*	Discuss nurse's responsibility toward patient's property	State usual disposition of personal effects in own facility	Arrange for safekeeping of patient's property	

5. Record keeping		List records required in own facility	Record observations, interview, disposition of personal property	Evaluate own performance using list of forms in Performance Checklist
Transfer				
1. Notify appropriate persons	List persons who should be made aware of transfer	Within the facility, note names and departments that should be contacted	Under the supervision of a staff nurse, make necessary calls	Check calls made against written hospital policy
2. Interaction with patient	Explore reason for visit and topics that might be discussed	Given a situation, discuss topics that may be discussed with patient before time of transfer	Visit a patient being transferred and identify information needed	Validate your assessment of needs with primary nurse
3. Care of personal property	State procedure for transfer of property with patient	Consult policy manual for places personal effects are stored	Review forms used in your facility for logging personal effects	Assess patient's completed forms before transfer
4. Communication to receiving staff	Discuss written and verbal communications to be transmitted to those who will be caring for the patient	List kinds of forms and other verbal information that should be communicated to receiving staff	Review policy of your facility regarding communicating patient data to receiving staff	Elicit primary nurse's evaluation of information you have communicated to receiving staff
Discharge				
1. Planning for continuity of care	State rationale for continuity of care. List resources for continuing care.	Given a situation, identify resources that would be needed for continued care	For a patient in the clinical area, plan appropriately for care after discharge from unit	
2. Patient teaching	List common learning needs for patients being discharged	Given a situation, identify learning needs	Teach patient in clinical area before discharge within limits of own ability	
3. Final assessment	Explain why final assessment is needed	Given a situation, list appropriate final assessment information for patient	Make complete final assessment of patient	Evaluate own performance using the Basic Data Gathering Guide in Module 5, Assessment

	Know Facts and Principles	Apply Facts and Principles	Demonstrate Ability	Evaluate Performance
4. *Care of personal property*	List places personal effects may be kept	List forms for own facility that must be completed at discharge regarding patient's belongings	Retrieve all of patient's personal effects and see that they accompany patient	Use Performance Checklist to see that all items are completed
5. *Business functions*	Discuss usual business functions for which nurse is responsible	List business functions required in facility	When discharging patient, see that financial arrangements are completed. Obtain medications and supplies if needed.	
6. *Record keeping*	Discuss usual records to be filled out	List discharge records required in facility	Record data on entire discharge procedure	Evaluate own performance using list of forms in Performance Checklist

LEARNING ACTIVITIES

1. Review the Specific Learning Objectives.
2. Read the section on threats to the patient's mental health (in the chapter on mental health) in Ellis and Nowlis, *Nursing: A Human Needs Approach,* or comparable material in another textbook.
3. Look up the module vocabulary terms in the Glossary.
4. Check the procedure book at your facility for the forms and processes required for admission, transfer, and discharge.
5. Assist a staff member or more experienced student with the admission of a patient. Discuss the procedure:
   a. Were all steps included?
   b. Did more than one person participate in the process?
6. With the supervision of your instructor, admit a patient. Evaluate your own performance using the Performance Checklist. Consult with your instructor regarding your performance.
7. Repeat steps 5 and 6 for the transfer of a patient.
8. Repeat steps 5 and 6 for the discharge of a patient.

VOCABULARY

A.M.A.
assessment
chart
nursing history
referral
urinalysis

ADMISSION, TRANSFER, AND DISCHARGE

Rationale for the Use of This Skill

W*henever a patient enters any health care facility, the nurse should always keep that person's possible transfer and eventual discharge in mind. For most patients, the nurse should begin planning for eventual transfer or discharge at the time the patient is admitted.*

For most people, entering a health care facility is a major crisis. Individuals have many needs and concerns that must be identified and for which action must be taken. In addition, each health care facility must maintain certain routine procedures and gather specific information about incoming patients that will help it perform its functions. Identifying and meeting both sets of needs is a challenging · task for the nurse.

Units within the hospital may be specialized, and this means that a patient may sometimes need to be transferred from one unit to another within the facility. Also, since the passage of the 1983 Medicare prospective reimbursement system, which limits the funding available for acute hospitalization, more older patients are being transferred to nursing homes for continued treatment and convalescence. Consequently, the transfer procedure is of growing importance. If it is done carefully, the relocation will have minimal impact upon the patient and the receiving staff will be provided with adequate knowledge upon which to base comprehensive nursing care.

When people are ready to leave the health care facility for home, the nurse has a similar responsibility. The patient should be instructed in any aspect of care that will be done on a continuing basis and that involves the patient or family. Questions should be answered to decrease anxiety, and resources that may be useful should be shared.[1]

Admission

When admitting a person to a health care facility, you have many responsibilities. They can be grouped under the following headings.

[1]You will note that rationale for action is emphasized throughout the module by the use of italics.

1. Immediate needs of the person
   a. Physical
   b. Emotional
2. Introduction and orientation
3. Baseline assessment
   a. Observations and physical examination
   b. Interview and history taking
4. Care of belongings
5. Record keeping

These activities will not always be done in the same order. For example, an item from baseline assessment may most conveniently be done at the same time that you begin record keeping. The needs of the individual patient and your own convenience will guide you.

Immediate Needs

A brief general assessment of a new patient *to ascertain immediate needs* is essential. This should be your first concern. *A person does not enter the hospital unless there is a health care problem.* This problem may not be causing any immediate distress, or it may be acute. A well-founded criticism of some health care workers is that they are so concerned about routines and forms that the patients' primary problems remain uncared for.

Immediate needs can be either physical or emotional. If a patient is in acute pain, contact the physician immediately regarding orders for medication and care; meanwhile, institute nursing measures to relieve pain. If a patient is upset or distraught, spend time listening and talking to the patient; this can facilitate the transition to the hospital environment. *If a patient feels that those around are concerned about his or her immediate needs and are taking action to meet them, a relationship of trust may well have begun.*

Introductions and Orientation

When you deem it appropriate, it is your responsibility to introduce the patient to people in the environment. This may be the very first thing you do, but it can wait until some immediate need has been met. Here you must use your judgment.

Your greeting should convey interest in and concern for the patient. A person just entering a hospital is really not concerned about your problems of staffing or time except as they directly affect his or her care. If it is necessary for a patient to wait, an explanation is appreciated.

Although you should not expect a patient to remember the names of all staff members initially, *introducing yourself and others by both name and position helps the patient to become oriented to what is happening.* Other patients who are in the same room should also be introduced.

Explain what will occur during the admitting process. *This relieves the anxiety created by fear of the unknown.*

A thorough patient orientation to the unit includes how all items for the patient's use work, which areas are for personal belongings, and the location of the bathroom. Especially important are directions on how to call a nurse.

Explain anything you expect a patient to do in detail, from exactly what to wear under the hospital gown to what activity is ordered. *A patient will be better able to participate in care if what is expected is clear.*

Baseline Assessment

The information to be gathered in baseline assessment varies from one facility to another. It almost always includes temperature, pulse, and respiration (TPR), blood pressure (BP), height, and weight. In some facilities, the nurse does a complete physical examination. In others, the nurse may do a thorough nursing assessment that does not encompass the traditional physical examination.

Laboratory values may become part of the baseline assessment. Depending on the diagnosis, some patients now have extensive lab work done the day before admission *to decrease costs and length of stay in the hospital.* In other cases, patients enter the hospital with little or no lab work and may be taken to the laboratory area on the way to the unit.

A nursing history is usually taken. Even if a formalized nursing history is not used, information relating to allergies, current medications, and the patient's perception of his or her entering problem (often called the *chief complaint*) is gathered. An interview is used to gather subjective information regarding the patient (see Figure 14.1).

These baseline data are necessary in order to evaluate future observations and other data gathered.

Personal Property

One of the more difficult problems in an institution, large or small, is keeping track of a patient's personal property. *The loss of valued items is upsetting to patients and can be costly to an institution.*

Most facilities have a routine for checking and noting all personal items a patient brings or wears to the facility. Items that are not needed can be sent home with family members. This is perhaps the best safeguard. Large sums of money and valuable items are usually kept in a safe in the business office with proper documents attesting to their location and their value. The amount of money that a patient should keep at the bedside depends on the policy of the facility and the patient's personal wishes and needs.

Items that are kept with the patient are less likely to get lost if they are marked with the patient's name, but this is not always possible. Arrange to keep these possessions together in a place that is accessible to the patient. A printed list of clothing and personal effects that you can quickly check off is often used to make an exact inventory. (See Figure 14.2 for an example of a clothing and personal effects list.)

Record Keeping

Recording all parts of the admission process is essential for legal records. The baseline assessment serves as a reference throughout the period of care, and frequently the record of care of personal effects must be consulted. In addition, you may be responsible for a variety of other records (notification of the dietary department, starting a Kardex card and medication record, filling out census forms).

Consult the procedure book at each facility to determine which forms are your responsibility.

Transfer

When you transfer a patient to another unit, to another hospital, or to a nursing home, you are responsible for carrying out certain procedures that will make the transition as smooth and nonstressful as possible for the patient and the receiving staff. These include:

1. Order for transfer

FIGURE 14.1 PATIENT CARE KARDEX

2. Notifying appropriate persons
3. Interacting with the patient, including reinforcement of any health teaching
4. Caring for the patient's personal property
5. Completing and/or duplicating assessment data and care plan
6. Arranging transportation
7. Giving report

Order for Transfer

A physician must write the order transferring a patient within the hospital or to another facility. If there is some nursing reason for transfer, such as inability to provide a room or equipment for a special patient need, notify the physician, who will then write the order.

Notifying Appropriate Persons

It is your responsibility to be sure that all persons involved have been notified of the transfer. These include the nursing supervisor, the admitting department, the patient's family, and the unit or facility that is receiving the patient. The discharge planner may already have made these contacts for you.

Interacting with the Patient

The patient probably knows of the plans for transfer, but you can clarify this and answer any questions the patient may have regarding the new environment. If you assess any signs of anxiety about the transfer, spend time with the pa-

NURSING ADMISSION DATA

Patient arrived via: Amb. (WC) Cart	TPR 99 ^{2} – 88 – 32	BP 140/82 WT. 63 k HT. 5'2"

From: (Home) ECF ER Other

Allergies: (drug, food, other) — *pollen, shellfish*

Reaction (describe):

Emergency Notification:

Phone No.

VALUABLES: DESCRIPTION	LOCATION
(Glasses) Contacts:	pt.
Hearing Aid:	
Mobility Aid:	
Prosthesis:	
Dentures: Upper (Lower) (Partial)	
Wallet:	
Money:	bus. off.
Watch:	pt.
Jewelry:	

Medications	Dose	Frequency	Last Dose	Location
Isoproterenol Inhaler	P.T. Dept.	B.I.D.	—	ordered
Aminophyllin gt. I.V.	25 mg/hr.	cont.	0900	—
Gentamycin I.V.	80 mg	q.8.h.		

ORIENTATION TO HOSPITAL: Visiting Hours ☑ Chaplaincy Service ☑ Hospital Educational TV ☑
Info Booklet ☑ Call System ☑ Bed Controls ☑ Bathroom ☑ Storage ☑ TV ☑ Telephone ☑

Date: 4/16/88   Time: 0915   Signature: B. Jordan, R.N.

NURSING DATA BASE

Significant Past Health History: NO/YES Cardiac/Respiratory/Neurological/ Muscular-skeletal/Endocrine/G.I./G.U./Liver Disease/Skin/Past Surgeries:

Long term emphysema (COPD)

Present Illness and Patient's Expectation of Hospitalization:

Asthma/pneumonia — improved breathing — decrease need for O₂

S L E E P / C O M F O R T

PAIN: NO/(YES) Location — breathing
Duration ___ - Type sharp
Intensity 1 2 3 (4) 5 6 7 8 9 10 Onset ___
Mild   Severe
Relieved by ___
Aggravated by resp.
SLEEP PATTERN: 7 – 9 hours
Aids for sleep: Quiet, door closed, cool room

N E U R O S E N S O R Y

LEVEL OF CONSCIOUSNESS: Alert/Lethargic/Restless/Agitated/ semi-coma/Coma
PUPIL STATUS: (when indicated) NA
ORIENTATION: Person/Place/Time/Situation oriented
SENSORY DISABILITY: (NO)/YES
CMS Parameter Flow Sheet started: YES/NO
NEURO Parameter Flow Sheet started: YES/NO

S O C I A L / E M O T I O N A L

AFFECT: Within normal limits/Angry/(Anxious)/Depressed/Flat/Hostile
LIVES: Alone/With family/With friends/ECF — husband
SUPPORT SYSTEMS: Describe minimal, husband also anxious at present

M O B I L I T Y / S A F E T Y

ACTIVITY LEVEL: bedrest until weakness improves
LIMITATIONS IN MOVEMENT: NO/YES Contractures/paralysis/Amputation/ Weakness/Gait/Balance/Cast
AIDS FOR MOBILITY: Cane/Crutches/Walker/Prosthesis/Wheelchair/ Other staff assist

---

C O M M U N I C A T I O N

PRIMARY LANGUAGE (If not English)
Trouble speaking/understanding English
Interpreter N/A
Phone Number
SPEECH: Clear/Slow/Slurred/Aphasic/Inappropriate/none
Describe: some hesitancy d/c resp.
HEARING: norm. — compromise
VISION: norm. corrective lenses.

S K I N

SENSITIVITIES: Soap/Tape/Lotion/Other none
CONDITION: Normal/Dry/Bruises/Abrasions/Open wounds/Ulcers/Rash:
Describe
USUAL BATHING PREFERENCES tub q.d. (a.m.)

N U T R I T I O N

RECENT WEIGHT CHANGE: Gain/Loss none Pounds
INTAKE: Normal/Nausea/Vomiting/Dysphagia/Malnourished/ Alternate Route 4 small meals
MEAL PATTERN: (resp. compromise
SPECIAL DIET: NO/YES Type
Dislikes fried foods.
ALCOHOL: Type and amount Ø

R E S P I R A T O R Y

QUALITY: Normal/Labored/Shallow/SOB/SOB c̄ exertion/Orthopnea/ Other
COUGH: Absent/Non-productive/Productive mod. amt. clear mucus
LUNG SOUNDS: dull in ↓ lobes, wheezes.
TOBACCO USE: (NO)/YES Type and amount
2 pkg./day 16 years — quit 3 yrs. ago

G I / G U

ABDOMEN: Normal/Tender/Rigid/Distended
BOWEL TONES: Normal/Hypo-active/Hyper-active/Absent
BOWELS: Usual Pattern q.o.d. Last BM 4/15
Laxatives/Enemas: NO/YES occasional
Diarrhea/Blood in stool/Constipation/Impaction/Incontinence/ Other
URINARY: No difficulty/Frequency/Urgency/Pain/Burning/Hematuria/ Nocturia/Catheter

---

C I R C U L A T O R Y

HEART RHYTHM: Regular/Irregular
PERIPHERAL PULSES (When indicated) present
Edema/Dehydration/Neither
SKIN COLOR: Normal/Cyanotic/Dusky/Jaundice mild
SKIN TEMPERATURE: Normal/Cold/Hot/Diaphoretic

R E P R O D U C T I O N / S E X U A L I T Y

LAST MENSTRUAL PERIOD NP   PAP SMEAR '86
Breast Exam
CONTRACEPTIVES: NO/YES
LAST TESTICULAR EXAM/PROSTATE EXAM NP
Discharge/Bleeding/Pain

DATE: 4/16/88   TIME: 0915   RN SIGNATURE: Beth Jordan

ROOM NO.: 811   NAME: Sutherland, Bella

NORTHGATE GENERAL HOSPITAL					Patient's Clothes List			Admission Data
AMT.	CLOTHING	AMT.	CLOTHING	AMT.	MISCELLANEOUS	AMT.	DENTURES	
	BATHROBE		NIGHTGOWN		CANE		UPPERS	ADM. TIME 4/16/88
	BED JACKET		PAJAMAS		CONTACT LENS	1	LOWERS	B.P. 140/82
	BELT		PANTI HOSE		ELECTRIC RAZOR	1	PARTIAL	T. 99 P. 88 R. 32
	BLOUSE		SCARF	1	GLASSES			WT. 63K HT. 5'2"
	BRA		SHIRT		HEARING AID			TRANSFUSIONS
1	COAT		SHOES (PAIR)		LUGGAGE		VALUABLES	ALLERGIES
1	DRESS		SKIRT		RADIO		BANK BOOK	pollen
1	GARTER BELT		SLACKS		T. V.	1	RING	shell fish
1	GIRDLE		SLIP				WALLET	
	GLOVES (PAIR)		SLIPPERS (PAIR)			1	WATCH	MEDICINES MED. DR.
	HANDKERCHIEF		SOCKS (PAIR)			1	PURSE	none
	HAT		SUIT				$11.20	
1	HOSE		SWEATER				VALUABLES ENVELOPE NUMBER 2748	
	JACKET		UNDERSHIRT					
	NECKTIE		UNDERWEAR					

ANY VALUABLES OR FUNDS NOT DEPOSITED WITH THE HOSPITAL ARE RETAINED AT MY OWN RISK AND ANY VALUABLES, ELECTRICAL APPLIANCES, RADIOS, T.V., ETC., BROUGHT TO ME WHILE A PATIENT WILL BE MY OWN RESPONSIBILITY.

DIET 2gm Na
DINNER DRINK tea
SNACK juice

1. SIGNATURE OF PATIENT _Bella Sutherland_

2. CHECKED IN BY (NURSE-AIDE) _Al Feldon, NA_   DATE _4/16/88_

3. SIGNATURE OF PERSON RECEIVING ITEMS ABOVE _____

4. SIGNATURE OF PERSON RECEIVING VALUABLES ENVELOPE _Flo Joiner, Bus. office_

5. CHECKED OUT BY (NURSE-AIDE) _____ DATE _____

PLEASE COMPLETE IN INK ONLY

DISCHARGED _____

FIGURE 14.2 PERSONAL PROPERTY LIST

tient and the family exploring details of the move.

Caring for Personal Property

Make sure that all the patient's personal property is checked and accompanies the patient being transferred.

Completing or Duplicating Records

If the patient is being transferred *within the hospital,* gather all assessment forms and care plans, bedside equipment, and plastic identification card. Review the assessment and care plan for completeness and accuracy. Make an appropriate entry in the record concerning the move.

Completing Assessment Data and Care Plan

Although you can begin preparing the documents that will accompany the patient a day or so before transfer, updating the data and plan of care just before the patient leaves is essential. This provides the receiving staff with a current assessment and identification of any unresolved patient problems. Remember that these documents are confidential and should be given only to authorized persons. (See Figure 14.3.)

Arranging Transportation

When the patient is being transferred to a nursing home or another facility, the business office or discharge planner often makes arrangements for an ambulance or Cabambulance (a specially fitted van that can transport patients who do not need close monitoring). When critical care is needed, the nurse may make arrangements, particularly when the patient needs special equipment, such as oxygen or maintenance of intravenous therapy, or specialized personnel, such as a respiratory therapist or critical care nurse. If the patient is going to another unit of the hospital, you may decide whether the patient can be transferred by wheelchair or stretcher.

Giving Report

When the patient is going to another unit of the hospital, call the new unit and go with the pa-

tient *so that you can give the nursing staff a verbal report and answer any questions.* When the patient is being transferred to another hospital or to a nursing home, duplicate the records and make a telephone call to the receiving staff, giving them a comprehensive report regarding the patient.

Discharge

When you are planning for a patient's discharge home, your responsibilities are similar to those in transfer to another unit. They include the following.

1. Planning for continuity of care
2. Patient teaching
3. Final assessment
4. Care of personal property
5. Business functions
6. Record keeping

Order for Discharge

An order is needed for the patient to be discharged. Although the nurse begins planning for the patient's discharge as early as admission, no business documents or final papers are started until the precise time of discharge is determined. However, if you have been told verbally that a patient is to be discharged but the order has not yet been written, you may sometimes complete such tasks as ordering take-home medications and making patient assessments before the actual discharge order is written *so that the patient's departure is not delayed.*

Continuity of Care

Your nursing responsibility does not end when the patient leaves the area in which you work. You have a responsibility to see that plans are made for continuing care as needed. If the patient is going home, this planning can be done with the patient and the family. You may have to consult the official discharge planner of your facility if home nursing care is needed.

Patient Teaching

Talk with the patient regarding the planned time of departure and how you might be useful in the discharge. Explain what will happen and

291

Original Copy Goes To Receiving Facility — Xerox Copy To Be Retained In Patient Record — **Attach Xerox Copy Of Patient Admittance Sheet.**

Patient's Last Name	First Name	MI
Sutherland,	_Bella_	_M._

Address, City, State, Zip Code   Phone
1018 Alder , Blaine, WA .788-1011

Date of Birth	Age	Sex	Marital Status	Church
_2-1-28_	_60_	_F_	S (M) W D Sep.	_C_

Relative or Guardian (specify relationship) name, address   Phone
Henry   PHYSICIANS ORDERS _husb. Same_

Name and Address of Facility Transferring:

From: _Swedish Hospital_
To: _Blaine Conval. center_   Pt. Hosp. No. _6402573_

Family Informed Of Transfer	Yes ☑	No ☐
Does patient know diagnosis	Yes ☑	No ☐
Does family know diagnosis	Yes ☑	No ☐

Date of telephone referral: _5/19_ Adm. Date: _4/16_ Discharge Date: _5/21/88_
Previous Hospitalization and/or Nursing Home Stay (Within last 90 days):

none

Health Insurance Info: Soc. Sec. No. _462-51-8717_

Medicare _____   Medicaid _✓_

Other _____

Attending Physician: _Wm. Hawkins, M.D._
Consulting Physician(s): _Tom Andrews, M.D._
Physician after transfer: _Jean Simpson, M.D._
Admitting Diagnosis: _asthma / pneumonia_

Discharge Diagnosis:
Primary: _asthma / pneumonia-resolving_

Secondary: _chronic respiratory desease_

Course of Treatment: attach copy of Physician's Discharge Summary.
   See attached

Any significant changes from initial H & P   ☐ Yes   ☑ No
If Yes, changes are:

MEDICATION ORDER FOR RECEIVING FACILITY (If PRN, state reason for giving and max. amt. to be given. List discontinuation date, if any, on all medications ordered) Note: Any brand or form of drug identical in form and content may be dispensed unless checked here: ☐

Theophylline 100 mg. q.c.h.
conjugated estrogen 0.625 mg. q.d.
multivitamin ÷ q.d.
Tums ÷÷ B.I.D.

DIET ☐ Regular   ☑ Sodium Restriction, _2_ gm.   ☐ Salt Substitute _____   ☐ Diabetic, ___ calories   ☐ Low Residue   ☐ Bland
☐ Mechanical   ☐ Soft   ☐ Tube, ___ cc per ___ hr   ☐ Dietary Supplement _____   ☐ Other _____

ALLERGIES ☐ No   ☑ Yes   Type: _pollen, shell fish_

SPECIAL TREATMENTS (Including Physical Therapy, Speech, O.T., etc.) Specify frequency.
   ↑ oral fluids to 2500 ml./day.   _I + O_
   O₂ PRN
   breathing and relaxation exercises.

ACTIVITY ORDERS (List activity level, restrictions and/or precautions, etc.) Note: If ordering restraints indicate reason for use.
   Increase activity level. Ambulation to tolerance c̄ assist.

REHABILITATION POTENTIAL   (Describe the highest level of independent, functioning the patient can be expected to achieve.)
☐ Independent   Semi-Independent: ☑ Assistance for few activities   ☐ Assistance for most activities

ADDITIONAL COMMENTS:

Certification ☑ I certify that post hospital skilled nursing care is medically necessary on a continuing basis for any of the conditions for which he/she received care during this hospitalization. ☐ I certify that my above orders regarding home health services (skilled nursing care, therapy, or others as defined) are medically necessary because my patient is confined to home. These services are related to the condition(s) for which he/she received inpatient hospital or SNF care.

Signature of Physician _William A. Hawkins_   MD   Phone: _____   Date: _____

This form has been approved by the Seattle Area Hospital Council and the Washington State Health Facilities Association. To re-order, call (206) 682-5995
Revised Date September 1981   **PATIENT TRANSFER FORM**   Seattle Area Hospital Council

FIGURE 14.3 PATIENT TRANSFER FORM

when it will happen. The patient may need information about medications, treatments, activity, diet, and continued health supervision. Ideally, teaching will have begun earlier so that the patient is not overwhelmed with stimuli and information at the time of discharge. Occasionally, however, teaching is not done in advance and must be done on the day of discharge. Often the family is also included in the teaching.

Final Assessment

Before a patient leaves your unit, you must prepare a final assessment. Include the patient's physical status, emotional status, and ability to continue or participate in care.

If data indicate that the patient is not ready for discharge (if the patient has an elevated temperature, for example), report the information to the physician immediately for evaluation.

Personal Property

Be sure that all personal belongings accompany the patient. Especially critical are dentures, glasses, and special appliances, such as crutches. If a list of personal effects was made on admission, this will help, but remember that items brought in after admission may not be on the list. Check your list with the patient. Do not forget that there may be items in the safe or in the medicine room.

The patient may also take home items that were purchased in the hospital and are billed to the patient. These might include an egg-crate mattress, a sheepskin mattress pad, or an admission kit.

Business Matters

Before a patient leaves a hospital, it is customary for either the patient or the family to consult with the business office regarding financial matters. This may have been taken care of on admission through identification of an insurance company or a third-party payer. Be sure you know the usual routine in your facility. You may have to get drugs from the pharmacy or supplies from somewhere else for the patient to take home. You should plan for these items when you consider continuity of care and patient teaching.

Record Keeping

Again, forms will vary from facility to facility. Record your final assessment, patient teaching, plans for continuity of care, disposition of personal items, and completion of business functions. Some facilities use a chart with a section that should help to remind you of all these points.

Delegation of Tasks

If a nursing assistant, a volunteer, or anyone else is able to assist with a patient's admission, transfer, or discharge, you must carefully evaluate which tasks require greater skill and judgment. For example, decision making and assessment are nursing functions that do not lend themselves to delegation to nonnursing personnel. A routine task such as orientation to the physical unit, however, can be delegated.

Many patients have shorter hospital stays than was previously common and need more post-discharge care. In hospitals that use primary care nursing, a current concept is for the primary nurse (the nurse who has total responsibility for the patient's care during the hospitalization) to see that individualized care takes place after discharge (Pilcher, 1986, p. 50).

REFERENCE

Pilcher, Mary W. "Post-Discharge Care: How to Follow Up." *Nursing '86,* 1, No. 8 (August 1986), 50–51.

PERFORMANCE CHECKLIST

Admission

	Unsatisfactory	Needs More Practice	Satisfactory	Comments
1. Check for orders.				
2. Meet immediate needs. a. Physical				
b. Emotional				
3. Make introductions and orient patient. a. Greet patient.				
b. Introduce self.				
c. Explain admission routine.				
d. Orient patient to individual unit: bed, bathroom, call light, supplies, and belongings.				
e. Orient patient to entire unit: location of nurses' station and day room or lounge.				
f. Explain expected behavior.				
g. Introduce other staff and roommates.				
4. Perform baseline assessment. a. Observation and physical examination. (1) TPR				
(2) BP				
(3) Weight and height				
(4) Total assessment				
b. Interview and history (1) Medications				
(2) Allergies				
(3) Entering complaints and concerns				
5. Take care of personal property. a. Items to be kept at bedside.				
b. Items to be put in safe or medicine room				
c. Items to be sent home				
6. Keep records. a. All data recorded				
b. Special forms for facility completed (add your own list of forms)				

Transfer

	Unsatisfactory	Needs More Practice	Satisfactory	Comments
1. Check for orders.				
2. Notify appropriate persons. a. Nursing supervisor				
b. Admitting office				
c. Unit or facility receiving the patient				
d. Family members				
3. Visit the patient. a. Answer any questions about the transfer.				
b. Allay anxiety by spending time with the patient.				
4. Take care of personal property: a. Items kept at bedside				
b. Items in safe or medicine room				
5. Complete or duplicate records. a. Complete basic assessment.				
b. Complete or duplicate care plan.				
6. If not already arranged, obtain transportation; within hospital, wheelchair or stretcher.				
7. Give report. a. If transferring to another unit in the hospital, accompany patient and give report.				
b. If transferring to another facility, call and give report by phone.				

Discharge

	Unsatisfactory	Needs More Practice	Satisfactory	Comments
1. Check for orders.				
2. Plan for continuing care. a. Referrals as needed.				
b. Information for new persons involved in care				
c. Contacting family or significant others if needed				
d. Transportation				
3. Teach patient. a. What to expect				
b. Medications				
c. Treatments				

	Unsatisfactory	Needs More Practice	Satisfactory	Comments
d. Activity				
e. Diet				
f. Needs for continued health supervision				
4. Perform final assessment. a. Physical status				
b. Emotional status				
c. Ability to continue own care				
5. Check and return personal property. a. Personal items on unit				
b. Items from safe or medicine room				
6. Perform business functions. a. Financial matters				
b. Obtaining supplies				
7. Keep records. a. Discharge note				
b. Special forms for facility (add your own list of forms)				

QUIZ

Multiple-Choice Questions

_____ 1. The first thing you should do when admitting a patient is

    a. orient the patient to the unit.
    b. ascertain and meet the patient's immediate needs.
    c. take TPR and BP.
    d. make a baseline assessment.

_____ 2. When orienting a patient to the environment, which of the following is not necessary?

    a. The location of the utility room and kitchenette
    b. How to call a nurse
    c. The location of the bathroom
    d. How to operate the bed

_____ 3. If a patient is very distraught on admission, you should

    a. hurry as quickly as possible.
    b. go slowly to provide calm as you follow the usual routine.
    c. temporarily omit routine items.
    d. continue with the regular admission procedure as usual.

_____ 4. If a volunteer is available to assist with admission, which task would it be most appropriate to delegate to him or her?

    a. Baseline assessment
    b. Ascertaining immediate needs
    c. Orientation to the unit
    d. Charting data

_____ 5. Which of the following should you consider if you are transferring a patient to another unit? (1) continuing care; (2) patient teaching; (3) care of belongings; (4) final assessment

    a. 1, 2, and 4
    b. 2, 3, and 4
    c. 1 and 2 only
    d. All of these

_____ 6. A patient has a very valuable jeweled ring. You would suggest

    a. that the patient wear it.
    b. that the patient hide it well in his or her suitcase.
    c. keeping it at the nursing station.
    d. putting it in the office safe.

_____ 7. Which of the following are usually nursing responsibilities related to transfer? (1) equipment for transfer; (2) teaching the patient about medications; (3) making a final assessment; (4) making sure the patient's property is also transferred

    a. 2 and 3
    b. 1 and 4
    c. 1, 3, and 4
    d. All of these

_____ 8. Which of the following are usually nursing responsibilities related to discharge? (1) planning for transportation; (2) teaching the patient about medications; (3) making a final assessment; (4) making sure that the patient's personal property is sent along

    a. 1, 2, and 3
    b. 2, 3, and 4
    c. 1, 3, and 4
    d. All of these

_____ 9. Which of the following patients are most likely to need a referral to provide continuing care after discharge? (1) one who had a routine appendectomy; (2) one who had a stroke and has right-sided paralysis; (3) one who had acute pneumonia; (4) one with a new colostomy

    a. 1 and 3
    b. 2 and 4
    c. 3 and 4
    d. All of these

Short-Answer Questions

10. The person within some facilities whose task it is to facilitate discharge is called _____.

11. One patient situation that may delay discharge and should be reported to the physician is _____.

MODULE 15

Intake and Output

PREREQUISITES

Successful completion of the following modules:

OVERALL OBJECTIVE

To be able to measure correctly and keep accurate records of patients' fluid intake and output.

SPECIFIC LEARNING OBJECTIVES

	Know Facts and Principles	Apply Facts and Principles	Demonstrate Ability	Evaluate Performance
1. *Initiating measurement*	State who may initiate measurement and reasons for measurement	Given a patient situation, state why measurement is important for that patient	Determine relationship of amounts measured to the patient's medical status	Evaluate with instructor
2. *What is measured*	State what items must be measured for intake and output	Given a sample patient diet, identify items to be measured. Given a patient situation, identify intake, other than dietary, that must be measured. Given a patient situation, identify which excretions must be measured for output.	Measure intake accurately. Measure output accurately.	With instructor, evaluate choices of what to measure
3. *Record-keeping forms*	List pertinent information that should be recorded at patient's bedside. List pertinent information that should be recorded on patient's chart.	Given a listing of information about patient's intake and output, record it on correct form in proper place	Record intake and output on proper forms	With instructor, evaluate use of forms
4. *Measurements used*	Identify when to add or subtract quantities to get correct totals	Given a patient situation with amounts of intake and output, figure correct totals	Total intake and output. Record totals on correct form.	Evaluate own performance using Performance Checklist

300

5. *Time periods for measurement*	Know variety of time periods that may be used for recording intake and output	Given patient's amounts of intake and output, calculate total for 8-hour and 24-hour systems	Calculate totals for 8- to 24-hour periods	Evaluate own performance using Performance Checklist
6. *Fluid balance*	Define fluid balance. Identify factors in addition to intake and output that must be considered in regard to fluid balance.	Given a patient situation, identify factors that relate to fluid balance. State additional data that may be needed for accurate assessment of fluid balance.	Determine whether patient is in fluid balance. Report instances of fluid imbalance to appropriate person.	
7. *Patient's participation*	Identify ways of explaining to patient need for measurement of intake and output, and method to be used	Given a patient situation, devise plan for measuring intake and output that includes patient participation	In the clinical setting, successfully maintain intake and output record on patient from patient's list	Compare own results with those of staff person also assigned to care of patient

LEARNING ACTIVITIES

1. Review the Specific Learning Objectives.
2. Read the section on fluids (in the chapter on nutrition and fluids) in Ellis and Nowlis, *Nursing: A Human Needs Approach,* or comparable material in another textbook.
3. Look up the module vocabulary terms in the Glossary.
4. Read through the module.
5. In the practice setting:
   Practice measuring, using containers showing metric measurement.
   Using the container measurements given on the sample form in Figure 15.2, calculate the intake and output for the following patient:

Mr. Denner, on rising, brushed his teeth. After rinsing his mouth, he drank half a glass (small) of water. Breakfast arrived and was composed of:

Fruit juice, small glass
Cereal bowl of hot oatmeal with a pitcher of
   cream
Bacon and soft-boiled egg
Pot of coffee with small cream
Glass of milk

Shortly after breakfast, he felt nauseated and vomited 75 ml semiliquid emesis. Throughout the morning, he voided two times: 50 ml and 225 ml.

By lunch, he was feeling much better and a light diet was ordered. When it arrived, he ate a small bowl of broth and half of a small bowl of gelatin.

He voided once more after lunch: 125 ml.

He was given oral medications twice, each time with 1 oz water.

At the end of the day shift, half of a 1,000-ml bottle of IV fluids had been absorbed.

Turn in the above computations. Have your instructor evaluate their accuracy.
6. In the clinical setting:
   a. Familiarize yourself with the various diets used in your facility and the fluid content of each.
   b. Check the form used by your facility for intake and output measurement.
   c. Keep an intake-output record on one of your assigned patients for one meal and for the time period you are on the unit. Have your instructor check your accuracy.
   d. For a patient in the clinical area who is on intake-output measurement, figure the last three 8-hour periods and total your figures for 24 hours.
   e. For the same patient, check the record and decide, based on recorded data, whether this patient is in fluid balance. Present your data and your decision to your instructor for verification.

VOCABULARY

catheter
diaphoresis
diarrhea
diuresis
diuretic
infusion
minibottle
parenteral fluid
piggyback
preformed water
profuse
pureed
water balance

INTAKE AND OUTPUT

Rationale for the Use of This Skill

Many illnesses cause changes in the body's ability to maintain fluid balance. Intake can be decreased as a result of anorexia, nausea, vomiting, and many other conditions. Output can be altered by various disease processes in the body, especially kidney and heart problems. There are a number of drugs in current use that alter urinary elimination. These and many other conditions make a careful measurement of both intake and output essential to total patient assessment. A record of this measurement is maintained for the use of all health team members.[1]

Initiating Measurement

A patient's fluid intake and fluid output (I and O) may be measured for a variety of reasons. For example, *you may initiate measuring to assess whether a patient is taking adequate fluids or to verify that the output is adequate for optimum kidney function.* This specific information may be important to a complete and accurate assessment. Patients taking drugs that may cause water retention as a side effect also may be placed on intake and output measurement. Urinary output may be measured to evaluate the effectiveness of a diuretic, a drug given to increase urinary output.

The physician may order that intake and output be measured for any of these reasons or *for diagnosis and treatment progress.* Most post-op patients and patients with indwelling catheters are routinely on intake and output measurement. For some patients whose water balance is crucial, daily weights are ordered as well.

Items Measured

Intake

Measure all items that are naturally fluid at room temperature. These include water, milk, juice, and all other beverages, as well as ice cream, gelatin, and soups. Do *not* measure pu-

reed foods; *they are simply solids that are prepared in a different form.*

Patients on intake and output measurement receive a full water pitcher of 1000 ml. When the water in the pitcher is changed, the amount remaining is measured in a container, the water is discarded, and the difference is "credited" to the patient's intake because the patient actually took this amount. Occasionally a patient on restricted fluids will not have a water pitcher at the bedside. For such a patient, the small amount of water needed to take oral medications should be calculated *because this amount will be deducted from the amount of fluid allowed the patient.*

Any solution that is infused intravenously, including blood products and irrigating solutions that are not returned, are included in intake.

Output

Urine is the major output item that is measured. In the healthy person, "the volume of urine excreted is approximately equal to the volume of oral fluid ingested, and water derived from solid food and from chemical oxidation in the body approximately equals the normal losses of water through the lungs and skin and in the stool" (Metheny and Snively, 1983, p. 11). If the losses of water through the skin and stool become excessive, they should be measured and added to the output. For example, this measurement is appropriate if the patient has diarrhea or profuse diaphoresis.

Vomitus, drainage from suction devices, wound drainage, and bleeding are abnormal losses of fluid. They should always be measured or estimated.

Units of Measurement

Depending on the hospital and the forms used, intake and output are measured in either cubic centimeters (cc) or metric liquid units called milliliters (ml). The cubic centimeter is a milliliter equivalent. It is far preferable to use the milliliter, which is the liquid unit, as a standard *because it lends itself more easily to calculations that require the conversion of liquid and weight measures. Intravenous fluids have been standardized in metric measurements for this reason also.*

Accurate intake and output records are greatly fa-

[1]You will note that rationale for action is emphasized throughout the module by the use of italics.

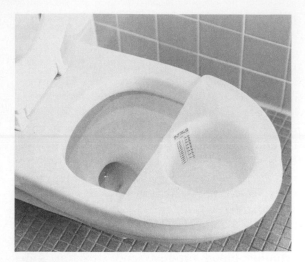

FIGURE 15.1 A "HAT" USED FOR URINE COLLECTION
Courtesy Ivan Ellis

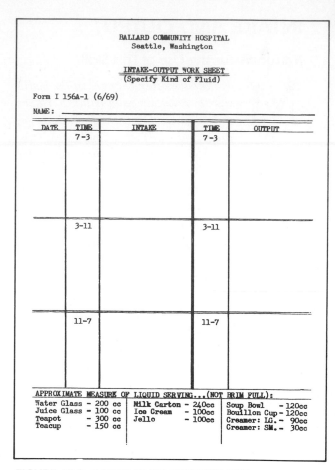

FIGURE 15.2 INTAKE-OUTPUT WORKSHEET

cilitated when the patient is involved in the process. Assess the patient's knowledge base. *If the patient understands what is to be done and the reasons for doing it,* he or she may even remind personnel of the need to measure intake and output. Also, the patient will be more conscientious in saving all urine for measurement and may even assist with recording intake.

A device that is helpful for measuring urine is a collection "hat" made of plastic. It resembles a hat which, when placed upside down, fits the seat of the toilet or commode so that urine can collect in it as the female patient urinates. A male patient can use a urinal for collection. (See Figure 15.1.)

Record Keeping

Bedside Records

First, a record must be kept at the patient's bedside or in the patient's room *so that measurements can be recorded immediately.* A form is often taped near the wash basin or on the door as a reminder to the health care team. Make a complete listing of the items measured and their quantities on this record. Many of these forms list the metric equivalents of the U.S. standard units of liquid measurement. (See Figure 15.2.)

Permanent Records

There is a special record form on the patient's chart for making a permanent record of the patient's intake and output (see Figure 15.3). Do not record individual items on this form, but do record totals for each 8-hour or 24-hour period (according to the hospital's procedure) for each category. Thus, the intake record might include a figure for oral intake, one for intravenous fluid intake, one for miscellaneous intake, and a *total* intake figure. The output is recorded similarly, with totals for each category and then a comprehensive total for all outputs.

Parenteral fluids (those given by infusion) may be recorded on an independent record (see Figure 15.4).

304

FLUID BALANCE RECORD

DATE	SHIFT	FLUID INTAKE				FLUID OUTPUT				
		ORAL	PARENTERAL	BLOOD	8 HR. TOTALS	URINE	GASTRIC	DRAINAGE	OTHER	8 HR. TOTALS
	11-7									
	7-3									
	3-11									
	24 HR. TOTAL									
	11-7									
	7-3									
	3-11									
	24 HR. TOTAL									
	11-7									
	7-3									
	3-11									
	24 HR. TOTAL									
	11-7									
	7-3									
	3-11									
	24 HR. TOTAL									

BALLARD COMMUNITY HOSPITAL
Seattle, Washington

FLUID BALANCE RECORD

FIGURE 15.3 *INTAKE-OUTPUT RECORD FOR PATIENT'S CHART*

PARENTERAL FLUID SHEET

DATE	TIME	NO.	SOLUTION	ADDITIVES	Amount Start	Time De'd	Amount Remaining	Total Amt. Given	Signature & Remarks

BALLARD COMMUNITY HOSPITAL
Seattle, Washington

PARENTERAL FLUID SHEET

FIGURE 15.4 PARENTERAL FLUID SHEET

Procedure

Assessment

1. Check the orders to learn whether the physician has ordered intake and output to be measured. If this has not been ordered, I and O may be initiated as a nursing action. Be sure to write this on the plan of care *so that others on the team are aware of measurement.*

2. Review the patient's status, including diagnosis, presence of intravenous infusions, medications being taken, the presence of an indwelling catheter, and other factors that would make the measurement of intake and output a helpful assessment tool for this patient.

3. Assess the patient's knowledge base concerning the procedure. Establish whether the patient will be able to participate in keeping accurate records.

Planning

4. Locate the intake-output worksheet at the patient's bedside. Some facilities attach these sheets above the bathroom sink; others, to the door of the room. Familiarize yourself with the location at your facility.

5. Determine the extent to which the patient will participate in keeping records.

Implementation

6. Explain or reinforce the reasons for accurate measurement to the patient.

7. Encourage the patient to participate. Helping you compute the values *makes some patients feel more involved in their own care.*

8. After a meal, record on the I and O sheet the amount of each fluid item taken. (Compute partial intake of any fluid item. This figure may have to be an estimate, except for a patient on very strict measurement for medical reasons.)

9. Add free water. Include any given with medications if indicated.

10. Add any nourishment given between meals.

11. To perform the following, put on a pair of clean gloves to protect yourself from contact with body fluids. With each voiding, use the measuring container to accurately measure the urine. Again, the patient may wish to do this for you and can be instructed to keep an accurate account. Any fecal material should be removed from the container for accuracy. Toilet tissue displacement can be approximated and is usually not removed. It is sometimes easier to pour off the urine from the bedpan in order to measure it. If the patient has an indwelling catheter, measure the contents of the drainage bag at the end of the shift or earlier, if it becomes full.

12. Record the output on the I and O sheet, using the proper column (see Figure 15.2).

13. On the parenteral fluid sheet, add any intravenous fluids given in the manner prescribed by your facility. Include "mini-bottles" of fluid given with medications as well as large bottles or bags ordered for fluid content (see Figure 15.3).

14. Using the permanent intake and output record for the patient's chart, fill in the totals from the intake-output worksheet and the parenteral fluid sheet (see Figure 15.4).

15. Add any other output, including liquid stools, emesis, and any drainage of considerable volume. The quantity of some of these items will have to be estimated; even so, they should be added.

16. Note any profuse diaphoresis.

17. Total all your eight-hour measurements at the end of your shift on the record in the chart.

Evaluation

18. Compare the intake and output figures for a general estimate of fluid balance. If there is a marked difference, review the intake and output balance for the last several days.

19. Compare the intake and output figures with the recommended norms for intake for a person of that age and health status.

REFERENCE

Metheny, Norma Millian, and W. D. Snively, Jr. *Nurses' Handbook of Fluid Balance.* 4th ed. Philadelphia: J.B. Lippincott Company, 1983.

PERFORMANCE CHECKLIST				

Intake and output	Unsatisfactory	Needs More Practice	Satisfactory	Comments
Assessment				
1. Check orders.				
2. Review the patient's status.				
3. Establish patient's ability to participate.				
Planning				
4. Locate intake-output worksheet.				
5. Decide extent to which patient may participate.				
Implementation				
6. Explain reasons for I and O to patient.				
7. Encourage the patient to participate.				
8. After meals, record intake and output.				
9. Add free water taken.				
10. Add between-meal nourishment.				
11. Each time patient voids, accurately measure amount of urine.				
12. Record output on I and O worksheet, using proper column.				
13. On parenteral fluid sheet, record any intravenous fluids.				
14. On permanent record in chart, fill in totals.				
15. Add any other output other than urinary totals.				
16. Note any profuse diaphoresis.				
17. Total all eight-hour measurements at the end of your shift.				
Evaluation				
18. Compare intake to output.				
19. Compare intake and output to norms for patient.				

QUIZ

Multiple-Choice Questions

_____ 1. Intake and output are measured in metric units because

a. metric weights and measures lend themselves to easier conversion from one to another.
b. metric measures are more accurate.
c. intravenous fluids are measured in metric units.
d. nursing is a science, and scientific disciplines use metric measures.

_____ 2. The intake-output worksheet is used primarily to

a. show the patient his or her fluid status.
b. total fluid intake and output.
c. record the various items of fluid intake and output at the bedside.
d. provide a permanent record of intake and output.

_____ 3. The permanent record of intake and output is usually kept

a. on the worksheet.
b. in the nurse's notes.
c. on a special form in the chart.
d. on the graphic record with temperature and vital signs.

_____ 4. The following items should be included in the total measurement of intake: (1) dietary fluids; (2) irrigation fluids returned; (3) gelatin; (4) fluids at bedside; (5) cereal; (6) ice cream; (7) intravenous fluids; (8) pureed fruits and vegetables.

a. 1, 4, 7, and 8
b. 1, 3, 4, 6, and 7
c. 1, 2, 4, 5, and 7
d. All of these

_____ 5. The following items should be included in the total measurement of output: (1) urine; (2) normal stools; (3) diarrheal stools; (4) vomitus; (5) normal perspiration; (6) excessive perspiration; (7) wound drainage.

a. 1, 3, 4, 6, and 7
b. 1, 4, 5, 6, and 7
c. 1, 3, and 4
d. All of these

6. In checking the I and O sheet for a certain elderly patient, Jane Smith, RN, noted that the 8-hour intake total was recorded as 720 ml, which was larger than usual. She then checked the worksheet on which the exact items taken were recorded. The following items were listed:

Breakfast	Snack
cereal, 60 ml	pureed peaches, 100 ml
half and half, 50 ml	
apple juice, 100 ml	Lunch
(water pitcher changed, 100 ml)	pureed peas, 60 ml
	pureed meat, 50 ml
	applesauce, 100 ml
	milk, 100 ml

Jane Smith determined that an error had been made. The error resulted from

  a. incorrect addition.
  b. including in the morning shift water that had actually been taken from the pitcher during the previous 8-hour shift.
  c. including amounts for things that should not have been included.

7. A patient has taken the following amounts during the day shift (7:00 a.m.–3:00 p.m.). This hospital records all intake and output for twenty-four-hour periods only. At the end of *your* shift, what will you record on the intake and output record?

Breakfast	Lunch	Snack
juice, 100 ml	milk, 240 ml	gelatin, 50 ml
milk, 90 ml	pureed peaches, 50 ml	
coffee, 150 ml		Water Pitcher
		500 ml

  a. 1080 ml
  b. 1130 ml
  c. 1180 ml
  d. Nothing should be recorded at that time.

8. Totals over 24-hour periods are helpful because

  a. intake and output balance usually cannot be identified over shorter time periods.
  b. they reduce the time needed for record keeping.
  c. physicians usually check them once every 24 hours.
  d. a 24-hour total is most accurate.

9. The following items were eaten by Mr. Jones. What is his total intake for the day shift?

Water Pitcher, 7:00 a.m.
100 ml

Water Pitcher Change, 2:30 p.m.
300 ml

Breakfast
coffee, 250 ml
juice, 90 ml

Dinner
coffee, 250 ml

Snack
juice, 100 ml

Water Pitcher Change
and Snack, 8:30 p.m.
broth, 150 ml
water, 350 ml

Lunch
milk, 240 ml

   a. 980 ml
   b. 1080 ml
   c. 1230 ml
   d. 1330 ml

10. If the facility in question 9 records intake every eight hours, the total recorded by the nurse working from 3:00 p.m. to 11:00 p.m. would be

   a. 450 ml
   b. 750 ml
   c. 1400 ml
   d. zero.

11. Mr. Jones had an output of 400 ml for the two shifts. This might indicate

   a. Not enough data is given to identify the problem.
   b. water intoxication.
   c. edema formation.
   d. kidney malfunction.

12. Mr. Ford is to have all intake and output measured. He is 45 years old, a truck driver, father of four, and he has been admitted with a possible kidney infection. In planning for accurate measurement, you would

   a. measure all urine yourself because this is a critical concern.
   b. see that urine is measured by a staff person (aide, LPN, RN), to guarantee accuracy.
   c. have Mr. Ford measure his own urine and record it.
   d. ask Mr. Ford if he would prefer to measure his output himself or have a staff person do it.

MODULE 16

Temperature, Pulse, and Respiration

MODULE CONTENTS

PREREQUISITES

Successful completion of the following modules:

OVERALL OBJECTIVE

To measure and record patients' temperature, pulse, and respiration accurately and safely, recognizing deviations from the norm.

SPECIFIC LEARNING OBJECTIVES

Know Facts and Principles	Apply Facts and Principles	Demonstrate Ability	Evaluate Performance
State normal oral, rectal, and axillary temperature range in both Celsius and Fahrenheit measurements	Give examples of factors that can cause variations in body temperature	Demonstrate taking patient's temperature, using both Fahrenheit and Celsius thermometers, observing proper technique and safety precautions. On both graphic and nurses' notes, record data clearly and accurately.	Evaluate own performance using Performance Checklist

1. *Body temperature*
   a. *Normal body temperature*
   b. *Methods of measurement*
   c. *Measurement procedures*
   d. *Documentation*

2. *Pulse*
  a. Normal pulse rate
  b. Pulse rate procedure
  c. Documentation
	Define normal pulse rates for different age groups	Identify factors that influence pulse rate	Count patient's pulse accurately, both radial and apical.
			On graphic, record pulse in proper location; on nurses' notes, record pulse in numerical and descriptive terms.
				Evaluate own performance using Performance Checklist

3. *Respiration*
  a. Normal respiratory rate
  b. Respiratory rate procedure
  c. Documentation
	Identify normal respiratory rates for different age groups	Relate factors that influence respiratory rates	Determine patient's respiratory rate using correct technique.
			Record rate and character of respiration on graphic and nurses' notes.
				Evaluate own performance using Performance Checklist

LEARNING ACTIVITIES

1. Review the Specific Learning Objectives.
2. Read the chapter on oxygenation, circulation, and neurological function in Ellis and Nowlis, *Nursing: A Human Needs Approach,* or a comparable chapter in another textbook.
3. Look up the module vocabulary terms in the Glossary.
4. Read through the module, taking note of the graphic chart used to record vital signs (see Figure 16.1).
5. Review the steps of the procedure in the Performance Checklist.
6. In the practice setting:
   a. Inspect and become familiar with the TPR equipment.
   b. Select a partner. Take your partner's oral and axillary temperatures and compare the two findings.
   c. Record the oral temperature reading on the vital signs graphic chart (see Figure 16.1).
   d. Have your partner drink a glass of cold water and retake the oral temperature in twenty minutes. How does this reading compare with the one taken previously?
   e. If an electronic thermometer is available, retake your partner's temperature and compare this reading with the reading from the conventional thermometer.
   f. With your partner in a supine position, count the radial pulse and record it. Record the quality of the pulse felt on a progress sheet or a piece of paper.
   g. After your partner has exercised briskly (running in place) for three minutes, retake the pulse and compare the rate and quality with that of the radial pulse taken previously.
   h. Choose another student in the practice setting. Then you and your partner take an apical-radial pulse on the student. What would you consider normal? Why?
   i. Repeat steps f, g, and h, this time measuring respiration.
   j. Complete the vital signs graphic and turn it in to your instructor.

7. In the clinical setting:
   a. Check the form used by your facility, the type of equipment being used, and the cleaning method for thermometers.
   b. Take a TPR on a patient. Follow the procedure with supervision and record your results.
   c. If possible, repeat the TPR procedure four hours later on the same patient · and compare the two readings. Which of the measurements has changed? What might this indicate about the patient's condition?

VOCABULARY

Temperature

   axilla
   Celsius
   centigrade
   circadian rhythm
   Fahrenheit
   febrile
   fever
   intermittent
   metabolism
   remittent
   Sims's position

Pulse

   apical pulse
   bounding pulse
   bradycardia
   carotid artery
   dorsalis pedis artery
   femoral artery
   midclavicular line
   pedal pulse
   pulse deficit
   pulse pressure
   radial artery
   tachycardia
   temporal artery
   thready pulse

Respiration

apnea
Cheyne-Stokes
dyspnea
Kussmaul's respirations
orthopnea
rhythm
stertorous
symmetry

TEMPERATURE, PULSE, AND RESPIRATION

Rationale for the Use of This Skill

*B*ecause temperature, pulse, and respiration (TPR)[1] are basic measurements that are helpful in assessing patients' conditions, it is essential that the practicing nurse be able to take and record them accurately. TPRs are taken by both professional and nonprofessional staff in health care settings. Both can perform the mechanics of the procedure equally well. The professional nurse, however, has the responsibility to understand the deviations from normal on which assessments and interpretations are based.

After completing this module, you should be able to accurately define, carry out, and record these signs. You should be able to adapt this procedure to both well and ill individuals of any age group and make appropriate interpretations of your findings. Then you will be able to move on to Module 17, Blood Pressure, which will complete the material on vital signs.[2]

General Considerations

The taking of TPR is important *because it serves as an indicator of a patient's health status.* Most institutions have routine times for taking TPR—often q.4h. (every four hours)—*but a patient's illness or certain other conditions may dictate more or less frequent measurement.* For example, you would make an independent nursing decision to take the temperature of a flushed patient who complains of feeling warm. Routine TPR is usually taken on a number of patients at one time, and the readings are recorded on paper at the bedside. These readings are then transcribed either to a central clipboard at the nurses' station or directly on the graphic record in the patient's chart (see Figure 16.1).

---

[1]TPR is the symbol for one procedure measuring temperature, pulse, and respiration. VS stands for *vital signs* and includes the measurement of blood pressure as well as TPR.

[2]You will note that rationale for action is emphasized throughout the module by the use of italics.

Temperature

Body temperature is the balance between heat produced and heat lost by the body. It is surprisingly consistent in healthy individuals; that is, a normal oral reading is 98.6° Fahrenheit or 37° Celsius (sometimes called *centigrade*). Actually, body temperature can register 97–99° F or 36.1–37.2° C and still be considered normal in healthy individuals.

There is also a normal daily temperature variation that results from circadian rhythm. The lowest temperature occurs between about 2 and 6 a.m., and the highest between about 4 and 8 p.m.

Many factors—age, presence of infection, temperature of the environment, amount of exercise, metabolism, and emotional status—can affect a patient's temperature and should be taken into consideration when evaluating a temperature reading. If the temperature is elevated, the patient is *febrile*, that is, has a fever. Depending on the fluctuations of the elevation, the temperature can be described as *remittent* or *intermittent*. (See Glossary.)

Types of Thermometers With a mercury-in-glass thermometer, temperature can be measured orally, rectally, or by placing the thermometer in the axilla. The mercury in the thermometer expands as it is heated. Therefore, when the mercury enclosed in the thermometer comes into contact with warm body tissues, it expands and registers a temperature on the glass tube in which it is housed.

The oral mercury thermometer has a slender bulb designed *to provide a large surface for exposure when it is placed under the tongue.* The rectal mercury thermometer has a pear-shaped bulb, and the multi-use thermometer has a blunt, stubby tip. This latter type of thermometer may be used in the oral, rectal, or axillary site, and is frequently used for children, *as it is considered the safest.* (See Figure 16.2.)

The obvious disadvantage of the glass thermometer is that it is breakable and could cause injury at any site, if not used with care. Although mercury can give off harmful vapors upon exposure to air, the amount of mercury in an individual thermometer is so small as to be of no consequence. If ingested, it oxidizes too slowly to be absorbed, and so it is not toxic.

Electronic thermometers (Figure 16.3) are available for oral and rectal use. These thermometers use a component called a thermister at the end

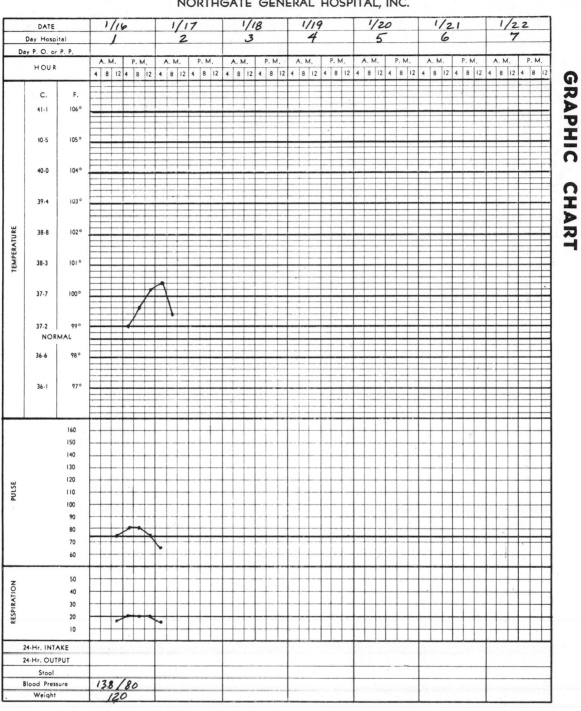

FIGURE 16.1 VITAL SIGNS GRAPHIC FORM

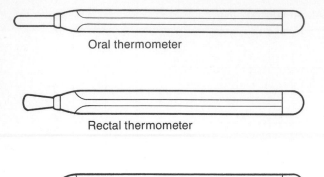

Oral thermometer

Rectal thermometer

Multi-use thermometer

FIGURE 16.2 ORAL AND RECTAL THERMOMETERS *A:* Oral thermometer; *B:* Rectal thermometer; *C:* Multi-use thermometer

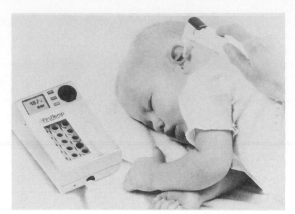

FIGURE 16.4 FIRST TEMP™ THERMOMETER
Courtesy Intelligent Medical Systems, Inc., Carlsbad, California

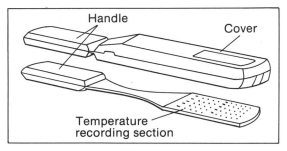

Handle Cover

Temperature
recording section

FIGURE 16.5 CHEMICAL THERMOMETER

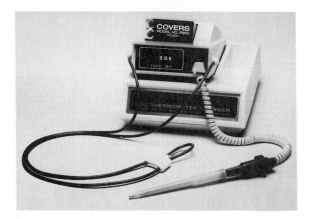

FIGURE 16.3 ELECTRONIC THERMOMETER IVAC 811 Electronic Clinical Thermometer System
Courtesy IVAC Corporation, San Diego, California

of a plastic and stainless steel probe to sense the temperature. While the temperature is being measured, the probe is covered with a disposable probe cover, which is discarded after each use. The temperature is read on a digital display that resets itself when the probe is replaced in the body of the battery-powered recording device. The electronic thermometer is carried from one patient to another, along with a sufficient supply of disposable probe covers. It therefore is not useful in cases of infectious disease, unless it can stay in the room and be used by one patient only. Most facilities do not own enough electronic thermometers to use them in this way, so mercury thermometers are commonly used in such situations.

FirstTemp™ is a new type of electronic thermometer that uses infrared technology to mea-

sure the temperature from the tympanic site. A covered probe is placed at the external opening of the ear canal, where it senses the infrared energy produced by the tympanic membrane. (See Figure 16.4.) The tympanic temperature is registered on a digital display in about one second. *Because the ear canal has no mucous membranes,* it is not easily influenced by evaporation or other ambient changes and has demonstrated reliable correlation with the body's core temperature. Cerumen does not affect the integrity of the readings, and if one ear shows evidence of otitis, the other can be used. The same nonintrusive probe covers may be used for both infants and adults.

Chemical dot thermometers are disposable and consist of a flat plastic device holding many temperature-sensing chemical "dots" that change color when they reach a certain temperature. (See Figure 16.5.) They are unbreakable and considered somewhat less precise than mercury or electronic thermometers.

Sites for Measuring Temperatures The best site for measuring the patient's temperature in the clinical setting is the oral site, with the ther-

320

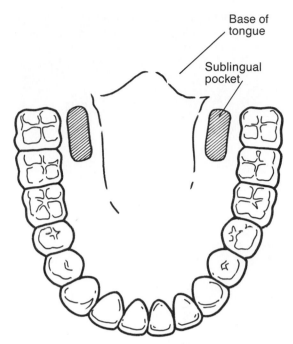

FIGURE 16.6 SUBLINGUAL POCKETS

TABLE 16.1 Approximate Pulse and Respiration Rates By Age		
	Pulse	**Respiration**
Newborn	120	35
4-Year-old	100	23
8-Year-old	90	20
14-Year-old	85	20
Adult	80	18

mometer placed in the left or right posterior sublingual pocket (Erickson, 1976, 1980). (See Figure 16.6.) The sublingual area has an abundant blood supply from the nearby carotid arteries and the central circulation at the heart. Contraindications to use of the oral site include pain or inflammation in the mouth, jaws being wired shut, or the inability of a small child or confused or unconscious patient to cooperate. Also, if a patient has recently ingested hot or cold food or beverages or has smoked, you should wait 20–30 minutes before taking an oral temperature *to ensure accuracy* (Erickson, 1983). Research indicates that oral temperatures may be taken in patients who are receiving oxygen by nasal cannula without concern about inaccuracy (Graas, 1974).

The rectal site may be used when the oral site is contraindicated. Although the rectal temperature is often higher than the oral, the rectum is farther from the central circulation, and so it is generally considered a less desirable site, in terms of both accuracy and acceptability to the patient. (A rectal temperature is usually about 0.7° F or 0.4° C higher than an oral temperature in a given individual.) The rectal site is frequently frightening to infants and small children, and there is danger of rectal ulceration or perforation because of the very small anal cavity.

Research indicates that, contrary to popular belief, the rectal site is safe as an alternative site for cardiac patients; there is little evidence to support the theory that reflex slowing of the heart occurs as a result of vagal stimulation (Earnest, 1969; Gruber, 1974).

The axilla is generally considered the least desirable site in the adult patient *because it is not close to major blood vessels and because it is more likely to be affected by the environmental temperature.* (An axillary temperature is usually lower than an oral one by 1° F or 0.6° C.) It is, however, recommended for infants and small children *because it is less frightening and safer.* Your facility may have policies concerning specific age groups and/or situations.

Pulse

When the left ventricle contracts, blood is pushed out into the arterial circulation. This can be felt in various places as the arterial pulse.

Pulse rates vary greatly among adults. A heart rate of around 70 is often considered "normal," although the American Heart Association states that a normal pulse rate may be 50 to 100 beats per minute. (See Table 16.1 for normal pulse rates for infants, children, and adults.) The pulse rate can increase or decrease *as a result of changes in body temperature.* Exercise, the application of heat or cold, medications, emotions, hemorrhage, and heart disease can all affect pulse rates as well. The term *bradycardia* describes an adult pulse rate below 60 per minute; *tachycardia* refers to an adult pulse rate above 100.

The quality and rhythm of the pulse must also be observed and described. Terms such as "full" or "bounding" are often used to describe

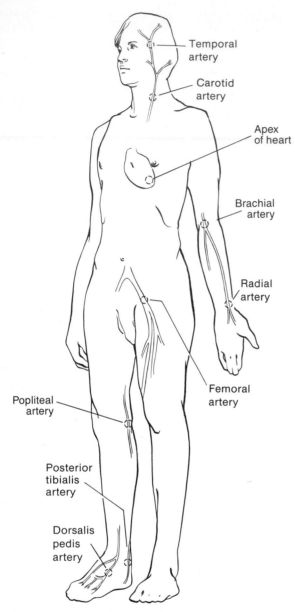

FIGURE 16.7 PULSE POINTS

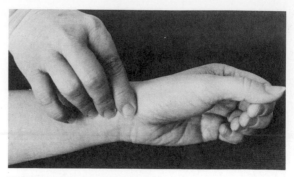

FIGURE 16.8 RADIAL PULSE
Courtesy Ivan Ellis

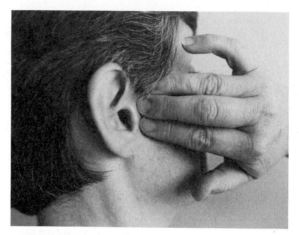

FIGURE 16.9 TEMPORAL PULSE
Courtesy Ivan Ellis

a strong pulse, and "thready" or "weak" might be used to describe a pulse of diminished strength.

A pulse is taken to evaluate the circulation distal to that point and to measure the rate, rhythm, and quality of the heartbeat. See Figure 16.7 for the location of various pulse points.

Peripheral Pulses Some of the peripheral pulses commonly assessed include the following:

Radial pulse Feel for the radial artery with the patient's arm positioned alongside the body, palm downward. Curl two or three of your fingers around the wrist on the thumb side and palpate gently. This site is used routinely to measure the pulse rate because of its convenience and accessibility. (See Figure 16.8.)

Temporal pulse Feel for the superficial temporal artery, which passes upward just in front of the ear. Palpate gently, using the tips of two or three fingers. This pulse is often used in infants and when the radial pulse is not accessible. (See Figure 16.9.)

Carotid pulse Feel for the carotid pulse by locating the larynx (voice box) and sliding two or three fingers off into the groove beside it. You should feel for the pulse on your side of the patient *to avoid compressing the other carotid artery*

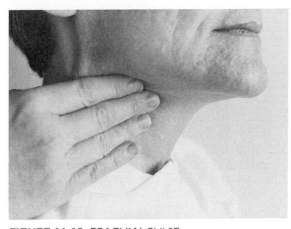

FIGURE 16.10 BRACHIAL PULSE
Courtesy Ivan Ellis

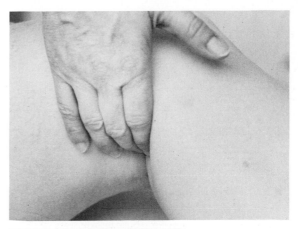

FIGURE 16.12 POPLITEAL PULSE
Courtesy Ivan Ellis

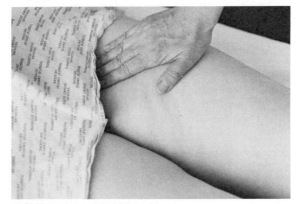

FIGURE 16.11 FEMORAL PULSE
Courtesy Ivan Ellis

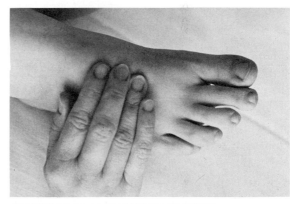

FIGURE 16.13 DORSALIS PEDIS PULSE
Courtesy Ivan Ellis

with your thumb. (See Figure 32.3.) The carotid pulse is used during adult CPR and to assess circulation to the head.

Brachial pulse Feel for the brachial artery, which is located near the center of the antecubital space, toward the little finger. Have the patient rest the arm palm upward, and use two or three fingers to locate the pulse. This pulse is commonly used to measure blood pressure. (See Figure 16.10.) See Module 32 for use of the brachial pulse during infant CPR.

Femoral pulse You may need to press harder to locate the femoral pulse, found about halfway between the anterior superior iliac spine and the symphysis pubis, below the inguinal ligament. Remember to respect the patient's privacy when attempting to locate this pulse. It is used to assess circulation to the leg and to evaluate chest compressions during CPR. (See Figure 16.11.)

Popliteal pulse With the patient's leg in a flexed position, feel behind the knee in the popliteal fossa. Again, you may need to press more deeply to locate this pulse. It is useful in assessing the circulation to the lower leg and when measuring the blood pressure using the leg. (See Figure 16.12.)

Pedal pulses Feel for the *dorsalis pedis pulse* on the dorsum (top) of the foot with the foot plantar flexed, if possible. This pulse is easily obliterated, so feel gently. You will find the pulse about halfway between the middle of the patient's ankle and the space between the great toe and the second toe. (See Figure 16.13.)

Feel for the *posterior tibial pulse* by curving your fingers behind and a little below the medial malleolus of the ankle. This pulse is often difficult to feel in the obese patient or the patient with considerable edema. (See Figure 16.14.)

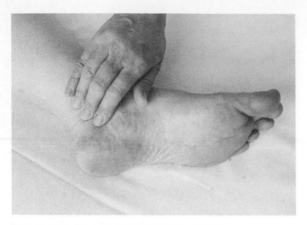

FIGURE 16.14 POSTERIOR TIBIAL PULSE
Courtesy Ivan Ellis

These last two pulses are used to assess circulation to the foot. If a patient has had surgery on blood vessels leading to the foot, you may be asked to mark the dorsalis pedis and/or the posterior tibial pulse with a marking pen so that these pulses can be located more easily.

Apical Pulse The apical pulse is measured by listening over the apex of the heart on the left side of the chest, using a stethoscope. The apex is usually found at the fifth intercostal space just inside the midclavicular line. You may need to move your stethoscope around in this general area to find the spot where the individual patient's apical pulse is heard most clearly. This pulse is often measured for a full minute before the administration of certain heart medications that might be withheld if the pulse is either too fast or too slow. The apical pulse is also used in infants, whose pulse rates are often difficult to determine using peripheral sites.

The *apical-radial pulse* is sometimes required when a patient has a cardiovascular disorder. Two persons are needed to take this pulse. Nurse 1 measures the pulse apically using a stethoscope, while at the same time nurse 2 takes the pulse by palpating the radial artery. The pulse is measured for a full minute, using a single watch that is placed in a convenient location where both nurses can see it. If the radial pulse is lower than the apical, the difference is called the *pulse deficit*. This means that some of the contractions of the heart are not strong enough to push a wave of blood that can be felt at the radial site.

Respiration

The act of breathing is involuntary but can be affected by voluntary control. Respirations are normally regular, even, and quiet, but they can be affected by all of the same factors that cause the pulse rate to vary. A rate of 16 to 20 is considered "normal" for the adult. (See Table 16.1 for the normal respiratory rates for infants, children, and adults.)

The depth and character of respirations must also be observed and described. Respiratory and metabolic disorders can cause variations, as can other acute and chronic problems. The sides of the chest may not rise and fall symmetrically. The term "dyspnea" can be used to describe any breathing difficulty, but a more specific description that includes both depth and any pattern that varies from normal should be included as well. The term "Cheyne-Stokes" respirations is used to describe a gradual increase and decrease in the rate and depth of respirations, usually including a period of apnea at the end of each cycle. Any periods of apnea noted should be timed. Check the vocabulary list and refer to the glossary for more terminology related to respiration.

In this module, the procedure lists the steps for taking the TPR of one patient. Blood pressure measurement is described in Module 17, Blood Pressure. If you are taking routine TPRs on several patients at once, adapt the steps below to accommodate more than one individual.

Procedure

Assessment

1. A doctor's order is not needed for the taking of TPR or vital signs. When a patient's condition is serious, however, the physician may order vital signs to be taken more frequently than normal. After surgery, when the patient is in the recovery phase, pulse, respirations, and blood pressure are taken every 15 minutes until the patient is alert or the signs are stable. The temperature of a patient with a fever should be checked hourly. The nurse can check TPR at his or her own discretion to assess the patient's health status. Find out the times at which routine vital signs are taken in your facility.

324

2. Assess the patient's readiness for the procedure. If the patient is smoking, eating, or drinking a hot or cold beverage, the reading will be altered, so wait at least 20–30 minutes before proceeding. Sometimes, because of a change in the patient's condition, you will have to change the route for taking the temperature. If you are taking TPRs on a number of patients at the same time, you may be carrying out this assessment as part of the procedure at the bedside of each.

Planning
3. Wash your hands *for asepsis.*
4. Choose the equipment you will need.
   a. Temperature: mercury or electronic thermometer from central storage area or from patient's bedside. If a rectal thermometer is to be used, obtain a lubricant.
   b. Pulse: a watch—digital or with a sweep second hand.
   c. Respirations: the watch described above.
   d. Vital signs board or paper and pencil from unit.

Implementation
5. Identify the patient *to be sure you are performing the procedure on the correct patient.*
6. Explain what you are going to do.
7. Be sure room lighting is adequate so that you can accurately read the thermometer.
8. Assist the patient to a position of comfort.
9. Proceed with the following:
   a. *Temperature*
      (1) *Oral*   Shake down the mercury thermometer with a quick snap of the wrist. It should register below 95°F, or 36°C, before you begin. Place the thermometer carefully in either the left or right posterior sublingual pocket at the base of the tongue. Ask the patient to hold his or her mouth open until you see that the thermometer is correctly placed, then instruct the patient to close the lips gently and breathe through the nose. Leave the thermometer in place for 8 minutes *to ensure accurate*

measurement (Nichols and Kucha, 1972). Some argue that although the difference between the temperature after 3 minutes and after 8 minutes is *statistically* significant, it is not *clinically* significant (Graves and Markarian, 1980; Baker, Cerone, Gaze, and Knapp, 1984). We urge you to consider the factors in each individual situation (such as time of day and temperature of the environment) when you decide how long to leave the thermometer in place, especially since temperature is often measured in the morning, when it is the lowest in its normal daily cycle.

   Remove the thermometer and wipe it, with a twisting motion, from your fingers to the bulb—*from clean to dirty.* Discard the tissue. Holding the thermometer at eye level, read it without touching the bulb end, and write down your finding on paper. Then shake down the thermometer.

      (2) *Rectal*   Shake down the mercury thermometer as you would an oral thermometer. Lubricate the clean rectal thermometer *to prevent damage to the rectal mucosa.* Insert the bulb end at least 1.5 inches into the rectum, with the patient lying on his or her side in Sims's position. Always hold the thermometer with your hand *to prevent displacement or breakage if the patient moves suddenly.* Leave the thermometer in place for a full three minutes (Nichols, 1972). Remove, clean, and read the thermometer as before. When you transfer the patient's temperature to the graphic form, mark (R) next to it, *to indicate that it was taken rectally.*
      (3) *Axillary*   Take axillary temperatures using the same general procedure. Place the tip of the thermometer in the center

of the armpit and keep the patient's arm held tightly against the side of the chest for 9 minutes in the adult (Nichols, Ruskin, Glor, and Kelly, 1966). One study indicated that 3 minutes may be adequate for infants weighing less than 6.5 pounds, 5 minutes for children weighing between 6.5 pounds and 13 pounds, and 7 minutes for children between 14 and 66 pounds (Hauck, 1984).

Again, when you transfer the patient's temperature to the graphic form, mark (*A*) next to it, *to indicate axillary measurement.*

(4) *Electronic thermometer* Follow the manufacturer's instructions that come with the device. A clean rigid plastic probe cover is used each time a temperature is measured. Push the probe into a cover (see Figure 16.3) and place the probe in the patient's mouth as described for mercury thermometers. The display panel will register the temperature reading in 30 to 50 seconds. Next, push the button on the probe to discard the probe cover, and replace the probe. This will automatically reset the thermometer, and it will be ready for the next use.

With an electronic thermometer there is a minimal effect on the result of the temperature measurement if the patient is unable to keep his or her mouth closed during the procedure. Therefore, you can obtain a valid reading with the patient's mouth either closed or open.

When the thermometer is used rectally, the oral probe is replaced by a rectal probe, which is covered with a probe cover and lubricated before use.

(5) Clean the thermometer according to the policy in your facility. If mercury thermometers are in use in the clinical setting, each patient often has an individual thermometer. After removing saliva or mucus, using a twisting motion toward the bulb end, wash the thermometer with soap and cool water. Then replace it in the holder by the bedside.

A thermometer sheath can be used *to keep the thermometer itself from direct contact with the patient.* The sheath is a tube of very thin plastic that comes wrapped in a paper strip. To use it, strip back the paper to expose the open end of the sheath. Insert the glass thermometer into the sheath and push down until it is completely protected except for the tip that you will hold in your hand. Then discard the paper covering. Insert the sheath-covered thermometer into the patient's mouth or rectum. Wait the appropriate time, then remove the thermometer. Pull the sheath down over itself and discard. Read the thermometer. Although most microorganisms are enclosed in the sheath, a simple washing with soap and cool water should be done *to ensure asepsis.*

b. *Pulse* You will use the radial artery for routine measurement of the pulse rate in most patients. In some patients, the radial pulse will not be discernible, so you will have to choose another site, such as the temporal or carotid artery. (See Figures 16.9 and 32.3.) Exert only light pressure, *so that the artery is never completely occluded. Because a patient's position can modify the pulse,* a resting pulse is usually taken with the patient in a supine position *for consistency.*

Count the pulse for 15 seconds, then multiply by four for a full minute count, if the pulse is regular. Any pulse that is irregular should be taken for a full minute. Also determine pulse rhythm and quality at this time.

326

Pulse rate using the ultrasound (Doppler) stethoscope This device is a battery-powered ultrasound instrument that detects blood flow through vessels. It is used commonly to determine blood pressure in unstable patients, but it also registers pulse rate very accurately and in a manner that is easy to hear.

You will need a Doppler instrument with stethoscope head or receiver probe, earpieces, headphones, or a speaker, and an electrode gel. The gel is placed on the end of the sound-sensitive probe. The probe is then placed over the artery while you listen with the stethoscope or headphones. The device may be adjusted to increase sensitivity. The pulse becomes audible and can be counted or simply reported as present or absent. (See Figure 17.4.)

c. *Respirations* It is best to count respirations after taking the pulse. If you use this sequence, you can keep your fingers on the patient's wrist and place the patient's arm across the chest. The patient should be unaware that you are doing another procedure and thus will continue to breathe naturally. Feeling the rise and fall of the patient's chest, count for the required 30 seconds. Multiply the result by two to determine the rate for a full minute. If a patient's respirations are very irregular, you may choose to count for a full minute *for accuracy.*

Remember to document breathing characteristics as well as rate and rhythm.

10. Wash your hands *for asepsis.*

☐ *Evaluation*

11. If the patient had any abnormal vital signs, consider retaking them if you think there is any possibility of inaccuracy.

☐ *Documentation*

12. When you are assigned to several patients, you will find that readings are sometimes difficult to remember. Keep a piece of paper in your pocket, so that after you have washed your hands, you can jot down the figures. Then transfer these numbers to a team vital signs clipboard or notebook and, later, to a graphic form in each patient's chart. Check with your facility for the routine to be used. If any of your readings are unusual or abnormal, notify the physician and make a note in the nurses' notes section of the chart.

Example of Charting   Progress Note

5/29/88
2015   Interim Note
           S "I feel like my heart is racing."
           O Radial pulse 96 and strong. Respirations 22 and deep. Has been walking in corridor for 10 minutes.
           P Return to bed. Recheck pulse and respirations in 15 minutes. Monitor closely when ambulates next.
                              C. Church, R.N.

REFERENCES

Baker, Nancy C., Sharon B. Cerone, Nancy Gaze, and Thomas R. Knapp. "The Effect of Type of Thermometer and Length of Time Inserted on Oral Temperature Measurements of Afebrile Subjects." *Nursing Research,* 33 (March–April 1984), 109–111.

Blainey, C. G. "Site Selection in Taking Body Temperature." *AJN,* 74 (October 1974), 1859–1861.

Earnest, D. L., and G. F. Fletcher. "Danger of Rectal Examination in Patients with Acute Myocardial Infarction—Fact or Fiction?" *The New England Journal of Medicine,* 281 (July 31, 1969), 238–241.

Erickson, R. "Oral Temperature Differences in Relation to Thermometer Technique." *Nursing Research,* 29 (May–June 1980), 157–164.

———. "Thermometer Placement for Oral Temperature Measurement in Febrile Adults." *International Journal of Nursing Studies,* 13 (1976), 199–208.

———. *A Sourcebook for Temperature Taking.* San Diego: IVAC Corporation, 1983.

Graas, Suzanne. "Thermometer Sites and Oxygen." *AJN*, 74 (October 1974), 1862–1863.

Graves, Ruby D., and Martha F. Markarian. "Three-Minute Time Interval when Using an Oral Mercury-in-Glass Thermometer With or Without J-Temp Sheaths." *Nursing Research*, 29 (September–October 1980), 323–324.

Gruber, P. A. "Changes in Cardiac Rate Associated with the Use of the Rectal Thermometer in the Patient with Acute Myocardial Infarction." *Heart and Lung*, 3 (March–April 1974), 288–292.

Hauck, M., K. Canclini, and B. Giordano. "The Influence of Selected Variables on Axillary Temperature Measurement in Children." Unpublished manuscript. Denver: The Children's Hospital, 1984.

Nichols, G. A. "Taking Adult Temperatures: Rectal Measurements." *AJN*, 72 (June 1972), 1092–1093.

———, and D. H. Kucha. "Taking Adult Temperatures: Oral Measurements." *AJN*, 72 (June 1972), 1091–1093.

———, R. L. Kulvi, H. R. Life, and N. M. Christ. "Measuring Oral and Rectal Temperatures of Febrile Children." *Nursing Research*, 21 (May–June 1972), 261–264.

———, M. M. Ruskin, B. A. K. Glor, and W. H. Kelly. "Oral, Axillary, and Rectal Temperature Determinations and Relationships." *Nursing Research*, 15 (Fall 1966), 307–310.

Torrance, J. T. "Temperature Readings of Premature Infants." *Nursing Research*, 17 (July–August 1968), 312–320.

PERFORMANCE CHECKLIST

Temperature, pulse, and respiration	Unsatisfactory	Needs More Practice	Satisfactory	Comments
Assessment				
1. Although a doctor's order is not needed for routine TPRs, check the policy of the facility.				
2. Assess patient's readiness.				
Planning				
3. Wash your hands.				
4. Choose equipment you will need. a. Type of thermometer				
(1) If rectal, obtain lubricant				
b. A watch—digital or with a sweep second hand— for taking pulse and respiration				
Implementation				
5. Identify patient.				
6. Explain what you are going to do.				
7. Be sure room lighting is adequate.				
8. Assist patient to a position of comfort.				
9. Proceed with the following: a. Temperature				
(1) *Oral* Shake down thermometer and place in left or right posterior sublingual pocket at base of tongue. Time for 8 minutes. Remove, wipe with tissue using a twisting motion from your fingers to the bulb, and read.				
(2) *Rectal* Shake down thermometer and lubricate bulb end. Insert at least 1.5 inches into rectum. Hold in place for three full minutes. Remove, clean, and read thermometer.				
(3) *Axillary* Place tip of thermometer in center of armpit and keep arm tight against side of chest for 9 minutes in adult patient. Remove and read.				

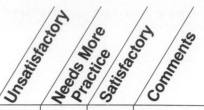

	Unsatisfactory	Needs More Practice	Satisfactory	Comments
(4) *Electronic thermometer* Cover oral or rectal probe with probe cover. For oral temperature, place in left or right posterior sublingual pocket at base of tongue. For rectal temperature, lubricate probe and insert at least 1.5 inches into rectum. Leave in place until final temperature registers on display panel—about 30 to 50 seconds. Discard probe cover and replace probe.				
(5) Clean mercury thermometer thoroughly. If washing, use cool water. Replace in holder.				
b. Pulse (1) *Radial pulse* Position patient's arm along side of body. Lightly place first fingers over radial pulse and count for 15 seconds, multiply by four, and record.				
(2) *Pedal pulse* Place first three fingers over the dorsalis pedis artery and count as you would a radial pulse.				
(3) *Apical/Radial pulse* Two nurses are required for this procedure. The first nurse takes the pulse radially at the same time that the second nurse is listening and counting the heart rate with a stethoscope over the apex of the heart. A single watch is used, and the count is for one full minute.				
(4) *Doppler pulse* Place electrode gel on end of sound-sensitive probe of Doppler device. Listen for pulse with stethoscope, earpieces, or headphones. Record rate and quality if audible.				
(5) *Newborns and infants* Take the pulse rate by listening over the apex of the heart with a stethoscope and counting the heart rate.				
c. Respiration With your fingers remaining on the patient's wrist and the arm across the chest, count the respirations for 30 seconds, multiply by two, and record.				
10. Wash your hands.				

	Unsatisfactory	Needs More Practice	Satisfactory	Comments
☐ *Evaluation*				
11. Retake any abnormal signs as necessary.				
☐ *Documentation*				
12. Record from your piece of paper to either the graphic form or the vital signs board, depending on the practice in your facility. You may have recorded directly on the board and need not record further unless there are any unusual findings to enter in the nurses' notes.				

QUIZ

Short-Answer Questions

1. The normal oral temperature for the average adult is _____ C or _____ F.

2. Four factors that may significantly change body temperature are

   a. _____

   b. _____

   c. _____

   d. _____

3. The bulb of the rectal thermometer should be lubricated in order to

   _____ .

4. The oral mercury thermometer should be held in place _____

   minutes; the rectal thermometer, _____ minutes; the axillary

   thermometer, _____ minutes; and the electronic thermometer, _____ .

5. Place a *1* beside the most accurate method of obtaining a temperature reading, a *2* beside the next most accurate method, and a *3* beside the least accurate method.

   _____ Axillary

   _____ Rectal

   _____ Oral

6. Normal pulse range for the adult at rest is _____ to _____ .

7. Four common factors that can alter pulse rate are

   a. _____

   b. _____

   c. _____

   d. _____

8. Three arteries that can be conveniently used for counting the pulse rate are

   a. _____

   b. _____

   c. _____

9. The normal rate of respiration for the adult at rest is _____ to _____ .

10. Four factors that cause changes in respiration are

    a. _____

    b. _____

    c. _____

    d. _____

MODULE 17

Blood Pressure

PREREQUISITES

Successful completion of the following modules:

OVERALL OBJECTIVE

To accurately measure and record blood pressure using a cuff, sphygmomanometer, and stethoscope.

SPECIFIC LEARNING OBJECTIVES

	Know Facts and Principles	Apply Facts and Principles	Demonstrate Ability	Evaluate Performance
1. *Definition* *a. Systolic BP* *b. Diastolic BP* *c. Norms* *d. Variables*	Define systolic and diastolic blood pressures. State norms for adults and children. List variables that affect blood pressure.	Given a patient situation, identify variables that might affect blood pressure. Given a patient situation, identify potential relationships between blood pressure and pulse. State rationale for taking blood pressure.	Promptly report blood pressures not within textbook norms as well as significant variations from baseline for particular patient	Evaluate with instructor
2. *Equipment* *a. Cuff* *b. Bladder* *c. Hand bulb and valve* *d. Sphygmomanometer (mercury gauge and aneroid gauge)* *e. Stethoscope*	Identify equipment involved in taking blood pressure. State use of equipment involved in taking blood pressure.	Identify missing or malfunctioning equipment		Evaluate own performance with instructor using Performance Checklist

336

3. *Procedure*
  a. Placement of cuff
  b. Estimation of systolic pressure
  c. Korotkoff sounds
  d. Systolic pressure
  e. Diastolic pressure
	State how blood pressure is correctly measured	Given a patient situation, identify correct and incorrect aspects of procedure	In the clinical setting, accurately measure patient's blood pressure	Blood pressure measurement by student is within 4 mm Hg of that taken by instructor

4. *Documentation*	Know how to record pressure on graphic and narrative records	Given a patient situation, identify correct recording of blood pressure	Accurately document blood pressure on appropriate records	Evaluate own performance with instructor

LEARNING ACTIVITIES	VOCABULARY

LEARNING ACTIVITIES

1. Review the Specific Learning Objectives.
2. Read the section on circulation (in the chapter on basic vital functions) in Ellis and Nowlis, *Nursing: A Human Needs Approach,* or comparable material in another textbook.
3. Look up the module vocabulary terms in the Glossary.
4. Read through the module.
5. In the practice setting:
   a. Look over and identify the parts of the blood pressure equipment in the practice setting and the clinical facility. How are they alike? Are there ways in which they differ?
   b. After reading over the procedure carefully, practice it, using another student as a patient, until you feel you can perform it adequately.
   c. Using a double, or "teaching," stethoscope (if one is available), measure your partner's blood pressure with your instructor. If no teaching stethoscope is available, have your instructor check your blood pressure measurement on the same arm two minutes later. Repeat, using palpation. Repeat again, measuring thigh pressure if suitable equipment is available.
   d. Record the arm blood pressure measurement on both a graphic and a narrative record, including some mock observations of your "patient." Have your instructor look over your work and make comments.
6. In the clinical setting:
   a. Under your instructor's supervision, measure a patient's blood pressure and record it appropriately.

VOCABULARY

aneroid manometer
antecubital space
auscultatory gap
brachial artery
dialysis cannula
diaphragm
diastolic blood pressure
intravenous infusion
Korotkoff sounds
palpation
popliteal artery
postural hypotension
radial artery
shock
sphygmomanometer
stethoscope
supine
systole
systolic blood pressure

MEASURING BLOOD PRESSURE

Rationale for the Use of This Skill

Blood pressure is the force exerted by the blood against the walls of the arteries of the body. It serves, in combination with other observations, as an indicator of the circulatory status of patients.

The nurse must be able to measure and record blood pressure accurately, and to interpret that measurement as it relates to particular patients. To do this effectively, the nurse must be aware of the norms and variables that affect blood pressure.[1]

Norms and Variables

Generally speaking, blood pressure increases with age, being lowest in the newborn (approximately 40/20) and gradually increasing during childhood and adolescence to the adult level (approximately 120/80). Blood pressure, however, varies considerably with the individual. Hence, a normal reading is usually identified as being within a certain range. For example, the normal range for adults is 110–140/60–90. A systolic blood pressure over 160 or a diastolic blood pressure over 100 is termed *hypertensive*; a systolic blood pressure below 100 is termed *hypotensive*. Blood pressure, however, is only one indication among many and must be evaluated in the context of an entire situation, not as an isolated event.

Many factors can affect blood pressure. Activity, anxiety, strong emotion, recent intake of food, disease, pain, and drugs can all cause a rise in blood pressure. A fall in blood pressure is caused by blood loss or anything that causes blood vessels to dilate. Postural, or orthostatic, hypotension is a sudden drop in blood pressure that is caused by a change in position, for example, from lying to sitting or standing. It may cause dizziness, fainting, or falling. When postural blood pressures are ordered, they should be recorded in the same order as they are taken: first lying, then sitting, then standing.

Equipment

What is commonly referred to as the *blood pressure cuff* really consists of an oblong rubber bag, or *bladder*, covered with a nonexpandable fabric called the *cuff* (see Figure 17.1).

The *hand bulb* is a device attached to the bladder by a rubber tube through which air is pumped. The hand bulb has a valve, regulated by a thumbscrew, that allows air to escape from the bladder at the desired rate.

Mercury manometers are manufactured in a variety of models, including a floor model (which can be moved from one place to another), a portable model (which comes in a box), and a wall model (which is probably the most common). The mercury rises in a calibrated glass tube as the cuff is inflated with air, then falls as the air is released. Rubber tubing connects the mercury reservoir with the cuff.

The *aneroid manometer* is an air pressure gauge that registers the blood pressure by a pointer on a dial. The dial generally attaches to the cuff by hooks that fit into a small pocket.

The *stethoscope* is an instrument used for listening to body sounds. The bell head of the stethoscope is usually used for listening when blood pressure is measured. (*Low-pitched sounds are heard more easily with the bell head of the stethoscope than with the diaphragm.*)

Width of the Cuff

The width of the blood pressure cuff is important. If the cuff is too narrow, it may yield a reading that is higher than the correct one; if it is too wide, it may yield a reading that is lower than the correct one. According to the American Heart Association, the cuff should be 40 percent of the circumference of the midpoint of the limb on which it is being used (AHA, 1980). Most facilities have at least three sizes: child, adult, and thigh (which is also used for arm pressures in obese persons). A child's cuff could be used for a very thin adult as well. *The circumference of the arm, not the age of the patient, is the factor that determines cuff size.*

---

[1]You will note that rationale for action is emphasized throughout the module by the use of italics.

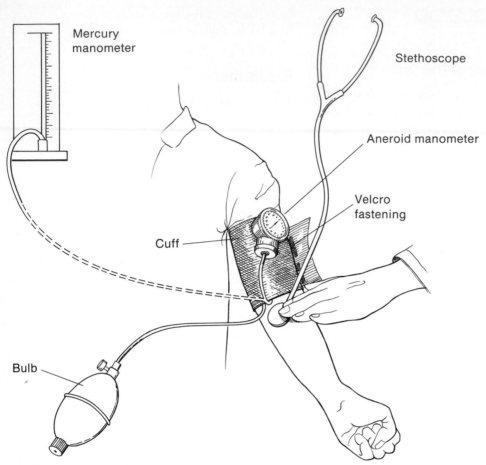

Mercury manometer

Stethoscope

Aneroid manometer

Velcro fastening

Cuff

Bulb

FIGURE 17.1 EQUIPMENT FOR MEASURING BLOOD PRESSURE

Procedure for Measuring Blood Pressure

Assessment

1. Check the orders to ascertain how frequently blood pressure is to be measured and also to see whether any special procedures—such as, for example, postural blood pressure measurements—are to be carried out.

2. Assess the patient to determine whether there are any factors present that might affect how the blood pressure is taken. For example, the presence of an intravenous infusion or a cannula for dialysis in one arm would indicate that the blood pressure should be taken in the other arm. In some patients there are anatomic or physiologic reasons why the blood pressure should not be taken on one arm or the other. This information may be found on the patient care plan, or it may even be a part of the physician's orders.

Planning

3. Wash your hands *for asepsis.*

4. Take the necessary equipment to the patient's bedside. Some facilities have a wall-mounted mercury gauge and a cuff, and sometimes even a stethoscope, at the bedside. In other places, you will have to bring all the necessary equipment with you.

Implementation

5. Identify the patient *to be sure you are performing the procedure on the correct patient.*

6. Introduce yourself to the patient and explain what you plan to do. Allow the patient to ask questions. Remember that

many variables can affect blood pressure. Be aware of such things as medications, recent activity, position, emotional state, recent meals, and pain.

7. Diminish room noise (radio, television, visitors' conversation). Also remind the patient not to talk to you while you are measuring the blood pressure.

8. Position the patient. Blood pressure is usually measured with the patient in the supine position, but it can be measured with the patient in the sitting or standing position if so ordered. The patient's arm should be fully supported on a flat surface at heart level. *There is an increase in blood pressure as the arm is lowered from heart level and a decrease as the arm is raised above this position.* Usually either arm can be used, although the presence of a cast, bandage, or intravenous infusion are some reasons why you might choose one arm over the other. In the rare cases where it is not possible to take an arm pressure, you can use the patient's leg instead of an arm. In any case, you should either remove any clothing in the way or roll up the patient's sleeves or pant legs. Do not attempt to apply the cuff over any bulky materials.

9. Wrap the blood pressure cuff around the arm above the elbow, making sure the rubber bladder is centered over the brachial artery. The lower edge of the cuff should be about 1 inch above the antecubital space (fossa). When the blood pressure equipment you are using is attached to the wall, the cuff may be inverted if the tubing is too short to allow you to wrap the cuff with ease. Wrap the cuff smoothly and snugly, and attach it securely. There are many ways to secure the cuff, but currently the most common method is a Velcro closure. If an aneroid gauge is attached to the cuff, place it where it can easily be read. The mercury manometer should be at eye level.

10. Feel for the brachial artery, which is located near the center of the antecubital space, toward the little finger. (The radial artery can also be used.)

11. Place the stethoscope earpieces in your ears. If you are not using your own stethoscope, wipe off the earpieces with alcohol *to prevent cross-contamination with other users of the same stethoscope.*

12. Keeping your fingers over the brachial artery, turn the valve on the hand bulb clockwise until it is tight.

13. Palpate the brachial artery while you pump the hand bulb to fill the rubber bladder in the blood pressure cuff with air. As you pump, the gauge will register. Pump until you no longer feel a pulse and continue for 30 mm Hg beyond that point. *This will prevent you from missing the top sound and so underestimating the systolic pressure as a result of the auscultatory gap,* which is present in some people, especially those with hypertension. In these cases, the sound is heard, but it fades out completely and is not heard again until 10 to 40 mm Hg lower.

14. Place the bell head of the stethoscope over the previously palpated brachial artery.

15. Open the valve on the hand bulb (turning it counterclockwise) gradually (no faster than 2 to 3 mm Hg per second), releasing the air from the rubber bladder, and watch the pressure registered on the gauge decrease.

16. Note the pressure at which you hear the first *regular* tapping sounds gradually getting louder (Korotkoff sounds; see Figure 17.2). Sometimes you will hear sounds that you think are first sounds, but that are not regular and do not get louder; they are considered extraneous. The pressure at which you hear the first sound is called the *systolic blood pressure,* the point at which the heart is beating (*systole*) and exerting its greatest force.

17. Continue to open the valve gradually, listening for a muffling sound. Note both the point of muffling and the point at which the sound disappears. Facilities differ as to which of these two sounds they consider the *diastolic pressure* (the point at which the heart is relaxing and filling with blood). The American Heart Association recommends that the onset of muffling (fourth phase) be regarded as the best index of diastolic pressure in children and that the fifth phase (when sounds become inaudible) be regarded as

As the pressure in the blood pressure cuff falls, the Korotkoff sounds become audible over the artery below the cuff and pass through the four phases until the sounds disappear.

Phase I That period marked by the first appearance of faint, clear tapping sounds which gradually increase in intensity.

Phase II The period during which a murmur or swishing quality is heard.

Phase III The period during which sounds are crisper and increase in intensity.

Phase IV The period marked by the distinct, abrupt muffling of sound so that a soft, blowing quality is heard.

Phase V The point at which sounds disappear.

FIGURE 17.2 KOROTKOFF SOUNDS Reprinted by permission of the American Heart Association, Inc. from "Recommendations for Human Blood Pressure Determination by Sphygmomanometer" published by the AHA, 1980.

the best index of diastolic blood pressure in adults.

18. If you want to double-check the blood pressure measurement, wait one to two minutes *to allow the release of blood trapped in the veins,* then repeat on the same arm.

19. Remove the stethoscope earpieces from your ears and remove the cuff from the patient's arm. (Wipe the earpieces with an alcohol swab unless it is your personal stethoscope. Wipe the bell head with an alcohol swab between patients *to maintain asepsis.*) Store the equipment properly.

20. Wash your hands *for asepsis.*

Evaluation

21. Evaluate using the following criteria:
    a. Blood pressure is within normal limits for the patient's age and usual blood pressure.
    b. Factors present that might affect the blood pressure have been taken into consideration.
    c. If there is reason to believe that the blood pressure recording is

inaccurate, it has been repeated after waiting one to two minutes.

Documentation

22. Record your findings on the patient's chart. In some facilities, only two numbers are recorded. In such instances, you will have to know which of the two lower sounds is considered the diastolic pressure and, hence, recorded. The American Heart Association recommends recording all three pressures, as follows:

      140 / 80 / 68

    If you do not hear all three points, use a dash to indicate the sound that was not heard, as follows:

      140 / — / 68

    If you hear beats all the way to zero, record your finding as follows:

      140 / 80 / 0

    The graph shown in Figure 17.3 demonstrates one method of display.

Measurement at the Thigh

There will be times when it is necessary to measure blood pressure using the thigh. In such instances, use an appropriately larger cuff (usually 18 to 20 cm, which is 6 cm wider than the arm cuff) and position the patient on the abdomen. A patient who cannot lie on the abdomen may be placed in the supine position, with the knee slightly flexed.

Place your stethoscope over the popliteal artery and measure the patient's blood pressure as before, but with the cuff applied at midthigh. "Comparison of intra-arterial blood pressures in the arms and legs in humans has shown that the femoral systolic pressure is only a few millimeters of mercury higher, and the diastolic a few millimeters lower than comparable arm pressures" (AHA, 1980, p. 13).

Measurement During Shock

It may be very difficult to hear Korotkoff sounds when a patient is in a state of clinical shock. When you cannot hear Korotkoff sounds, measure systolic blood pressure by palpation. (The diastolic pressure cannot be measured in this manner.) The procedure is the same except that no stethoscope is used and the pressure shown when the first pulsation is felt is considered the

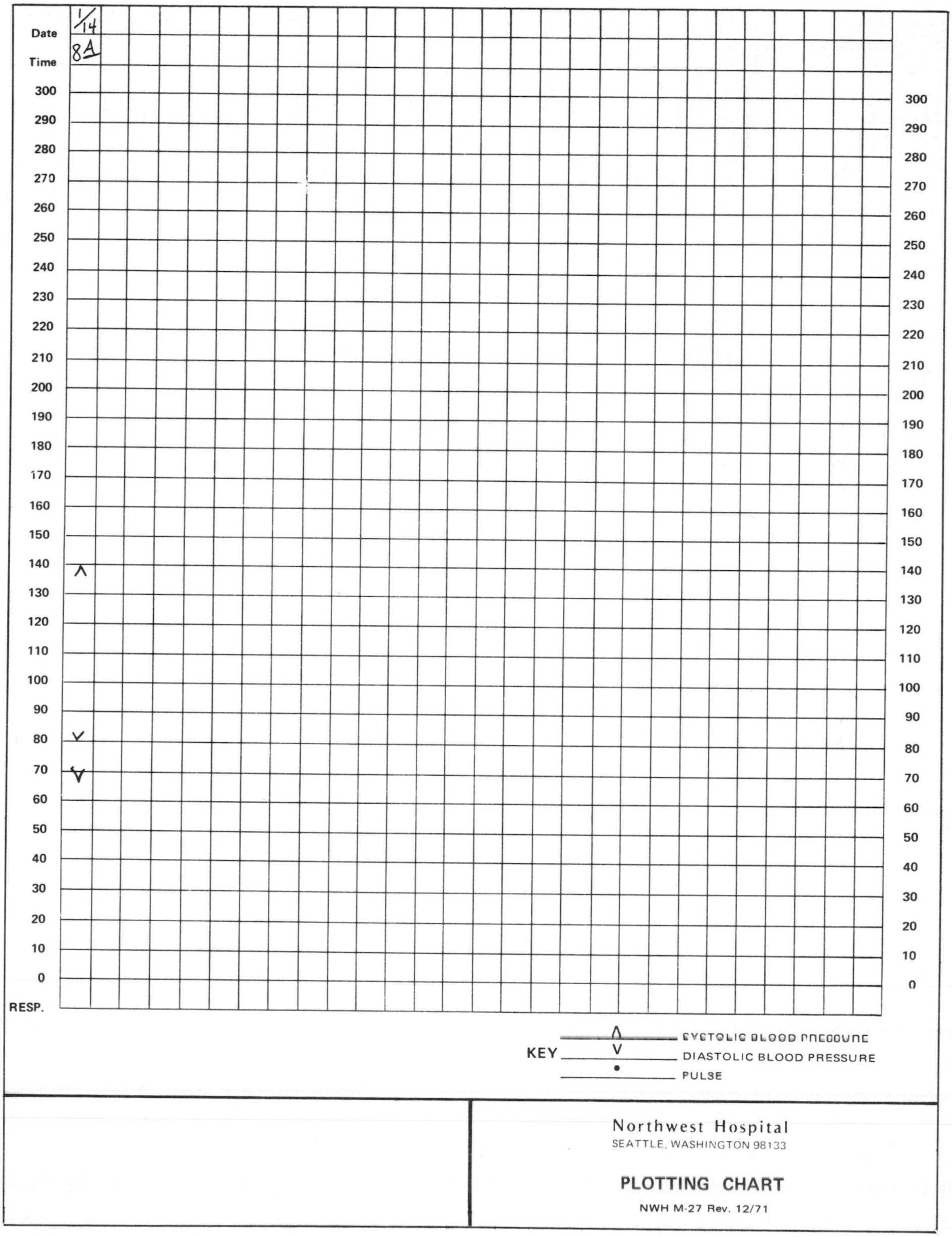

FIGURE 17.3 BLOOD PRESSURE GRAPH

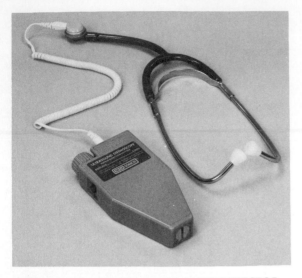

FIGURE 17.4 DOPPLER BLOOD-FLOW DETECTOR ULTRASOUND STETHOSCOPE
Courtesy Meda Sonics, Inc.

systolic pressure. A palpated blood pressure may be recorded as, for example, 80/P. Direct arterial blood pressure monitoring is also appropriate in these cases. This type of blood pressure monitoring requires sophisticated equipment, which is usually available only in intensive care settings.

Where Korotkoff sounds are difficult to hear (as, for example, in cases of shock, or with obese patients, with infants, and so on) a Doppler ultrasound stethoscope can be used. The Doppler, which is used to detect flow, consists of a stethoscope or headset attached to a battery-operated ultrasound unit (see Figure 17.4). To measure systolic blood pressure, locate the brachial or other pulse desired, apply electrode or contact gel, and gently place the instrument over the pulse point. Volume is adjustable. When the pulse is heard, the systolic blood pressure is measured as above. A Doppler blood pressure may be recorded as, for example, 80/D.

REFERENCES

American Heart Association. *Recommendations for Human Blood Pressure Determination by Sphygmomanometers.* Dallas: American Heart Association, 1980.

Birdsall, Carole. "How Accurate Are Your Blood Pressures?" *American Journal of Nursing,* 84 (November 1984), 1414.

PERFORMANCE CHECKLIST

Measuring blood pressure

	Unsatisfactory	Needs More Practice	Satisfactory	Comments
Assessment				
1. Check orders.				
2. Assess patient.				
Planning				
3. Wash your hands.				
4. Gather equipment.				
Implementation				
5. Identify patient.				
6. Explain procedure to patient.				
7. Diminish room noise.				
8. Position patient.				
9. Apply blood pressure cuff.				
10. Place stethoscope earpieces in your ears.				
11. Locate patient's brachial artery.				
12. Tighten valve on hand bulb.				
13. Pump hand bulb to 30 mm Hg above last pulse felt.				
14. Place bell head of stethoscope over brachial artery.				
15. Release valve.				
16. Note pressure at point where you first hear regular sound.				
17. Note pressure at point of muffling and point at which sound disappears.				
18. Wait two minutes to double-check, if necessary.				
19. Remove earpieces from your ears and cuff from patient's arm. Clean bell head between patients. Clean earpieces, if appropriate.				
20. Wash your hands.				

	Unsatisfactory	Needs More Practice	Satisfactory	Comments
☐ *Evaluation*				
21. Evaluate using the following criteria: a. Blood pressure within normal limits for patient's age and usual blood pressure				
b. Factors present that might affect blood pressure taken into consideration				
c. If there was reason to believe that blood pressure recording was inaccurate, it was repeated after one to two minutes.				
☐ *Documentation*				
22. Record appropriately, including narrative as necessary.				

QUIZ

Multiple-Choice Questions

_____ 1. Factors that can affect blood pressure include (1) age; (2) height; (3) recent activity; (4) position; (5) recent meals; (6) pain.

    a. 1 and 3
    b. 1, 2, 3, and 5
    c. 1, 3, 4, 5, and 6
    d. 3, 4, 5, and 6

_____ 2. The usual position for a hospitalized patient to assume during blood pressure measurement is

    a. sitting.
    b. prone.
    c. supine.
    d. lateral.

_____ 3. The bell head of the stethoscope should be placed over which artery to measure blood pressure in the arm?

    a. Radial
    b. Brachial
    c. Femoral
    d. Carotid

_____ 4. The first sound you hear on release of the hand bulb valve indicates

    a. systolic pressure.
    b. diastolic pressure.
    c. pulse pressure.
    d. You cannot tell by one sound.

_____ 5. The point at which the heart is beating and exerting its greatest force is called

    a. systolic pressure.
    b. diastolic pressure.
    c. pulse pressure.
    d. basal pressure.

_____ 6. If you want to double-check a blood pressure measurement, how long should you wait before you remeasure on the same arm?

    a. 30 seconds
    b. One to two minutes
    c. Three minutes
    d. It makes no difference.

Short-Answer Questions

7. The systolic pressure is heard at 140, the point of muffling is heard at 80, and the last sound heard is at 70. Document appropriately. _____

8. Why is the bell head of the stethoscope preferred to the diaphragm for measuring blood pressure? _____

_____

9. a. What is the auscultatory gap? _____

_____

   b. How can you prevent underestimation of the systolic pressure as a result of this phenomenon? _____

_____

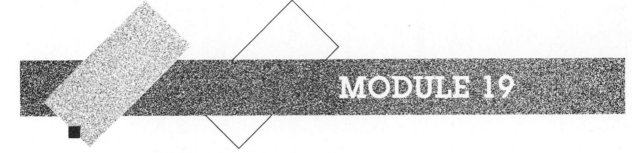

MODULE 19

Assisting with Examinations and Procedures

<table>
<tr><td>

MODULE CONTENTS

Rationale for the Use of This Skill
Physical Examinations
  Sequence
  Nurse's Role
    Psychological Factors
    Assisting the Examiner
General Procedure for Assisting with the
      Physical Examination
  Assessment
  Planning
  Implementation
  Evaluation
  Documentation
Diagnostic and Therapeutic Procedures
General Procedure for Assisting with
     Diagnostic and Therapeutic Procedures
Modifications of General Procedure
  Thoracentesis
  Paracentesis
  Lumbar Puncture
  Liver Biopsy
  Bone Marrow Biopsy
  Proctoscopy and Sigmoidoscopy

</td><td>

PREREQUISITES

Successful completion of the following modules:

VOLUME 1

Module 1 / An Approach to Nursing Skills
Module 2 / Medical Asepsis
Module 3 / Safety
Module 5 / Assessment
Module 6 / Documentation

The following modules may be necessary for some selected situations:

Module 8 / Moving the Patient in Bed and
  Positioning
Module 13 / Inspection, Palpation,
  Auscultation, and Percussion
Module 16 / Temperature, Pulse, and
  Respiration
Module 17 / Blood Pressure
Module 18 / Collecting Specimens

VOLUME 2
Module 35 / Sterile Technique

</td></tr>
</table>

OVERALL OBJECTIVE

To assist the examiner with the physical examination and with diagnostic and therapeutic procedures, with emphasis on the preparation and support of patients.

SPECIFIC LEARNING OBJECTIVES

	Know Facts and Principles	Apply Facts and Principles	Demonstrate Ability	Evaluate Performance
Assisting with a physical examination				
1. Equipment	List common equipment used to perform physical examinations	Identify each piece of equipment for part being examined	Gather appropriate equipment for examination	Evaluate own performance using Performance Checklist
2. Nurse's role in assisting	State two responsibilities of the nurse toward patient and examiner when performing physical examination		Demonstrate ability to assist with an examination or specific procedure	Evaluate with instructor
3. Physical and psychological preparation of patient	Explain methods for preparing patient physically and psychologically	In the practice setting, prepare partner physically and psychologically	In the clinical setting, prepare patient physically and psychologically for test	Evaluate preparation through patient interview after procedure
4. Procedure *a. Positioning for system being examined* *b. Sequence of physical examination*	Name usual sequence for carrying out physical examination and position used with each step	With partner, simulate physical examination, using sequence and position variations	Under supervision, assist examiner in performing physical examination on patient	Evaluate with instructor
c. Findings	Briefly describe several findings from each part of examination		In the clinical area, relate to instructor signs and symptoms found	Evaluate with instructor

d. *Recording*	List observations to be recorded	Practice recording of assisting with physical examination	Document correctly on chart	Evaluate own performance using Performance Checklist
Assisting with diagnostic and therapeutic procedures				
1. Equipment	Name equipment needed for six procedures described	Identify equipment needed for each of six procedures	In the clinical setting, select appropriate equipment for procedure to be performed	Evaluate own performance using Performance Checklist
2. Nurse's role in assisting	State the role of the nurse in each procedure			
3. Procedure a. *Positioning* b. *Observation* c. *Specimen collection* d. *Recording*	With each of six procedures, describe procedure, including position, necessary observation, specimen collection, and recording	In the practice setting, carry out nurse's role in simulated situation	Under supervision in the clinical setting, assist examiner with any of six procedures. Collect specimens and record correctly.	Evaluate performance with instructor

LEARNING ACTIVITIES

1. Review the Specific Learning Objectives.
2. Read the section on performing treatments (in the chapter on direct care skills) in Ellis and Nowlis, *Nursing: A Human Needs Approach,* or comparable material in another textbook.
3. Look up the module vocabulary terms in the Glossary.
4. Review the anatomy and physiology of the system being studied. This can be very helpful.
5. Read through the module.
6. Become familiar with the equipment that is available in the practice laboratory.
7. In the practice setting:
   a. Using a partner for a patient, simulate the sequence of the physical examination, reassuring and explaining as you proceed. You may leave out the genital portion of the examination, but be sure to include it in your explanation.
   b. Reverse roles, and you take the role of the patient.
   c. Evaluate each other's performance. Were the explanations sufficient? Was emotional support offered? Did you have any feelings about the experience?
   d. Practice the various positions for diagnostic procedures with your partner.
   e. Form groups of three students, and take turns being the person performing the procedure, the patient, and the assisting nurse. The student simulating the role of the physician will simply ask for equipment while standing in position as if to use it.
      (1) Set up for and perform a thoracentesis.
      (2) Set up for and perform a paracentesis.
      (3) Set up for and perform a lumbar puncture.
      (4) Set up for and perform a liver biopsy.
      (5) Set up for and perform a bone marrow biopsy.

For each of these procedures, discuss the things that made it easier for you as a patient, the concerns you felt, and how the nurse assisted with these concerns. Note how the equipment was set up. What things made it convenient and what aspects were awkward? How could you reorganize the physical environment so that it would be more convenient?

   f. Using a practice mannequin, set up for a sigmoidoscopy and/or proctoscopy. Consider the same questions raised above.

8. In the clinical setting:
   Consult with your instructor about opportunities to assist with a physical examination or a diagnostic or therapeutic procedure. Do this under supervision.

VOCABULARY

antecubital fossa
asymmetry
bone marrow
bruit
caries
cerumen
concurrent
cranium
dorsal recumbent position
dorsiflexion
edema
gooseneck lamp
Homan's sign
hypovolemic shock
lesion
lithotomy position
liver biopsy
lumbar puncture (spinal tap)
manometer
nares
nasal speculum
ophthalmoscope
otoscope
paracentesis
patellar tendon
pectoralis muscles
periphery

pinwheel
proctoscope
ptosis
reflex hammer (percussion hammer)
sigmoidoscope
stab wound
stethoscope
stopcock

stylet
thoracentesis
trocar
tuning fork
turgor
uvula
vaginal speculum

ASSISTING WITH EXAMINATIONS AND PROCEDURES

Rationale for the Use of This Skill

A*lthough the sophistication of laboratory and radiological tests has increased remarkably in recent years, the foundation of diagnosis remains the patient's history. The physical examination, however, is essential to support the history. The two are commonly referred to as the* H&P, *or* history and physical. *Examinations are also used to establish a baseline for patients' health status and to rule out concurrent disease. The nurse who has special training in primary care may perform a physical examination as an important part of assessment. In most facilities, however, this remains the responsibility of a physician.*

Assisting with procedures is an extension of this skill, in that preparation, providing comfort for the patient, and carrying out the procedure require many of the same principles as physical examinations. The nurse, therefore, has an important obligation to be a skillful and effective assistant.[1]

Physical Examination

The physical examination is one of the most valuable data-gathering procedures. By using methods of inspection, palpation, auscultation, and percussion, often with the help of instruments, *the examiner can obtain an overview of the patient's general health as well as data concerning specific systems.* An examination can be performed as part of a yearly checkup, or it can be performed when a person has sought help because of signs or symptoms of illness. In the latter case, the physical assessment *may suggest or even establish a diagnosis.* Abnormal findings in other related or nonrelated systems *may confirm the extent of the presenting illness or reveal a different, concurrent disease process altogether.*

Usually a physical examination is the second part of a standard two-part procedure called the H&P, or history and physical. First, the examiner takes a detailed verbal history from the patient that consists of demographic information,

[1]You will note that rationale for action is emphasized throughout the module by the use of italics.

family medical history, and the patient's past history of injury or illness. A description by the patient of the current signs and symptoms completes the history. In some facilities, the history is taken and the physical is done by a skilled nurse.

Sequence

Before the physical examination is begun, the vital signs have usually been taken and recorded by the nurse. Some examiners, however, will retake the pulse, respiration, and blood pressure. Physicians rarely measure a patient's temperature themselves but may ask the nurse for the information. It is best to take the vital signs shortly before the physical examination, *so that this information is at hand.* Follow the procedure in the facility or office where you work.

Most examiners perform the physical examination in approximately the same sequence—from head to toe—*perhaps because this is the way it is taught. More importantly, the sequence lends a structure to the examination; thus, you can assist more effectively by anticipating the sequence, and other health personnel can read the written data more easily that way.* Occasionally, one part of an examination is more detailed or lengthy *because specific pathology has been found that needs closer inspection.*

Nurse's Role

The nurse fulfills two major functions: (1) meeting the psychological and physical needs of the patient throughout the examination, and (2) obtaining the necessary equipment and assisting the examiner.

Psychological Factors Most people have experienced a physical examination in a doctor's office, clinic, or hospital. Nevertheless, most patients commonly experience a degree of embarrassment or fear that brings about anxiety.

Certainly embarrassment can arise from having the entire body inspected. You can help overcome this by exposing the patient no more than is necessary. The element of fear is also understandable: a patient may worry that a disease process will be discovered. Most people greet the completion of a physical examination in which no disease is found with great relief.

You can help by clearly explaining to the patient what is about to take place and, in general terms, the parts of the examination. Use words the patient can understand. Your presence during the examination—and assuring the patient of it—*also provides a degree of comfort.* In fact, most male examiners request that a female nurse be present when they perform a vaginal examination, *both for the patient's comfort and to forestall possible legal complications.*

Assisting the Examiner   Your presence as an assistant to the examiner during a physical examination or the performance of procedures is important, *because you know what is physically expected of and psychologically comforting for the patient.* For example, if the examiner is using sterile technique, you must provide items to the sterile field. *Also, certain procedures can be performed more quickly and effectively with your help.* It falls to you, the nurse, to make the examination as comfortable as possible for the patient and as effective as possible for the examiner.

General Procedure for Assisting with the Physical Examination

> *Assessment*

1. Assess the patient for any undue anxiety and lack of knowledge about the examination. In general terms, explain the steps of the examination *to allay any undue anxiety.*

> *Planning*

2. Wash your hands *for asepsis.*
3. Gather the equipment. You will find it convenient to assemble the items on a tray. The specific items may vary: some physicians carry certain instruments in their bags; whereas others do not. You will have to obtain any additional instruments needed from a storage area on the unit. The following are the most commonly used; delete or add to this list as the examiner indicates (see Figures 19.1 through 19.8). Look up in the Glossary any items with which you are not familiar.
   a. Tongue depressor or tongue blade.
   b. Ophthalmoscope (check that the batteries and bulb are working)
   c. Otoscope (check that the batteries and bulb are working)

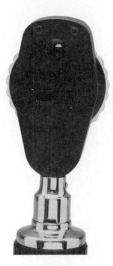

FIGURE 19.1 OPHTHALMOSCOPE HEAD
Courtesy Burton Division/Cavitron Corp., Van Nuys, California, and American Hospital Supply Corp., McGaw Park, Illinois

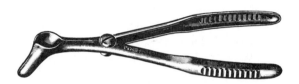

FIGURE 19.2 NASAL SPECULUM
Courtesy SKLAR Manufacturing Co., Long Island, New York, and American Hospital Supply Corp., McGaw Park, Illinois

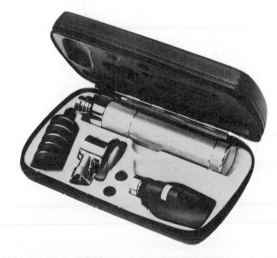

FIGURE 19.3 COMBINATION OTOSCOPE-OPHTHALMOSCOPE
Courtesy of Welch Allyn, Inc., Skaneateles Falls, New York, and American Hospital Supply Corp., McGaw Park, Illinois

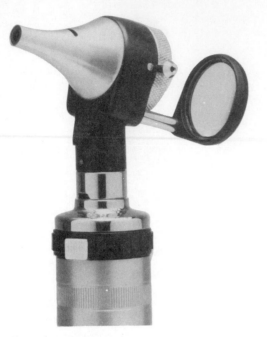

FIGURE 19.4 OTOSCOPE HEAD
Courtesy Burton Division/Cavitron Corp., Van Nuys, California, and American Hospital Supply Corp., McGaw Park, Illinois

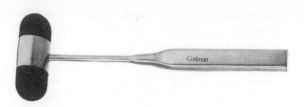

FIGURE 19.6 REFLEX HAMMER
Courtesy Codman & Shurtleff, Inc.

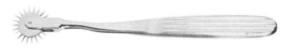

FIGURE 19.7 PINWHEEL
Courtesy Codman & Shurtleff, Inc.

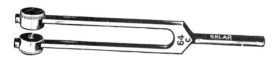

FIGURE 19.5 TUNING FORK
Courtesy SKLAR Manufacturing Co., Long Island, New York, and American Hospital Supply Corp., McGaw Park, Illinois

FIGURE 19.8 VAGINAL SPECULUM
Courtesy SKLAR Manufacturing Co., Long Island, New York, and American Hospital Supply Corp., McGaw Park, Illinois

d. Flashlight (check that the batteries and bulb are working)
e. Reflex hammer, or percussion hammer
f. Pinwheel
g. Tuning fork
h. Nasal speculum
i. Vaginal speculum
j. Clean gloves
k. Lubricating jelly
l. Gooseneck lamp
m. Bath blanket (for draping)

> **Implementation**

4. Identify the patient *to be sure the procedure will be performed for the correct patient.*
5. Answer any questions the patient may have about the examination.

6. Close the door of the room and pull the curtains, if present, *for privacy.*
7. Raise the bed to the high position, *so that the examiner has a good working level.* If the patient is immobile or not totally responsible, keep the side rails up until the examiner is ready to begin the examination, *for reasons of safety.*
8. Help the patient into a clean gown with the ties toward the front, *to allow for easier access to the chest.* In a clinic or office, you may use a special examination cover-up. Usually this is a straight piece of fabric or soft paper material with an opening for the head that drapes poncho-style over the patient, covering the patient's chest and back.
9. Help the patient into a sitting position on

376

the side of the bed. Cover the lower body with a sheet.

10. It is useful for you to know the signs for which the patient is being examined. Review the material given in the summary in Module 5, Assessment. During the examination, your functions are to give psychological support to the patient, assist him or her to the various positions needed, and make equipment easily available to the physician.

11. If a lab. specimen is taken, label it and send it to the laboratory.

12. *For reasons of safety,* after the examination, return the bed to the low position, and help the patient to a position of comfort.

13. Provide a period of rest. *Undergoing a complete physical examination is both anxiety-producing and tiring, especially for an ill person.*

14. Dispose of the equipment properly. Wash, soak, or disinfect each item used according to the policy of your facility.

15. Wash your hands *for asepsis.*

Evaluation

16. Return to the patient and ask if you can assist him or her in any way.

17. Answer any questions about the examination.

Documentation

18. Record the procedure. The examiner may have a form on which you should record findings. If not, they should be on an admission or progress note sheet in standard sequence. You should also make a brief notation on the nurses' notes.

Diagnostic and Therapeutic Procedures

It is essential to obtain a patient's signed permission before diagnostic and therapeutic procedures are performed *to protect the physician and the hospital against legal action.* In some facilities, the more general consent-for-medical-treatment form, signed on admission, suffices. In other facilities, each procedure requires an individual consent. Know the policy of the facility in which you practice.

Throughout all these procedures, give the patient psychological support. If a patient is un-comfortable, assure him or her that it will only be for a short time. Let the patient know what is about to take place, and give clear instructions about ways to help. ("Please try not to move for the next few minutes so that we can get the test over with quickly.") *All this adds to the patient's psychological comfort. Remember that patients feel less anxious if they know what is going to happen and what they should do.* You may want to hold the patient's hand *for reassurance.*

You must observe the patient for untoward signs or reactions to the procedure. *Many times the physician is preoccupied with performing the test, and it is you, the nurse, who can see early signs of impending problems.* During any procedure, check the patient's pulse and respiration two or three times. Notify the physician promptly of any unusual signs.

General Procedure for Assisting with Diagnostic and Therapeutic Procedures

For each of these diagnostic and therapeutic procedures, the same general approach is needed.

Assessment

1. Check the physician's order *to be sure of the exact procedure to be done and to identify the purpose of the procedure.*

2. Check to be sure that a permission form has been signed, if this is necessary. *A patient must give informed consent for any procedure, and when the procedure is invasive and has possible adverse consequences, most facilities require that a written form be signed and placed in the patient's record. Although informing the patient is the physician's responsibility, in many facilities the nurse obtains the signature on the form and witnesses it. This does not transfer the responsibility for informed consent from the physician to the nurse. In other facilities the nurse prepares the form and presents it to the physician when information is being given. Follow the procedure in your facility.*

3. Assess the patient for the ability to assume and maintain the appropriate position for the procedure *in order to plan alternatives if necessary.*

Planning

4. Wash your hands *for asepsis.*
5. Obtain the equipment available in your facility and check the contents of any prepared tray *to identify what items must be obtained separately.*

Implementation

6. Identify the patient *to be sure that you are performing the procedure on the correct patient.*
7. Discuss the procedure with the patient. At this time you will need to find out what the patient understands, clarify concerns, and give explicit information about the way the procedure will affect the patient *to relieve anxiety and facilitate patient participation.* Do not increase the patient's anxiety with graphic descriptions of the procedure, but rather focus on how the patient will be positioned, what the patient will be asked to do, and what the patient will experience during the procedure. You might also emphasize that part of your role is to help the patient in whatever way is possible.
8. Prepare the unit:
   a. Provide privacy
   b. Set up a table for equipment. You may need to clean the surface of the table *for asepsis.*
9. Prepare the patient by positioning and draping as needed *to facilitate the procedure and provide privacy.*
10. Assist with the procedure, assessing and reassuring the patient throughout and providing equipment as needed.
11. Conclude the procedure:
    a. Restore the patient to a position of comfort or to a therapeutic position.
    b. Restore the unit by clearing away equipment and placing the call bell within reach.
    c. Label and properly care for any specimen obtained.
    d. Dispose of equipment.
    e. Wash your hands.

Evaluation

12. Establish specific criteria for evaluation based on the procedure. Include:
    a. Patient's comfort
    b. Patient's physiological response, such as bleeding, TPR, and BP
    c. Patient's psychological response, such as anxiety, distress, or relaxation

Documentation

13. Although the physician will document that the procedure was performed, the nurse briefly documents the procedure, the patient's response, and the disposition of any specimen in the progress notes of the record. In some facilities, there is a place on a flow sheet for this brief documentation.

Modifications of General Procedure

For each procedure discussed, the steps in the general procedure that must be modified are presented. The detailed procedures, which include all the steps of the General Procedure as well as those steps that need modification, are given in the Performance Checklist. Table 19.1 provides a quick overview of the special considerations for each of the procedures.

Thoracentesis

A thoracentesis is the insertion of a large bore needle or a trocar (a large, sharp metal device) into the pleural space of the chest. This can be done to remove air or fluid from the pleural space or to enable a chest tube to be inserted. You will need an understanding of sterile technique to assist appropriately with this procedure.

Assessment

3. The patient must sit upright during the procedure *so that the pull of gravity will consolidate the chest fluid in the lower portion of the affected lung.* He or she may sit on the edge of the bed leaning on an overbed table or may straddle a chair and lean on its back. Pad the back of the chair or the overbed table *for comfort.* Pillows on either side of the patient on the edge of the bed *may provide needed support.* If the patient is weak, you may need to have a person supporting the patient at all times. The back is exposed *for access to the intercostal spaces.*

TABLE 19.1   COMMONLY PERFORMED DIAGNOSTIC PROCEDURES

	Asepsis	Position	Specific Observations or Concerns	Specimen
Thoracentesis	Sterile	Sitting upright	Pallor, sudden pain, cough, dyspnea, diaphoresis	Chest fluid
Paracentesis	Sterile	After voiding, sitting upright	Signs of hypovolemic shock: fall in blood pressure, dyspnea, diaphoresis, pallor	Abdominal fluid
Lumbar puncture	Sterile	Side-lying, with neck and legs flexed	Sharp back pain, pain radiating to legs, or numbness or tingling in feet or legs; have patient lie flat—to 24 hours afterward	Cerebrospinal fluid
Liver biopsy	Sterile	Supine	Have patient hold breath for ten seconds during puncture; check vital signs during procedure; watch for internal bleeding or bleeding from site	Liver tissue
Bone marrow biopsy	Sterile	Supine	Bleeding from site or hematoma formation	Bone marrow
Proctoscopy or sigmoidoscopy	Nonsterile	Knee-chest	Sudden abdominal pain or shock symptoms from perforation (rare)	Small fragments of lesions in colon if present

Planning

5. Equipment needed includes a sterile thoracentesis set. These are usually disposable sets that contain all needed equipment. Read the label to determine if any items are not included. You may need to add sterile gloves in the size appropriate for the physician doing the procedure, a basin to receive large quantities of fluid being removed, and an injectable local anesthetic. If a chest tube is to be inserted, you will need a chest drainage set and a chest tube. (See Module 44, Caring for Patients with Chest Tubes.)

Implementation

10. Assess the patient especially for skin color, respirations, chest pain, and diaphoresis.

The sudden appearance of pallor (seen as a greying in those with dark skin), dyspnea, cough, chest pain, or diaphoresis may indicate that the needle is irritating or even puncturing the pleura. Inform the physician immediately if these signs are identified.

Open the sterile set on a convenient table. Open the glove package in an accessible location, and be prepared to hold the basin or set up the chest drainage if that is indicated. Because the equipment is sterile, the physician will handle it personally to avoid contamination. The physician will cleanse the insertion area with antiseptic, anesthetize the area using the local anesthetic, and insert a 16 or 17 gauge needle with a stylet into the pleural space at the level of the seventh intercostal space. The stylet is then removed, and a large syringe with a three-way stopcock is attached to the needle. This is used to aspirate fluid from the chest. When all the fluid has been removed, the needle is withdrawn and an impervious dressing is placed over the thoracentesis site. If a chest tube is being inserted, a large trocar is used; the chest tube is threaded through the trocar, the trocar is removed, and the chest drainage set is attached.

11. When restoring the patient to a position of comfort, plan for a period of undisturbed rest *because the removal of large amounts of fluid from the chest can result in weakness and fatigue owing to the shift in fluid distribution.*

Evaluation

12. Particular attention to evaluation of respiratory status is needed *because these procedures are performed to facilitate effective respiration.* Evaluation of pulse and blood pressure is also important *because changes in chest pressures may affect cardiac function, especially in the person of advanced age or with existing cardiac disease.*

Example of Charting   POR Style

7/6/88
0730   Interim note: Thoracentesis performed by Dr. Kraft. 450 ml. serosanguinous fluid removed. Specimen to lab.
Respiratory Status after procedure:

S "I feel weak and shaky but I can take a deeper breath. I just want to sleep."

O Breathing regular at 20/min. Site of thoracentesis clean and dry.

P 1) Allow to rest for remainder of morning.
2) Assess respiratory status and wound site q 15 min × 4, then q h × 3, then q4h. See flow sheet.

D. Chaney, N.S.

Paracentesis

A paracentesis is the insertion of a large bore needle or a trocar through the wall of the abdomen into the abdominal cavity for the purpose of removing fluid or instilling a solution. You will need an understanding of sterile technique.

Assessment

3. The patient is often placed sitting on the edge of the bed for this procedure. Devising a back support from pillows may decrease tiring. If that is not possible, the patient may be able to remain in a supine position with the head of the bed elevated. These positions consolidate the fluid in the lower portion of the abdomen. If the patient is unable to be upright, consult the physician about possible modifications of this position.

Planning

5. A disposable paracentesis set is usually used for this procedure. You may need to add sterile gloves in the appropriate size for the physician, a large basin or container for fluid to be removed, and a topical anesthetic agent.

Implementation

9. Have the patient void before beginning the procedure *so that the bladder is empty and confined to the pelvis to prevent accidental bladder perforation during the procedure.* Then position the patient as described and drape the patient's back and legs *to provide warmth and comfort.*

10. The physician will sit facing the patient to perform the procedure. You will set up the equipment. Observe the patient particularly for pallor, dizziness, faintness, diaphoresis, and rapid pulse and respirations, *which could indicate an adverse response to the sudden removal of abdominal pressure from the fluid and the consequent movement of a large quantity of blood into the abdominal circulation. This change in blood flow creates a systemic lack of blood supply and the condition called hypovolemic shock.*

11. After the paracentesis is complete and the patient is back in bed, allow a rest period *because the removal of large amounts of fluid from the abdomen can result in weakness and*

fatigue owing to the shift in body fluid distribution.

☐ *Evaluation*

12. Evaluation of physiologic response will include observation of respiratory status and pulse and blood pressure.

Example of Charting   Narrative Style

7/6/87
7:30 am   Paracentesis performed by Dr. Kraft. 1200 ml. cloudy fluid obtained. Specimen to lab. States no pain at site. Site clean and dry. Dry drsg. applied. Resting comfortably at this time. P-82, R-20, BP 126/84

D. Chaney, S.N.

Spinal Tap (Lumbar Puncture)

A spinal tap is the introduction of a large needle through the intervertebral space into the sub-arachnoid space of the spinal canal. This is done to measure the pressure in the spinal fluid and to collect specimens of the fluid. The tap is most commonly performed in the lumbar area, but on occasion it is done at the top of the spinal canal in the cisternal space. A cisternal tap is per-formed more frequently on children.

☐ *Assessment*

3. The patient will be positioned on the side in a very flexed position. If the patient has arthritis or some other condition that limits the ability to assume this position, consult with the physician regarding an alternative position.

☐ *Planning*

5. A disposable tray labeled "Lumbar puncture" or "Spinal" is used for this procedure. Sterile gloves in the size appropriate for the physician and a local anesthetic agent may be obtained separately.

☐ *Implementation*

9. The patient is positioned on the side with a flat support under the head *so that the spinal column is in horizontal alignment and the flow of spinal fluid is not impeded.* Flex the legs and neck, bowing the back toward the side of the bed where the physician will sit. *This position of flexion widens the intervertebral space.* (See Figure 18.4.) Drape the patient so that the lower spine is exposed, but the rest of the patient is covered *for warmth and privacy.*

10. The physician will anesthetize the site and then introduce the spinal needle into the spinal subarachnoid space. This procedure is uncomfortable, and the patient may need assistance to remain still and in the proper position. When the physician attaches the manometer to the needle to measure the pressure, you may be asked to support the top of the manometer to maintain its alignment. If so, be sure you touch only the very top *so that you do not contaminate the area that the physician must handle when disconnecting the manometer.* If specimens of fluid are needed, three separate specimens are usually obtained *because the first may be contaminated with blood from the puncture itself.* You may be asked to hold the tubes. If so, you should wear clean gloves *for asepsis* and keep your hands well away from any sterile area *to avoid contamination.* You may also be responsible for correctly labeling the specimens as #1, #2, and #3 in the order in which they were collected. Assessment during the procedure includes particular attention to comments indicating pain radiating to a leg; sharp, severe back pain; or sudden numbness or tingling of the feet or legs. The puncture is usually performed below the area where the actual cord is located, but *irritation of spinal tissue may create adverse neurological responses.*

11. The patient is usually advised to remain flat immediately after the procedure and for a period of from 8 to 24 hours, depending on the physician. *This is to allow the restoration of spinal fluid before the patient assumes an upright position. This may help to prevent post-spinal headache.* The provision of increased fluids also *helps the person to restore spinal fluid volume.*

☐ *Evaluation*

12. Evaluation should include information regarding lower-extremity neurological response—i.e., pain, numbness, and tingling—and the presence of headache.

Example of Charting   Narrative Style

7/3/88
7:20 am   Lumbar puncture performed by Dr. Kraft. Initial pressure 140 mm. Final pressure 90 mm. Three specimens of clear fluid sent to lab. Resting comfortably c̄ bed flat.

D. Chaney, S.N.

Liver Biopsy

A liver biopsy is the removal of a specimen of liver tissue for laboratory examination. A liver biopsy may be done during a surgical procedure when the abdominal cavity is open. The procedure discussed here is for a needle biopsy, in which a very large bore needle is inserted through the abdominal wall and a core of tissue is obtained for examination. The local anesthetic agent numbs only surface tissue, and the entry of the needle into the liver and removal of the liver tissue does cause pain. Acknowledging the discomfort and offering support and comfort measures are important.

☐ *Assessment*

1. There may be an order for Vitamin K to be given several days before the liver biopsy *in order to enhance the body's clotting ability and decrease the chance of bleeding. Because Vitamin K is a component of prothrombin, which contributes to clotting, its effect does not occur immediately, but rather after the body has had an opportunity to produce the prothrombin from Vitamin K.*

3. The patient will need to lie flat in a supine position *to help flatten and expose the liver tissue.* If the patient cannot lie flat, consult with the physician regarding an alternative position.

☐ *Planning*

5. A disposable liver biopsy tray is used for this procedure. Sterile gloves in the appropriate size for the physician and a local anesthetic agent may be obtained separately if they are not included in the set.

☐ *Implementation*

9. Position the patient supine with the lower portion of the chest and the abdomen exposed. The patient's gown may be left in place if it is folded so that it cannot drop onto the work area during the procedure.

10. The physician will anesthetize a small right subcostal area. The patient is instructed to take a deep breath, *which lowers the diaphragm and pushes the liver toward the abdomen,* then hold it while the actual biopsy is being done *to ensure that the liver does not move during insertion.* After insertion the needle is rotated *to create a core of tissue,* which is withdrawn. Pressure is exerted over the site *to stop bleeding,* and a small dressing is applied. The specimen is usually placed in a preservative solution to be sent to the laboratory.

11. After the procedure, the patient is usually placed on the *right side so that the body weight provides continuing pressure to the site to prevent bleeding.*

☐ *Evaluation*

12. In order to evaluate the patient's response to the procedure, establish a plan for observation and assessment of the patient for internal bleeding. *The liver is a very vascular tissue, and internal bleeding may occur from the trauma of the biopsy. This complication is rare but potentially serious.*

Example of Charting (SOAP)

7/3/88
0830   Interim note: Liver biopsy by Dr. Kraft. Spec. to lab.
S Expressed concern over pain and possible result of biopsy.
O BP 130/82, P 88, R 26
A Anxiety related to procedure. Potential for bleeding.
P Vitals q15 min. × 4 then q4h for 24 hrs. Encourage to voice concerns.

D. Chaney, N.S.

382

Observation of pulse, respiration, blood pressure, and the biopsy site every 15 minutes for an hour is a wise practice. If your facility has a policy requiring a specified observation schedule, follow that policy.

Bone Marrow Biopsy

A bone marrow biopsy is the removal of a specimen of bone marrow tissue for laboratory examination. A large-bore needle is inserted into the bone over a site known to have a large supply of marrow. The iliac crests and the sternum are the most common sites for bone marrow biopsy. The surface tissue is anesthetized, but the patient does feel pain when the bone marrow is aspirated into the syringe. In addition, the puncturing of the bone sounds distressing and is accompanied by strong pressure, which the patient may find uncomfortable. Acknowledging the discomfort, and not attempting to minimize or trivialize it, provides support to the patient and sustains a trust relationship.

Planning

5. Obtain a bone marrow biopsy tray. Most facilities use completely disposable equipment. In some facilities a reusable metal bone marrow biopsy needle with stylet and a glass aspiration syringe are used. These are obtained separately.

Implementation

9. Assist the patient to the supine position if a sternal tap is to be done. The prone position is used for an iliac crest tap.

10. Open the pack and supply sterile gloves. You may be requested to pour antiseptic solution into a container. A small area in the midsternum or over the iliac crest is anesthetized. A short, large-gauge needle with a stylet is inserted. There may be a soft, crunching sound as it punctures the bone tissue. The stylet is removed, a syringe is attached, and 1 to 2 ml bone marrow are aspirated. The patient may feel some mild discomfort when the bone marrow is aspirated. The needle is removed, pressure is applied *to stop the bleeding that occurs,* and a small dressing is applied.

Evaluation

12. Observe the patient for persistent bleeding. If this occurs, apply pressure for five minutes and apply a clean dressing.

Example of Charting   Narrative Style

7/23/88
8:30 am   Bone marrow biopsy performed by Dr. Kraft. Spec. sent to lab. Site covered by dry dressing. No bleeding at site. Pt. crying and states she is afraid of results. R.N. spent 15 min. with pt. for reassurance. Currently resting quietly.

D. Chaney, S.N.

Proctoscopy, Sigmoidoscopy, and Colonoscopy

A proctoscopy is the examination of the interior surface of the rectum, using a hollow tube with a light attached. A sigmoidoscopy uses the same principle to examine the interior surface of the bowel as high as the sigmoid colon. A colonoscopy involves examination of structures throughout the large intestine. During these examinations, small samples of tissue may be removed (biopsy) for laboratory examination, bleeding vessels may be cauterized, and the bowel can be visually examined for abnormalities. A rigid metal tube is most commonly used when only the rectum is being examined. When high structures are to be examined, a flexible fiber optic scope is used. (See Figures 19.9 and 19.10.) This permits the examiner to see higher bowel areas with less discomfort to the patient than would result from the use of a rigid scope. Nevertheless, the procedure is uncomfortable, the position used is uncomfortable, and both are considered embarrassing by most individuals.

For all these procedures, thorough cleansing of the bowel is essential. If feces are present in the bowel, the examiner is unable to visualize the tissue. See Module 28, Administering Enemas, and Module 50 regarding the use of suppositories and for other procedures frequently used to cleanse the bowel.

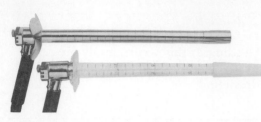

FIGURE 19.9 SIGMOIDOSCOPE

Courtesy Welch Allyn, Inc., Skaneateles Falls, New York, and American Hospital Supply Corp., McGaw Park, Illinois

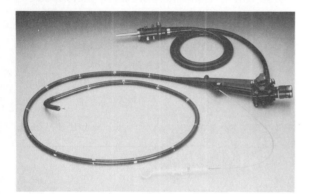

FIGURE 19.10 FLEXIBLE FIBER OPTIC COLONOSCOPE

Courtesy Olympus Corporation

⬛ *Assessment*

3. Check to see that the appropriate bowel cleansing plan has been completed. If it has not been completed or if it has been unsuccessful, notify the physician before proceeding. Some physicians prefer that the patient have nothing by mouth (NPO) before the examination *to decrease bowel activity.* Check the physician's order.

⬛ *Planning*

5. Obtain the appropriate scope and a suction machine. Also obtain clean towels, lubricating jelly, long cotton-tipped swabs, and slides or containers for tissue specimens. Special drapes or draw sheets and examination gloves are also needed.

⬛ *Implementation*

8. *For convenience,* arrange the scope and other items on a clean towel placed on a table.

9. Position the patient on a special examination table that "breaks" at the hips and has a kneeling platform at the end. This allows the patient to be placed in a knee-chest position, *which is best for visualization, and provides support to help the patient maintain the position.* If a special examination table is not available, the patient is placed in a knee-chest position, and pillows may be used *to help support the patient.*

   Drape the patient *to expose the rectal area but provide maximum protection of modesty. Anxiety often causes vasoconstriction and makes patients feel cold, and the drapes will also help to minimize this.*

10. The physician lubricates the scope and inserts it through the anus. Encouraging the patient to focus on breathing deeply through the mouth *assists in relaxation of the anal sphincter.*

    If the physician requests suction, attach the tubing from the scope to the suction apparatus and provide suction as needed.

12. Evaluate the patient's response to the procedure. Discomfort is common but not usually acute. Sudden, acute abdominal pain may indicate the rare complication of perforation of the colon.

Example of Charting   Narrative Style

7/23/88	
8:30 am	Proctoscopy performed by Dr. Kraft. Pt. expressed relief that it was over and not as uncomfortable as feared. Late breakfast tray ordered and pt. comfortable.
	D. Chaney, S.N.

PERFORMANCE CHECKLIST

General procedure for assisting with the physical examination	Unsatisfactory	Needs More Practice	Satisfactory	Comments
☐ *Assessment*				
1. Assess patient for anxiety and lack of knowledge concerning procedure and explain, if necessary.				
☐ *Planning*				
2. Wash your hands.				
3. Gather examination equipment.				
☐ *Implementation*				
4. Identify patient.				
5. Answer any questions patient may have.				
6. Provide for privacy.				
7. Raise bed to high position.				
8. Help patient into clean, front-tying gown and drape appropriately.				
9. Have patient sitting on side of bed.				
10. Know signs for which patient is being examined. Assist physician and offer psychological support to patient.				
11. Label any lab. specimens and send to lab.				
12. After examination, return bed to low position and patient to position of comfort.				
13. Provide period of rest.				
14. Send specimen to lab., and dispose of equipment.				
15. Wash your hands.				
☐ *Evaluation*				
16. Return to patient and ask how you might assist.				
17. Answer any final questions.				
☐ *Documentation*				
18. Record procedure on chart.				

General procedure for assisting with diagnostic and therapeutic procedures

	Unsatisfactory	Needs More Practice	Satisfactory	Comments
Assessment				
1. Check the physician's order.				
2. Check for signed permission form.				
3. Assess patient's physical abilities.				
Planning				
4. Wash your hands.				
5. Obtain equipment.				
Implementation				
6. Identify patient.				
7. Discuss procedure with patient.				
8. Prepare unit. a. Privacy				
b. Equipment				
9. Prepare patient. a. Positioning				
b. Draping				
10. Assist with procedure. a. Assess.				
b. Reassure and support.				
c. Provide equipment.				
11. Conclude the procedure a. Restore the patient.				
b. Restore the unit.				
c. Label and care for specimen.				
d. Dispose of equipment.				
e. Wash your hands.				
Evaluation				
12. Establish specific criteria. a. Comfort				
b. Physiological response				
c. Psychological response				

386

	Unsatisfactory	Needs More Practice	Satisfactory	Comments
☐ *Documentation*				
13. Record the procedure.				

General procedure for assisting with thoracentesis

	Unsatisfactory	Needs More Practice	Satisfactory	Comments
☐ *Assessment*				
1. Check the physician's order.				
2. Check for signed permission form.				
3. Assess patient's ability to sit upright.				
☐ *Planning*				
4. Wash your hands.				
5. Obtain thoracentesis set and gloves.				
☐ *Implementation*				
6. Identify patient.				
7. Discuss procedure with patient.				
8. Prepare unit. a. Privacy				
b. Equipment				
9. Prepare patient. a. Positioning				
b. Draping				
10. Assist with procedure. a. Assess for skin color, diaphoresis, respirations, chest pain.				
b. Reassure and support.				
c. Provide equipment.				
11. Conclude the procedure. a. Restore position of comfort and plan for rest period.				
b. Restore the unit.				
c. Label and care for specimen.				
d. Dispose of equipment.				
e. Wash your hands.				

	Unsatisfactory	Needs More Practice	Satisfactory	Comments
☐ *Evaluation*				
12. Establish specific criteria. a. Comfort				
b. Physiological response, especially respiratory status, pulse, and blood pressure				
c. Psychological response				
☐ *Documentation*				
13. Record the procedure.				
General procedure for assisting with paracentesis				
☐ *Assessment*				
1. Check physician's order.				
2. Check for signed permission form.				
3. Assess patient's ability to sit upright.				
☐ *Planning*				
4. Wash your hands.				
5. Obtain paracentesis set and sterile gloves.				
☐ *Implementation*				
6. Identify patient.				
7. Discuss procedure with patient.				
8. Prepare unit. a. Privacy				
b. Equipment				
9. Prepare patient. a. Have patient void.				
b. Position sitting on edge of bed.				
c. Drape.				
10. Assist with procedure. a. Assess for pallor, dizziness, faintness, diaphoresis, rapid pulse, rapid respirations.				
b. Reassure and support.				
c. Provide equipment.				

388

	Unsatisfactory	Needs More Practice	Satisfactory	Comments
11. Conclude the procedure. a. Restore the patient and plan rest.				
b. Restore the unit.				
c. Label and care for specimen.				
d. Dispose of equipment.				
e. Wash your hands.				
☐ *Evaluation*				
12. Establish specific criteria. a. Comfort				
b. Physiological response, especially respiratory status, pulse, and blood pressure				
c. Psychological response				
☐ *Documentation*				
13. Record the procedure.				

General procedure for assisting with spinal tap

	Unsatisfactory	Needs More Practice	Satisfactory	Comments
☐ *Assessment*				
1. Check physician's order.				
2. Check for signed permission form.				
3. Assess patient's ability to lie in flexed position.				
☐ *Planning*				
4. Wash your hands.				
5. Obtain equipment (disposable set, sterile gloves, local anesthetic).				
☐ *Implementation*				
6. Identify patient.				
7. Discuss procedure with patient.				
8. Prepare unit. a. Privacy				
b. Equipment				

	Unsatisfactory	Needs More Practice	Satisfactory	Comments
9. Prepare patient.				
a. Position on side in flexed position.				
b. Drape.				
10. Assist with procedure.				
a. Assess.				
b. Reassure and support in position.				
c. Provide equipment, hold manometer, and hold tubes for specimen.				
11. Conclude the procedure.				
a. Restore the patient (place in flat position if ordered by physician).				
b. Restore the unit.				
c. Label and care for specimen.				
d. Dispose of equipment.				
e. Wash your hands.				
Evaluation				
12. Establish specific criteria.				
a. Comfort, especially pain in back and lower extremities and/or headache				
b. Physiological response, especially abnormal neurological response in lower extremities				
c. Psychological response				
Documentation				
13. Record the procedure.				

General procedure for assisting with liver biopsy

Assessment				
1. Check physician's order and note whether Vitamin K was ordered and given previously.				
2. Check for signed permission form.				
3. Assess patient's ability to lie flat.				
Planning				
4. Wash your hands.				

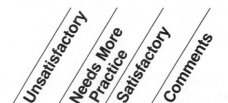

	Unsatisfactory	Needs More Practice	Satisfactory	Comments
5. Obtain liver biopsy tray and sterile gloves.				
Implementation				
6. Identify patient.				
7. Discuss procedure with patient.				
8. Prepare unit. a. Privacy				
b. Equipment				
9. Prepare patient. a. Position patient supine.				
b. Drape with upper right abdomen exposed.				
10. Assist with procedure. a. Assess.				
b. Reassure and support.				
c. Provide equipment.				
11. Conclude the procedure.				
a. Position patient on right side.				
b. Restore the unit.				
c. Label and care for specimen.				
d. Dispose of equipment.				
e. Wash your hands.				
Evaluation				
12. Establish specific criteria. a. Comfort				
b. Physiological response, especially signs of internal bleeding (i.e., pulse, blood pressure, skin color, respiratory rate)				
c. Psychological response				
Documentation				
13. Record the procedure.				

General procedure for assisting with bone marrow biopsy

	Unsatisfactory	Needs More Practice	Satisfactory	Comments
Assessment				
1. Check physician's order.				
2. Check for signed permission form.				
3. Assess patient's physical abilities.				
Planning				
4. Wash your hands.				
5. Obtain bone marrow biopsy tray and sterile gloves.				
Implementation				
6. Identify patient.				
7. Discuss procedure with patient.				
8. Prepare unit. a. Privacy				
b. Equipment				
9. Prepare patient. a. Position for sternal or iliac crest biopsy.				
b. Drape.				
10. Assist with procedure. a. Assess.				
b. Reassure and support.				
c. Provide equipment.				
d. Apply pressure after needle is withdrawn.				
11. Conclude the procedure. a. Restore the patient.				
b. Restore the unit.				
c. Label and care for specimen.				
d. Dispose of equipment.				
e. Wash your hands.				
Evaluation				
12. Establish specific criteria. a. Comfort				
b. Physiological response, especially local bleeding at site				

	Unsatisfactory	Needs More Practice	Satisfactory	Comments
c. Psychological response				
Documentation				
13. Record the procedure.				

General procedure for assisting with proctoscopy, etc.

	Unsatisfactory	Needs More Practice	Satisfactory	Comments
Assessment				
1. Check physician's order regarding bowel cleansing, intake status, and procedure to be done.				
2. Check for signed permission form.				
3. Assess patient's physical abilities.				
Planning				
4. Wash your hands.				
5. Obtain scope, suction machine, towels, lubricating jelly, long swabs, slides or containers, exam gloves.				
Implementation				
6. Identify patient.				
7. Discuss procedure with patient.				
8. Prepare unit. a. Privacy				
b. Equipment				
9. Prepare patient. a. Position on special table or in knee-chest position.				
b. Drape with anus exposed.				
10. Assist with procedure. a. Assess.				
b. Reassure and support.				
c. Provide equipment.				
11. Conclude the procedure. a. Restore the patient.				
b. Restore the unit.				
c. Label and care for specimen.				

	Unsatisfactory	Needs More Practice	Satisfactory	Comments
d. Dispose of equipment.				
e. Wash your hands.				
☐ *Evaluation*				
12. Establish specific criteria. a. Comfort				
b. Physiological response, especially acute abdominal discomfort				
c. Psychological response				
☐ *Documentation*				
13. Record the procedure.				

QUIZ

Short-Answer Questions

1. What are two important functions of the nurse when assisting with a physical examination or a diagnostic procedure?

   a. _____

   b. _____

2. What is the best position for a patient having a physical exam?

   _____

3. An ophthalmoscope is used to examine the _____ .

4. An otoscope is used to examine the _____ .

5. Heart sounds should be heard with the patient in the _____ position.

6. During a thoracentesis, the patient should be observed carefully for such signs as _____ , _____ , _____ , _____ , or _____ .

7. Vitamin K is sometimes given to the patient who is to have a liver biopsy in order to _____ .

Multiple-Choice Questions

_____ 8. The signs listed in Question 6 could indicate

   a. infection.
   b. respiratory arrest.
   c. pleural irritation or puncture.
   d. all of the above.

_____ 9. The patient about to undergo a paracentesis should be instructed to void first so that

   a. there will be no discomfort from distention.
   b. the urine can be tested.
   c. the bladder will not be punctured.
   d. the bladder will not be in the way of the intestines.

_____ 10. The reason for positioning the patient having a lumbar puncture in the flexed position is to

   a. widen the intervertebral spaces to allow entrance of the needle.
   b. attain a position of comfort.
   c. gain exposure of the back.
   d. relax the musculature.

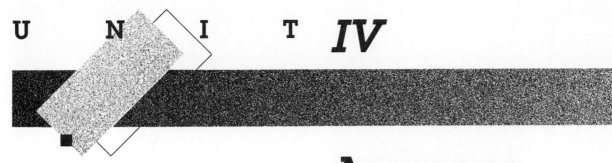

U N I T *IV*

ASSISTING WITH ACTIVITY AND REST

MODULE 21

Applying Restraints

MODULE CONTENTS

Rationale for the Use of This Skill
Nursing Diagnoses
General Considerations
Knots Used with Restraints
General Procedure for Applying Restraints
  Assessment
  Planning
  Implementation
  Evaluation
  Documentation
Specific Restraints
  Wrist or Ankle Restraints
  Belt Restraints
  Vest Restraints
  Elbow or Knee Restraints
  Soft-Tie Restraints
  Mitt Restraints

PREREQUISITES

Successful completion of the following modules:

VOLUME 1
Module 1 / An Approach to Nursing Skills
Module 2 / Medical Asepsis
Module 3 / Safety
Module 4 / Basic Body Mechanics
Module 5 / Assessment
Module 6 / Documentation
Module 8 / Moving the Patient in Bed and Positioning
Module 12 / Basic Infant Care
Module 24 / Range-of-Motion Exercises

OVERALL OBJECTIVE

To apply a variety of restraints, taking into account the comfort and safety of the individual patient.

SPECIFIC LEARNING OBJECTIVES

	Know Facts and Principles	Apply Facts and Principles	Demonstrate Ability	Evaluate Performance
1. *Reasons for physical restraint*	List two reasons for applying restraints	State reason in a given situation	In the clinical situation, understand reason for application	
2. *Legal implications*	State reason for obtaining order		Check order before applying, or take steps to obtain order	
3. *Choice of restraint*	Know various restraints used. State factors to consider in use of particular restraint.	Adapt choice to patient's needs	With an individual patient, choose appropriate restraint	Evaluate own performance with instructor
4. *Application of restraints*	Explain how to apply particular restraints		Apply restraint chosen, taking into account comfort and safety factors	Evaluate own performance using Performance Checklist
5. *Safety*	Give rationale for releasing restraints at intervals		Remove restraints at proper intervals, and turn or exercise patient	Evaluate own performance using Performance Checklist
6. *Documentation*	List data to be recorded		Make complete record of entire procedure, including assessment demonstrating need for restraint, time applied or removed, and condition of skin and circulation	Evaluate own performance using Performance Checklist

428

LEARNING ACTIVITIES

1. Review the Specific Learning Objectives.
2. Read the section on the effects of immobility (in the chapter on activity and rest) in Ellis and Nowlis, *Nursing: A Human Needs Approach,* or comparable material in another textbook.
3. Read through the module.
4. In the practice setting:
   a. Inspect the various physical restraints.
   b. Have a partner apply various restraints to you. Answer the following questions:
      (1) Which are the most comfortable?
      (2) Which are the least comfortable?
      (3) Why?
   c. Apply the various restraints to your partner. Check them for comfort and safety.
5. In the clinical setting:
   a. Observe any restraints being used. Have they been applied correctly and safely?
   b. When the opportunity arises, apply an appropriate restraint with your instructor's supervision.
   c. Using the Performance Checklist, evaluate your performance with the help of your instructor.
   d. Record pertinent data regarding the application of the restraint. Check recording with your instructor.

APPLYING RESTRAINTS

Rationale for the Use of This Skill

Physical restraints are applied in most cases for the safety of patients and occasionally for the protection of staff. All restraints must be applied with care to avoid damaging tissue and causing undue discomfort to patients. The nurse must use discretion in deciding when restraints should be applied and know the proper application of any restraints used.[1]

Nursing Diagnoses

Examples of some nursing diagnoses that might indicate a need for restraints include:

Injury, potential for, related to confusion
Injury, potential for, related to unsteady gait
Violence, potential for, related to suicidal· behavior

General Considerations

Restraints are used to restrict movement in the adult or child for a variety of reasons: to protect the patient from falling (out of bed, off a stretcher, out of a chair or wheelchair); to prevent the removal of tubes or other equipment (either as a result of excessive movement or in a confused or uncooperative moment); to prevent the patient from scratching rashes or other areas of irritation; and to prevent the patient from injuring himself or herself or members of the staff. Restraints can limit motion in a single limb, or they can immobilize the patient almost completely. The nurse selects the appropriate device on the basis of the nursing diagnosis that has been identified. Information specific to the use of restraints with infants and toddlers can be found in Module 12, Basic Infant Care. Remember that restraints should be used only when absolutely necessary. Sometimes the presence of a family member or friend makes restraining the patient unnecessary, at least for a time.

[1]You will note that rationale for action is emphasized throughout the module by the use of italics.

Knots Used with Restraints

Two knots that are commonly used with restraints are the clove hitch and the square knot. The *clove hitch* allows the patient some movement. *Because this knot is relatively loose* and does not tighten with movement of an extremity, circulation to the part is not restricted. The *square knot* is used more often to secure a tie to the bed frame or back of a wheelchair *because it will not slip* (see Figures 21.1 and 21.2).

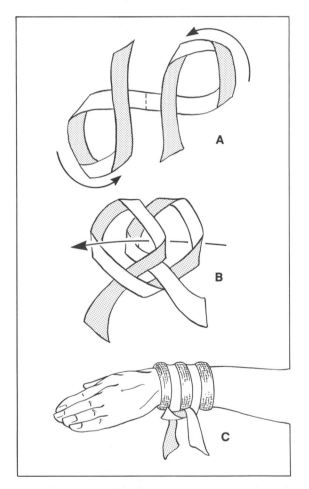

FIGURE 21.1 CLOVE HITCH Pad wrist or ankle with gauze, cloth, or ABD pad cut to size. Using a 1½-yd. strip of gauze or muslin, make two loops as in A. Place loops together and put wrist or ankle through loops as in B. Allowing ½" for comfort, tie a half hitch (C) to secure. Tie free ends to bedframe using a square knot.

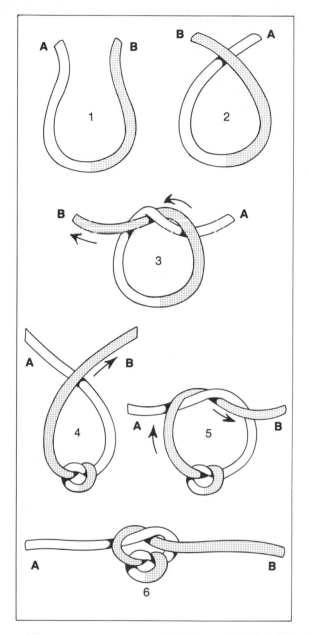

FIGURE 21.2 SQUARE KNOT

is not needed. *If the immediate safety of a patient or of the staff is in question,* apply restraints at once, and secure an order at the earliest possible moment. If this procedure is not followed, *the patient could take legal action against you.* You should be aware of state law in your locale and hospital policy regarding the use of restraints.

2. If the patient already has a restraint or restraints in place, assess the current need for them. *The situation that made the restraints necessary may have changed, or the patient may need a different degree of restraint.* The decision to restrain a patient physically must always be made after careful assessment. Restrain the patient as little as possible to accomplish your purpose.

3. Find out what types of restraints are available in your facility. In some facilities, restraints are referred to as *protective devices.* In others they are commonly called *Poseys,* after a leading manufacturer of restraints.

Planning

4. Wash your hands *for asepsis.*

5. When possible, provide for the patient's elimination needs before applying the restraint. *This adds to the patient's comfort and lessens the chance that you will have to remove the restraint to provide for elimination immediately after it is in place.*

6. Plan for any assistance that may be needed. You may need help with positioning or perhaps to subdue the confused or irrational patient.

7. Choose a restraint that fits the needs of the patient. Use the minimum restraint necessary to protect the patient or staff effectively. For example, if a patient is attempting to remove a nasogastric tube with the left hand, and the right upper extremity is paralyzed, you need use only a wrist restraint on the left wrist. You might leave the restraint loose enough *to allow some flexion of the elbow,* though not enough to let the patient reach the nasogastric tube. You can always modify a restraint later if necessary.

General Procedure for Applying Restraints

Assessment

1. Check the physician's orders. For routine restraining, such as securing a patient to a chair or stretcher *to prevent a fall,* an order

Implementation

8. Identify the patient *to be sure you are carrying out the procedure for the correct patient.*

9. Regardless of how irrational a patient might be, always explain what you plan to do and why. Never convey the impression that restraints are a punishment. For example, you might say that the restraint is to "remind" the patient not to lean too far forward in the chair. *This often makes the procedure more acceptable.* Showing the restraint to the patient *sometimes helps to allay the patient's fears.*

10. Apply the appropriate restraint, using a clove hitch or square knot. If the patient is in bed, never knot the ties to the side rails. *(If the rails were suddenly lowered, the patient could be injured.)* Knot them to the frame of the bed instead. Be careful not to secure any restraint too tightly *so that you do not cause the patient discomfort, impair circulation, or restrict function. For example, a too tight vest restraint could restrict breathing.*

11. If the patient is extremely restless or has fragile skin, add extra padding to the restraint *to protect the tissues.* You can use clean rags, washcloths, or gauze padding.

12. Reassure the patient.

13. Remove restraints every two hours or less, *so that the patient's position can be changed and the body part under restraint can be inspected and exercised. Never* leave a restraint on for longer than two hours without checking and moving it.

14. Reapply the restraint if necessary.

15. Wash your hands *for asepsis.*

Evaluation

16. Evaluate using the following criteria:
    a. Patient comfort
    b. Effectiveness of the restraint

Documentation

17. Record on the nurses' notes the type and location of the restraint, the time, and the reason for application. If you do not yet have a physician's order, note that the physician has been notified of your action. Include condition of skin under restraints, circulation distal to a restraint, and removal of restraints for skin care and ROM as appropriate. There may be a flow sheet for this purpose.

Specific Restraints

Wrist or Ankle Restraints

Commercial wrist or ankle restraints are cloth straps with a thread-through buckle device or Velcro cuff that are usually used to restrict motion of a limb for therapeutic reasons, such as to maintain an IV or to prevent the patient from pulling out a tube (see Figure 21.3). Slip the restraint on the patient's wrist or ankle, thread it, and tie it to the bed frame (never to a side rail). Attach wrist and ankle restraints to the movable portion of the bed frame *so that if the head of the bed is raised, the ties will not be pulled.*

Disposable wrist and ankle restraints, which are made of fabric or soft but strong paper, are also available. For severely disturbed and active psychiatric patients, leather straps locked with a key (which is in the nurse's possession at all times) are still sometimes used.

Belt Restraints

Belt restraints are threaded at the back (see Figure 21.4) and are used to keep the patient from falling out of bed or out of a chair. The smaller top belt is fastened around the patient's waist, and the lower belt is fastened to the bed frame. Disposable belt restraints are also available.

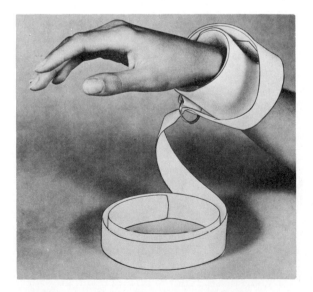

FIGURE 21.3 WRIST OR ANKLE RESTRAINT
Courtesy J. T. Posey Company, Arcadia, California

432

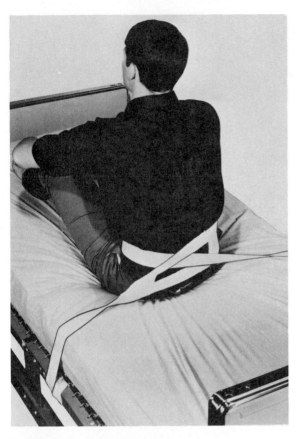
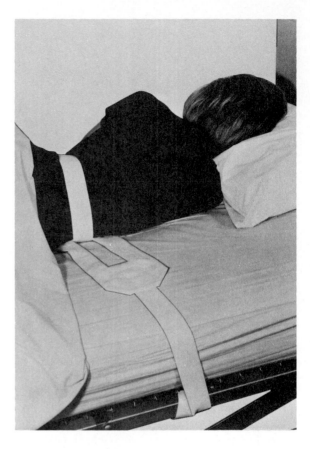

FIGURE 21.4 BELT RESTRAINT
Courtesy J. T. Posey Company, Arcadia, California

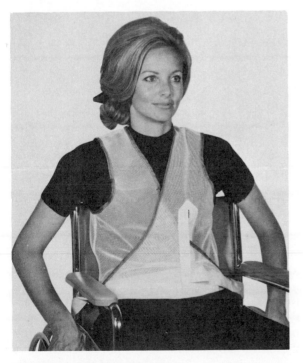
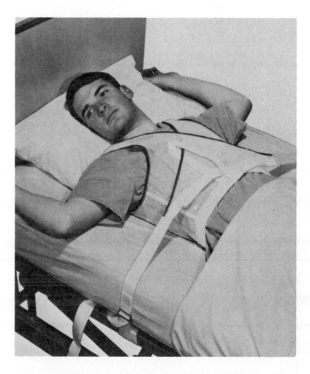

FIGURE 21.5 VEST RESTRAINT
Courtesy J. T. Posey Company, Arcadia, California

433

Examples of Documentation

12/3/88
1430
1. Injury, potential for, related to confusion
S "I don't remember trying to get out of bed"
O Found attempting to climb over side rail
A Risk of falling
P Have belt restraint in place at all times when patient is unattended. Check patient q.2.h. and reposition.

S. Atherton, S.N.

12/3/88
1430

Responding to name. Restless, grasping IV tubing with right hand. Wrist restraint applied.

D. Andrews, S.N.

Vest Restraints

These canvas or mesh vests have tails that are secured to the bed frame (see Figure 21.5). The tails may cross at the front or back, depending on the design of the vest. Vest restraints are used when the patient needs more support or a stronger reminder than a simple belt restraint provides. As with wrist and ankle restraints, make sure you attach the ties to the movable part of the bed.

Elbow or Knee Restraints

These are canvas or mesh wraparound restraints that have lengthwise rigid stays *to prevent joint flexion* (see Figure 21.6). They are used most often to prevent the pediatric patient from disturbing a tube or dressing, or from scratching a rash.

Soft-Tie Restraints

Some facilities make their own restraints. One of the most common is a soft tie, a long, narrow (3 inches × 5 to 8 feet) piece of fabric. It is often made from a worn bedspread or other heavy fabric.

The soft tie is used in a variety of ways. For a *waist restraint,* place it across the patient's lap

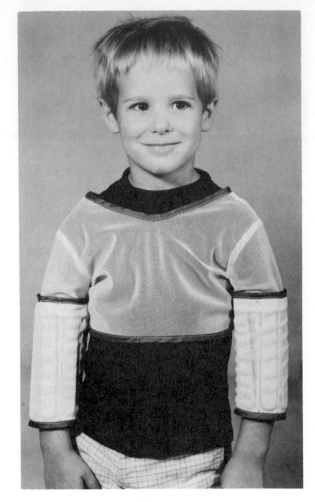

FIGURE 21.6 ELBOW RESTRAINT
Courtesy J. T. Posey Company, Arcadia, California

and under the arms of the chair; then tie it securely behind the chair. If necessary, wrap the tie around the arm of the chair before tying it or wrap it around the back legs of the chair and tie it under the chair *to keep the knot out of the patient's reach* (see Figure 21.7).

This long tie may also be used as a figure-8 restraint. *The purpose of this restraint is to keep a patient from sliding, feet first, from under the restraint and out of the chair.* Instead of the soft tie, you can also use a large sheet twisted from opposite corners into a long tie for a figure-8 restraint. Place the center of the tie across the top of the patient's thighs, just above the knees. Pass the ends behind each leg and bring them up between the legs at the knees. Then cross the two long ends and put them under the arms of the chair and

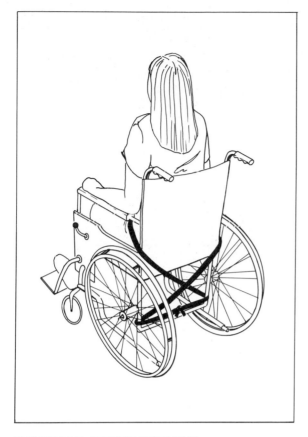

FIGURE 21.7 SOFT-TIE RESTRAINT

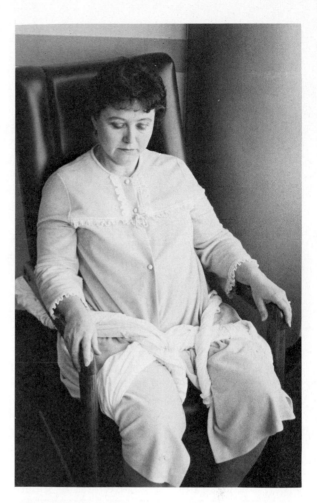

FIGURE 21.8 FIGURE-8 RESTRAINT
Courtesy Ivan Ellis

around to the back of the chair, where they are tied together. Take care not to pull this restraint too tight, and check the inner aspects of the thighs and knees carefully *for skin abrasion.* This restraint is useful in maintaining a correct sitting posture (see Figure 21.8).

Mitt Restraints

Mitt restraints (see Figure 21.9) are used for patients who absentmindedly pull at tubes or appliances or who may injure themselves by scratching a rash or picking at a wound. They restrict only the hand and fingers and *allow the arm to move freely.* Mitts are available commercially, or they can be made by wrapping the hands loosely with strips of soft fabric or rolls of dressing material. Secure the wrapping with paper tape *to prevent skin irritation and allow easy removal.* Remove the mitts periodically, as you would other restraints, *to clean and exercise the hands and fingers.*

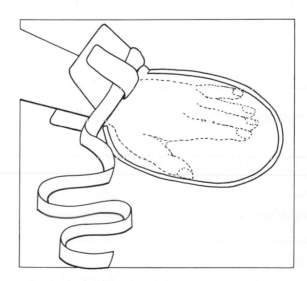

FIGURE 21.9 MITT RESTRAINT

PERFORMANCE CHECKLIST

General procedure for applying restraints	Unsatisfactory	Needs More Practice	Satisfactory	Comments
Assessment				
1. Check physician's orders for restraint. If need is immediate, proceed.				
2. Assess patient's current need for restraint.				
3. Find out types of restraints available.				
Planning				
4. Wash your hands.				
5. Provide for patient's elimination needs.				
6. Plan any assistance needed.				
7. Choose appropriate restraint.				
Implementation				
8. Identify patient.				
9. Explain what you plan to do and why. Elicit patient's cooperation.				
10. Apply restraint using clove hitch or square knot.				
11. Add extra padding, if needed.				
12. Reassure patient.				
13. Remove restraints at least every two hours, and inspect and exercise part.				
14. Reapply restraint if necessary.				
15. Wash your hands.				
Evaluation				
16. Evaluate using the following criteria: a. Patient comfort				
b. Effectiveness of the restraint				
Documentation				
17. Record: a. Type and location of restraint				
b. Time and reason for application				
c. Condition of skin, circulation, skin care				

QUIZ

Short-Answer Questions

1. List two reasons why physical restraints are applied to patients.

    a. _____

    b. _____

2. To restrain a patient who is trying to remove a tube, such as a catheter, you could apply either a(n) _____ or _____ restraint.

3. For a patient who is attempting to get up and out of bed, you would apply a(n) _____ or _____ restraint.

4. List two reasons why restraints should be removed every two hours or less.

    a. _____

    b. _____

5. Correctly state one nursing diagnosis that would be appropriate as the title of a SOAP note regarding the application of restraints to a patient who is confused and at risk of falling if up unassisted.

    _____

    _____

    _____

Multiple-Choice Question

_____ 6. A major reason a nurse should obtain a physician's order after restraining a patient is to

    a. determine the type of restraint to be used.
    b. determine the length of time to apply the restraint.
    c. legally protect the physician.
    d. legally protect the nurse.

MODULE 22

Transfer

MODULE CONTENTS

Rationale for the Use of This Skill
Safety
General Procedure for Transfer
  Assessment
  Planning
  Implementation
  Evaluation
  Documentation
Specific Transfer Techniques
  Bed to Chair: One-Person Maximal Assist
  Bed to Chair: One-Person Minimal Assist
  Bed to Chair: Two-Person Maximal Assist
  Chair to Chair: Two-Person Lift
  Bed to Chair: Two-Person Lift
  Bed to Chair: Hydraulic Lift
  Horizontal Lift: Three or Four-Person Assist

PREREQUISITES

Successful completion of the following modules:

VOLUME 1
Module 1 / An Approach to Nursing Skills
Module 2 / Medical Asepsis
Module 3 / Safety
Module 4 / Basic Body Mechanics
Module 5 / Assessment
Module 6 / Documentation
Module 8 / Moving the Patient in Bed and
  Positioning
Module 21 / Applying Restraints

OVERALL OBJECTIVE

To transfer a patient from a bed to a chair, wheelchair, commode, or stretcher, with a maximum of comfort and safety for both patient and nurse.

SPECIFIC LEARNING OBJECTIVES

	Know Facts and Principles	Apply Facts and Principles	Demonstrate Ability	Evaluate Performance
1. Reasons for transfer	List four reasons for patient's activity	Given a patient situation, state purpose of activity	In clinical setting, state reasons for patient's activity	Determine that patient was not injured in transfer
2. Safety	List common hazards	Recognize hazards in a particular situation	Provide safe setting for transfer	
3. Assessment of patient	State reasons for knowing patient's diagnosis and capabilities	Give examples of how different diagnoses and capabilities would affect plans for transfer	Gather data on patient's abilities and diagnoses before moving patient	After transfer, review procedure to find whether more data would have helped. Validate with instructor.
4. Transfer of patient a. Bed to chair b. Bed to stretcher c. Chair to chair	List steps of usual transfer procedures	Plan modification of procedures for particular patient situation. Identify best procedure to use in specific situation.	Successfully transfer patient a. from bed to chair or commode b. from bed to stretcher c. from chair to chair or commode	Evaluate own performance using Performance Checklist

LEARNING ACTIVITIES	VOCABULARY

LEARNING ACTIVITIES

1. Review the Specific Learning Objectives.
2. Read the section on posture and body mechanics and ambulation (in the chapter on activity and rest) in Ellis and Nowlis, *Nursing: A Human Needs Approach,* or comparable material in another textbook.
3. Look up the module vocabulary terms in the Glossary.
4. Read through the module.
5. In the practice setting:
   a. Place a colored tie or scarf around your partner's left arm and another on the left leg (or right arm and right leg). This will be the nonfunctional side.
   b. Transfer your partner from a supine position in bed to an upright position sitting on the side of the bed.
   c. Transfer your partner from the bed to a chair using a one-person, minimal-assist transfer.
   d. Transfer your partner using a one-person, maximal-assist transfer.
   e. With a third person, transfer your partner using a two-person, maximal-assist transfer.
   f. Transfer your partner using a two-person lift transfer.
   g. Transfer your partner from a bed to a stretcher using a three-person horizontal lift.
   h. Change roles as "patient" and nurse, and repeat all of the transfers until each person participating has had an opportunity to be in each role.
   i. If a hydraulic lifting device is available:
      (1) Obtain the lift.
      (2) Review the specific directions for its use.
      (3) Practice pumping up and lowering the device without a person in it.
      (4) Using the directions in this module, transfer another student from a bed to a chair and back to the bed using the lift.
      (5) Ask the student who was transferred to describe how it felt.

VOCABULARY

horizontal
hydraulic
supine
weight-bearing

TRANSFER

Rationale for the Use of This Skill

M*oving patients out of bed has proved very beneficial to them. The movement maintains and restores muscle tone and also stimulates the respiratory and circulatory systems and improves elimination. Patients need only dangle their legs over the side of the bed or sit in a chair at the bedside for a few minutes to improve their well-being. Many patients are unable to move at all or need some assistance in moving. It is the nurse's responsibility to help by moving patients, by directing them in the best techniques for self-movement, and by seeing that enough people are on hand to ensure their safety during transfer.*

Properly helping a patient from the bed to a chair is an important nursing function, in which you play a vital role by giving the patient physical support and encouragement. Pay special attention to safety precautions, as well as to the basics of body mechanics, to ensure both your safety and the patient's.

The level of activity is usually determined by a physician's orders, but nursing assessment is necessary to determine the best method for carrying out the order.[1]

Safety

Falls are the most common hazard to a patient being transferred. The patient may become dizzy or have less strength than expected, or the nurse may not be strong enough to accomplish the task. Consider these possibilities carefully before beginning. If a patient begins to fall, he or she should be lowered to the bed, the chair, or the floor in such a way as to prevent injury.

Another hazard in moving patients is the pull on indwelling tubings (such as catheters or IV tubing). Take care to move tubings as necessary without dislodging them. Position the patient carefully *so that he or she will not strike against side rails or furniture.* Be sure the patient is wearing shoes or slippers (with firm soles) *to prevent sliding or bruising the feet.*

---

[1]You will note that rationale for action is emphasized throughout the module by the use of italics.

General Procedure for Transfer

Assessment

1. To facilitate a transfer, you must know the patient's diagnosis and any restrictions to be observed. For example, a patient with a recently repaired fractured hip may be allowed to rest only 25 percent of his or her weight on the affected side, whereas a post-op patient who has had an appendectomy may not be restricted in any way.
2. In addition, you should assess the capabilities of the patient. Is the patient capable of moving all extremities? If the patient is partially incapacitated, which is the stronger side? How was the patient transferred before? Asking the patient is not always the best way to get this information; some patients may not be able to provide accurate information. You should check with other nurses and consult the record and Kardex.
3. Find out what equipment is available for moving patients, as well as who is available to assist you.

Planning

4. With the data in hand, devise a plan to transfer the patient, in the safest and most convenient manner, taking into account proper body mechanics for both you and the patient. Be realistic: you may need more than one person to transfer a heavy or severely disabled patient.
5. Wash your hands *for asepsis.*
6. Obtain any equipment that you or the patient will need.

Implementation

7. Identify the patient *to be sure you are carrying out the procedure for the correct patient.*
8. Lower the bed itself as well as the head of the bed. *The position of the bed can help greatly in transfer.* Some beds are lowered by an electrical control at the side or foot of the bed, and some are lowered manually by crank. Make these mechanical devices work for you.
9. Foot coverings are essential. *Firm-soled shoes give the patient a sense of security and prevent slipping.* If shoes are not available, leather-soled slippers can be used. Always

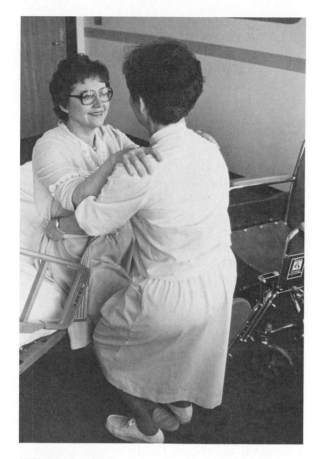

FIGURE 22.1 BED TO WHEELCHAIR: ONE-PERSON MAXIMAL ASSIST
Courtesy Ivan Ellis

put braces and appliances on a patient before he or she is transferred.

10. Transfer and ambulation belts are very useful assistive devices. The belt is made of heavy twill with a buckle that stays fastened when pressure or force is applied. It is placed around the patient's waist *to give those assisting with the activity a way to hold onto the patient firmly.* The belt must be applied snugly enough *to hold the patient in a secure fashion* but not so snugly *as to be uncomfortable.* (See Figure 22.1.) In the past, these belts were available only in physical therapy departments, so many nurses are not familiar with their use. Once you have used one, you will be convinced of their value.

Use a transfer belt for all transfers except those in which you lift the patient. When a belt is not available, devise a substitute from items on hand. A drawsheet can be folded and wrapped around the patient's waist. If the sheet is thin enough to permit tying it, do so. If it is too bulky to tie, cross it in back and grasp the ends along with the side when you use it for lifting. A patient's gown can be another substitute. Tie it around the patient's waist and use it as you would a transfer belt. A patient may even have a regular leather belt that can be used, but be careful that a narrow belt does not cut into the patient.

11. As simply as possible, explain to the patient what you intend to do or how you intend to help, as well as how he or she is expected to participate. Ask if there are any questions.

It is essential that you appear confident. It is also important not to rush the patient.

12. Carry out the specific procedure as outlined.

Evaluation

13. Evaluate using the following criteria:
    a. Patient's body alignment
    b. Patient's comfort
    c. Safety for the patient
    d. Safety and proper body mechanics for the nurse(s) involved

Documentation

14. Keep a record for other members of the health care team of the best means of transfer, the number of people needed to help, the patient's ability to cooperate, and any aids or devices needed. The Kardex or nursing care plan is usually used for this purpose.

15. Each time a transfer is carried out, note on the patient's record the exact nature of the activity, the time it was carried out, and the patient's response to it. Evaluate the patient's response in terms of pain, fatigue, pulse and respiration rate, blood pressure changes, and dizziness.

Specific Transfer Techniques

Be sure to review the module on Basic Body Mechanics *in order to understand the rationale for the way you move patients.*

Bed to Chair: One-Person Maximal Assist

For each transfer technique discussed, step 12 of the General Procedure is presented specific to that technique. The detailed procedures, which include all the steps of the General Procedure as well as the individualized step 12, are given in the Performance Checklist.

Implementation

12. Transfer the patient from bed to wheelchair or armchair.
    a. Angle the wheelchair or armchair to the bed so that the chair is on the patient's stronger side. If the footrests are removable, remove them at this time; otherwise, fold them out of the way. *This arrangement will allow the patient to pivot on the stronger leg.*
    b. Lock the bed and wheelchair. *This prevents the wheelchair from moving during transfer.* Be sure the patient sees the chair and its position.
    c. Begin with the patient in a supine position, with the hips placed where the bed will bend as the head of the bed is raised, and close to the edge of the bed.
    d. Raise the head of the bed so that the patient is in a sitting position. *(This decreases the effort for both you and the patient.)* Raise the bed slowly *so that the patient does not get dizzy.*
    e. Slide one arm under the patient's legs and place the other arm behind the patient's back. Swing the patient's legs over the side of the bed while pivoting the patient's body, so that he or she ends up sitting on the edge of the bed with the feet hanging down.
    f. Allow the patient to sit for a few minutes *to prevent lightheadedness or orthostatic hypotension,* which can occur with any sudden change in circulation caused by lowering the legs. Support the patient if he or she feels dizzy.
    g. Position the patient's feet firmly on the floor and slightly apart, with the patient's hands on the bed or on your shoulders. *To protect yourself from injury,* do not let the patient hold you about the neck.
    h. Take a wide stance, bend your knees, and grasp the patient at the sides of the belt. You may want to straddle the patient's weaker leg with your own legs, or to stabilize the patient's knees by supporting them with your own knees (see Figure 22.1).
    i. Inform the patient that he or she will be assisted to a standing position on a count of "one, two, three, *stand!*"
    j. On the count, straighten your knees, assisting the patient to a standing position.
    k. Stand close to the patient and pivot to the chair.
    l. Instruct the patient to place both hands on the arms of the chair.
    m. Lower the patient to the seat.
    n. Be sure the patient's body is positioned firmly back in the seat *for good posture.*

This same technique can be used to transfer a patient from one chair to another.

Bed to Chair: One-Person Minimal Assist

Proceed as you would for the one-person, maximal-assist transfer described above, with two exceptions. It is not necessary to brace the patient's knees, nor is a transfer belt usually necessary. *You will be primarily providing balance, not lifting the patient's weight* (see Figure 22.2).

Bed to Chair: Two-Person Maximal Assist

Implementation

12. Transfer the patient from bed to wheelchair or armchair.
    a. Put the bed flat.
    b. Position the wheelchair or armchair next to the bed, at a 45-degree angle, with the seat facing toward the bed. Secure the brakes.
    c. Help the patient to a sitting position on the edge of the bed as described in the one-person maximal assist, step 12e and f.
    d. Have the patient place his or her hands on the bed or on the shoulders of Nurse 1.

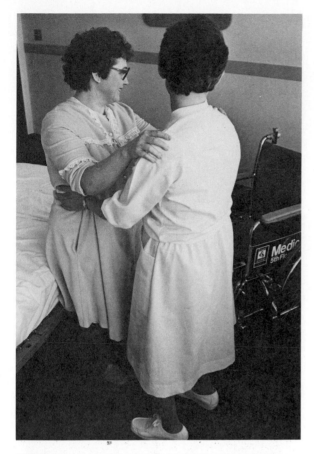

FIGURE 22.2 BED TO WHEELCHAIR: ONE-PERSON MINIMAL ASSIST
Courtesy Ivan Ellis

Chair to Chair: Two-Person Lift

`_____` *Implementation*

12. Transfer the patient from chair to chair or commode. The transfer belt is not used for this transfer technique.
    a. Place the chairs (or commode and chair) side by side, facing in the same direction.
    b. Remove the footrests from the wheelchair or fold them out of the way, and lock or brace the chair (or commode).
    c. The taller nurse (1) stands behind the chair.
    d. The shorter nurse (2) stands facing the patient.
    e. Nurse 1 folds the patient's arms across the patient's chest. The nurse then reaches under the patient's arms from behind the patient and grasps the opposite wrists.
    f. Nurse 2 bends knees and hips, adopting a squatting position, and grasps the patient under the knees to support the legs (see Figure 22.4).
    g. Nurse 1 informs the patient that he or she will be moved on a count of "One, two, three, *lift!*"
    h. Nurse 1 counts ("One, two, three, *lift!*"), and both lift at the same time. Nurse 1 controls the timing because he or she will bear the greatest weight.
    i. When the word "lift" is said, both nurses lift the patient and move over to the second chair (or commode), lowering the patient immediately, slowly and smoothly.

Bed to Chair: Two-Person Lift

`_____` *Implementation*

12. Transfer the patient from bed to chair, wheelchair, or commode. The transfer belt is not used for this transfer technique.
    a. Put the bed flat in the low position and lock it.
    b. Set the wheelchair parallel to the bed and secure its brakes. If the armrests

e. Nurse 1 stands in front of the patient (one-person maximal assist, step 12g and h), grasping the belt at the sides.
f. Nurse 2 stands between the wheelchair and the bed, with one knee on the bed, and grasps the transfer belt at the patient's back (see Figure 22.3).
g. Nurse 1 informs the patient that he or she will be moved on a count of "One, two, three, *lift!*"
h. Nurse 1 signals, "One, two, three, *lift!*" Both assistants lift and pivot the patient at the same time, then lower the patient into the wheelchair.
i. Be sure the patient's body is positioned straight and firmly back in the wheelchair *for good posture.*

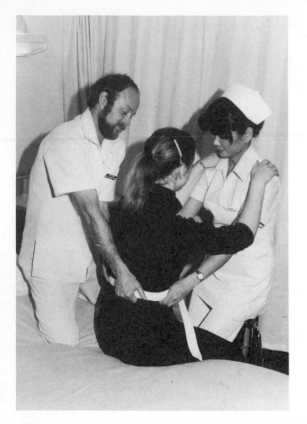
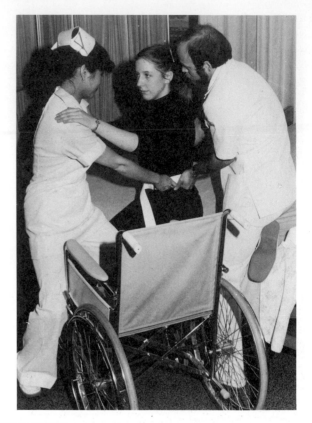

FIGURE 22.3 BED TO WHEELCHAIR: TWO-PERSON MAXIMAL ASSIST
Courtesy Ivan Ellis

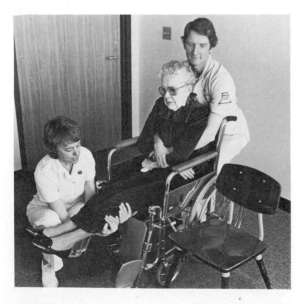

FIGURE 22.4 CHAIR TO CHAIR: TWO-PERSON LIFT
Courtesy Ivan Ellis

are removable, remove the one next to the bed.

c. Slide the patient to the edge of the bed.

d. Nurse 1 slides one arm under the patient's arms and begins lifting the shoulders. The nurse places one knee on the bed and slides his or her arms around the patient until both arms are under the patient's arms and the patient is sitting, leaning on the nurse's chest.

e. Nurse 1 crosses the patient's arms on the chest, grasping the opposite wrists in front of the patient.

f. Nurse 2 squats beside the bed and slides both arms under the patient's thighs from the same side (see Figure 22.5).

g. Nurse 1 informs the patient that he or she will be moved on a count of "One, two, three, *lift!*"

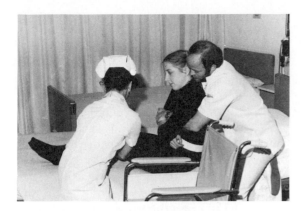 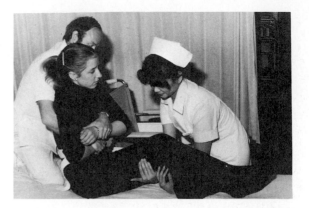

FIGURE 22.5 BED TO CHAIR: TWO-PERSON LIFT
Courtesy Ivan Ellis

h. Nurse 1 counts ("One, two, three, *lift!*"), and both nurses lift the patient onto the wheelchair (or commode).

A third person can help in this lift, sliding his or her arms under the patient's buttocks *so that the three people can lift at one time.*

Bed to Chair: Hydraulic Lift

The hydraulic lift enables a nurse to lift a very heavy patient or one who is badly incapacitated without relying on personal strength. (The Hoyer is one brand of hydraulic lift.) All lifts have a sturdy frame that supports the patient's weight; a canvas or nylon sling of some type, which is positioned under the patient; and a hydraulic pump. Consult the literature for specifics about the particular brand and model used in your facility, but the following should serve as a general outline of the procedure. Two people are usually needed *to ensure the patient's safety.* Two are essential for incapacitated patients who cannot support their own heads. The transfer belt is not used for this transfer technique.

☐ *Implementation*

12. Using the hydraulic lift, transfer the patient.
 a. Explain to the patient what the lift is for and how it works. Emphasize the safety of the procedure *because the patient may be frightened by the large mechanical device.*
 b. Raise the bed to a comfortable working position.
 c. Place the patient in the supine position.

d. Place the sling by rolling the patient side to side and slipping it under the body in the same way you would place a sheet under a patient in bed. If the patient is not clothed (as in a transfer to a tub, for example), cover the patient with a bath blanket.

For the patient's safety, the sling must be positioned correctly. *If the lower edge of the sling is too high, the patient could slip feet first out of the sling. If the lower edge is too low (on a two-piece sling), the patient could "fold up" and slip out of the sling.*
 (1) *One-piece sling* Place the bottom edge just above the knees. The top edge can extend behind the shoulders or to the head.
 (2) *Two-piece sling* Place one of the canvas strips behind the patient's thighs, *so that it forms a seat for the sling.* Position the second canvas strip under the patient's shoulder blades, *so that it supports the patient's trunk in a semireclining position.*
 e. Lower the bed.
 f. Position the lift by the bed, *so that the lifting arm extends above the patient.* If the support legs are adjustable, they should be in their widest, *most stable position.*
 g. Place the patient's arms across his or her chest, *keeping them out of the way during the lift.*
 h. Fasten the chains of the lift to the sling. The chains to the seat section

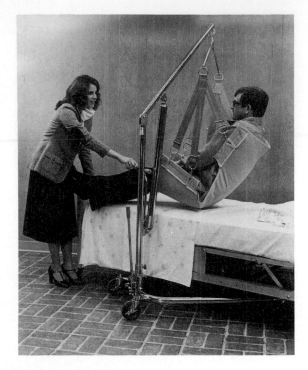

FIGURE 22.6 HYDRAULIC LIFT
Courtesy Ted Hoyer & Company, Inc., Oshkosh, Wisconsin

should be slightly longer than the chains to the trunk section, *to create a semireclining position when the sling is lifted.* When you fasten the chains, make sure that the hooks are pointed *away* from the patient *to prevent them from jabbing him or her.* Be careful not to catch skin folds in the metal edges and chains.

i. Nurse 1 stands at the patient's head, *to support the head and guide the patient during the lift.*

j. Nurse 2 makes sure the valve on the hydraulic pump is closed and begins pumping, gradually lifting the patient off the bed. Lift until the patient just clears the bed and no higher. *The higher the lift, the less stable its balance.*

k. Nurse 1 guides the patient and nurse 2 guides the lift as the lift is maneuvered away from the bed (see Figure 22.6).

l. Double-check the position of the bath blanket if you are transporting a patient to a tub. You may want to place additional coverings around the patient's buttocks and shoulders *to keep the patient warm and to provide for modesty.*

m. Slowly, keeping careful balance, move the lift to the chair, tub, or other bed.

n. Position the patient above the next resting place, with special attention to the correct positioning of the hips.

o. Release the hydraulic valve carefully and lower the patient very slowly, correcting the positioning as the patient moves downward. Be careful not to open the valve too far, *which would cause the patient to move down too abruptly.*

p. Close the valve as soon as the patient's weight is on the chair. Otherwise *the support arm will lower onto the patient.*

q. Detach the chains from the sling and remove the lift. The sling usually remains under the patient in the new position, so that the reverse procedure, back to the bed, is easy. If you have transferred the patient to another bed, remove the sling by turning the patient from side to side.

Horizontal Lift: Three- or Four-Person Assist

⬜ *Implementation*

12. Transfer the patient as outlined below. The transfer belt is not used for this transfer technique.

a. Place the stretcher at the foot of the bed, at a right angle to it, with the brakes secured.

b. Move the patient to one side of the bed.

c. Nurse 1, the tallest, stands at the patient's head and slides his or her arms under the patient's neck and shoulders.

d. Nurse 2, the next tallest nurse, stands at the patient's waist and hips and slides both arms under the patient.

e. The shortest nurse, nurse 3, stands at the patient's knees and slides both arms under the lower legs and thighs. If a fourth nurse is used, nurse 2 is at the waist and chest, nurse 3 is at the

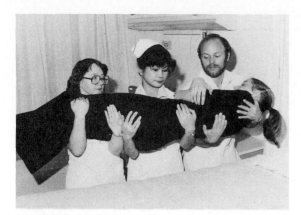

FIGURE 22.7 HORIZONTAL LIFT: THREE-PERSON ASSIST
Courtesy Ivan Ellis

hips, and nurse 4 is at the knees and legs.

f. Nurse 2 instructs the patient that he or she will be lifted on a count of "One, two, three, *lift*!"

g. Using the elbows as levers, all nurses roll the patient toward themselves in a hugging motion. Then the patient is lifted on the count "One, two, three, *lift*!"

h. Holding the patient against their bodies, the nurses walk together, with synchronized steps, to the side and backward, until they are parallel to the stretcher (see Figure 22.7).

i. At the count ("One, two, three, *down*!"), the patient is placed on the stretcher.

PERFORMANCE CHECKLIST

General procedure for transfer

	Unsatisfactory	Needs More Practice	Satisfactory	Comments
Assessment				
1. Check patient's diagnosis and restrictions.				
2. Assess capabilities of patient.				
3. Identify equipment and help available.				
Planning				
4. Devise plan for transfer.				
5. Wash your hands.				
6. Obtain equipment needed.				
Implementation				
7. Identify patient.				
8. Lower the entire bed.				
9. Place shoes or slippers on patient.				
10. Put transfer belt on patient if needed for the transfer technique being used.				
11. Explain method of transfer to patient.				
12. Carry out specific procedure.				
Evaluation				
13. Evaluate using the following criteria: a. Patient's body alignment				
b. Patient's comfort				
c. Safety for the patient				
d. Safety and proper body mechanics for the nurse(s) involved				
Documentation				
14. Record on Kardex or nursing care plan: a. Best method and aids to use				
b. Number of people needed to help				
c. Patient's ability to participate				
15. Record on patient's chart: a. Time of activity				

	Unsatisfactory	Needs More Practice	Satisfactory	Comments
b. Activity carried out				
c. Patient's response				

Bed to chair: One-person maximal assist

☐ *Assessment*

1. Follow Checklist steps 1–3 of the General Procedure for Transfer (check patient's diagnosis and restrictions, assess capabilities of patient, and identify equipment and help available).

☐ *Planning*

2. Follow Checklist steps 4–6 of the General Procedure (devise plan for transfer, wash your hands, and obtain equipment needed).

☐ *Implementation*

3. Follow Checklist steps 7–11 of the General Procedure (identify patient, lower the entire bed, place shoes or slippers on patient, put transfer belt on patient if indicated, and explain method of transfer to patient).

4. Transfer the patient from bed to wheelchair as outlined below:
   a. Angle chair to bed on patient's stronger side.

   b. Lock or brace bed and chair.

   c. Have patient in supine position.

   d. Raise head of bed slowly.

   e. Swing patient's legs over side of bed while pivoting patient's body to achieve sitting position.

   f. Allow patient to sit for a few moments.

   g. Place patient's feet slightly apart and position patient's hands on your shoulders.

   h. Straddle patient's knees with your own, keeping wide stance and knees bent, and grasp belt.

   i. Inform patient of signal.

   j. On the count, straighten your knees, lifting patient to a standing position.

	Unsatisfactory	Needs More Practice	Satisfactory	Comments
k. Stand close to patient and pivot to chair.				
l. Place patient's hands on armrests.				
m. Lower patient to seat.				
n. Be sure patient's buttocks are positioned in back of seat.				
☐ *Evaluation*				
5. Evaluate using the criteria in Checklist step 13 of the General Procedure (patient's body alignment, patient's comfort, safety for the patient, and safety and proper body mechanics for the nurse(s) involved.)				
☐ *Documentation*				
6. Record as in Checklist steps 14 and 15 of the General Procedure (on the Kardex or nursing care plan, best method and aids to use, number of people needed to help, and patient's ability to participate; and on the patient's chart, time of activity, activity carried out, and patient's response).				
Bed to chair: Two-person maximal assist				
☐ *Assessment*				
1. Follow Checklist steps 1–3 of the General Procedure for Transfer (check patient's diagnosis and restrictions, assess capabilities of patient, and identify equipment and help available).				
☐ *Planning*				
2. Follow Checklist steps 4–6 of the General Procedure (devise plan for transfer, wash your hands, and obtain equipment needed).				
☐ *Implementation*				
3. Follow Checklist steps 7–11 of the General Procedure (identify patient, lower the entire bed, place shoes or slippers on patient, and explain method of transfer to patient).				
4. Transfer the patient from bed to wheelchair or armchair as outlined below: a. Put bed flat and lock it.				

	Unsatisfactory	Needs More Practice	Satisfactory	Comments
b. Assist patient to sit.				
c. Position wheelchair at 45-degree angle and lock.				
d. Nurse 1 stands in front of patient and grasps belt at sides. Patient has hands on bed or on shoulders of nurse 1.				
e. Nurse 2 stands between chair and bed, with one knee on bed, and grasps belt at back.				
f. Nurse 1 informs patient of signal.				
g. Nurse 1 signals, and both lift.				
☐ *Evaluation*				
5. Evaluate using the criteria in Checklist step 13 of the General Procedure [patient's body alignment, patient's comfort, safety for the patient, and safety and proper body mechanics for the nurse(s) involved].				
☐ *Documentation*				
6. Record as in Checklist steps 14 and 15 of the General Procedure (on the Kardex or nursing care plan, best method and aids to use, number of people needed to help, and patient's ability to participate; and on the patient's chart, time of activity, activity carried out, and patient's response).				
Chair to chair: Two-person lift				
☐ *Assessment*				
1. Follow Checklist steps 1–3 of the General Procedure for Transfer (check patient's diagnosis and restrictions, assess capabilities of patient, and identify equipment and help available).				
☐ *Planning*				
2. Follow Checklist steps 4–6 of the General Procedure (devise plan for transfer, wash your hands, and obtain equipment needed).				

	Unsatisfactory	Needs More Practice	Satisfactory	Comments
Implementation				
3. Follow Checklist steps 7–11 of the General Procedure (identify patient, lower the entire bed, place shoes or slippers on patient, and explain method of transfer to patient).				
4. Transfer the patient from chair to chair or commode as outlined below:				
a. Place chairs (chair and commode) side by side.				
b. Remove footrests from chair, and lock or brace chair (commode).				
c. Taller nurse (nurse 1) stands behind chair with patient.				
d. Shorter nurse (nurse 2) stands facing patient.				
e. Nurse 1 crosses patient's arms and grasps wrists from behind.				
f. Nurse 2 squats and grasps patient around knees.				
g. Nurse 1 informs patient of signal.				
h. Nurse 1 counts.				
i. On "*lift*," both nurses lift patient and move to second chair (or commode).				
Evaluation				
5. Evaluate using the criteria in Checklist step 13 of the General Procedure [patient's body alignment, patient's comfort, safety for the patient, and safety and proper body mechanics for the nurse(s) involved].				
Documentation				
6. Record as in Checklist steps 14 and 15 of the General Procedure (on the Kardex or nursing care plan, best method and aids to use, number of people needed to help, and patient's ability to participate; and on the patient's chart, time of activity, activity carried out, and patient's response).				

Bed to chair: Two-person lift

	Unsatisfactory	Needs More Practice	Satisfactory	Comments
☐ *Assessment*				
1. Follow Checklist steps 1–3 of the General Procedure for Transfer (check patient's diagnosis and restrictions, assess capabilities of patient, and identify equipment and help available).				
☐ *Planning*				
2. Follow Checklist steps 4–6 of the General Procedure (devise plan for transfer, wash your hands, and obtain equipment needed).				
☐ *Implementation*				
3. Follow Checklist steps 7–11 of the General Procedure (check patient's diagnosis and restrictions, assess capabilities of patient, and identify equipment and help available).				
4. Transfer the patient from bed to chair, wheelchair, or commode as outlined below: a. Put bed flat and lock it.				
b. Position chair parallel to bed and secure brakes.				
c. Slide patient to edge of bed.				
d. Nurse 1 slides arm under patient's shoulders and maneuvers patient to sitting position.				
e. Nurse 1 crosses patient's arms over chest and grasps opposite wrists.				
f. Nurse 2 squats beside bed and slides arms under patient's thighs.				
g. Nurse 1 informs patient of signal.				
h. Lift at nurse 1's signal.				
☐ *Evaluation*				
5. Evaluate using the criteria in Checklist step 13 of the General Procedure [patient's body alignment, patient's comfort, safety for the patient, and safety and proper body mechanics for the nurse(s) involved].				

	Unsatisfactory	Needs More Practice	Satisfactory	Comments
Documentation				
6. Record as in Checklist steps 14 and 15 of the General Procedure (on the Kardex or nursing care plan, best method and aids to use, number of people needed to help, and patient's ability to participate; and on the patient's chart, time of activity, activity carried out, and patient's response).				

Bed to chair: Hydraulic lift

	Unsatisfactory	Needs More Practice	Satisfactory	Comments
Assessment				
1. Follow Checklist steps 1–3 of the General Procedure for Transfer (check patient's diagnosis and restrictions, assess capabilities of patient, and identify equipment and help available).				
Planning				
2. Follow Checklist steps 4–6 of the General Procedure (devise plan for transfer, wash your hands, and obtain equipment needed).				
Implementation				
3. Follow Checklist steps 7–11 of the General Procedure (identify patient, lower the entire bed, place shoes or slippers on patient, put transfer belt on patient if indicated, and explain method of transfer to patient).				
4. Using the hydraulic lift, transfer the patient as indicated below: a. Explain lift to patient.				
b. Raise bed to comfortable working position.				
c. Place patient in supine position.				
d. Position sling correctly, and drape patient if necessary.				
e. Place bed in low position.				
f. Position lift over patient.				
g. Place patient's arms across chest.				
h. Fasten lift's chains.				
i. Nurse 1 at patient's head.				

	Unsatisfactory	Needs More Practice	Satisfactory	Comments
j. Nurse 2 begins pumping.				
k. Nurse 1 guides and supports patient's head while nurse 2 moves lift away from bed.				
l. Double-check draping.				
m. Slowly move lift to new position.				
n. Position patient above chair.				
o. Release valve and lower patient slowly.				
p. Close valve promptly.				
q. Detach chains from sling.				
Evaluation				
5. Evaluate using the criteria in Checklist step 13 of the General Procedure [patient's body alignment, patient's comfort, safety for the patient, and safety and proper body mechanics for the nurse(s) involved].				
Documentation				
6. Record as in Checklist steps 14 and 15 of the General Procedure (on the Kardex or nursing care plan, best method and aids to use, number of people needed to help, and patient's ability to participate; and on the patient's chart, time of activity, activity carried out, and patient's response).				

Horizontal lift: Three- or four-person assist

	Unsatisfactory	Needs More Practice	Satisfactory	Comments
Assessment				
1. Follow Checklist steps 1–3 of the General Procedure for Transfer (check patient's diagnosis and restrictions, assess capabilities of patient, and identify equipment and help available).				
Planning				
2. Follow Checklist steps 4–6 of the General Procedure (devise plan for transfer, wash your hands, and obtain equipment needed).				

	Unsatisfactory	Needs More Practice	Satisfactory	Comments
Implementation				
3. Follow Checklist steps 7–11 of the General Procedure (identify patient, lower the entire bed, place shoes or slippers on patient, and explain method of transfer to patient).				
4. Transfer the patient as outlined below: a. Place stretcher at right angle to bed.				
b. Move patient to edge of bed.				
c. Tallest nurse (1) stands at patient's head and shoulders.				
d. Second tallest nurse (2) stands at patient's waist and hips.				
e. Shortest nurse (3) stands at patient's legs.				
f. Nurse 2 informs patient of signal.				
g. Using elbows as levers, roll and lift at signal.				
h. Nurses hold patient and walk to stretcher.				
i. At signal, nurses place patient on stretcher.				
Evaluation				
5. Evaluate using the criteria in Checklist step 13 of the General Procedure (patient's body alignment, patient's comfort, safety for the patient, safety and proper body mechanics for the nurses involved).				
Documentation				
6. Record as in Checklist steps 14 and 15 of the General Procedure (on the Kardex or nursing care plan, best method and aids to use, number of people needed to help, and patient's ability to participate; and on the patient's chart, time of activity, activity carried out, and patient's response).				

QUIZ

Short-Answer Questions

1. List four reasons for patient activity.

   a. _____

   b. _____

   c. _____

   d. _____

2. State two reasons for having the patient wear shoes or slippers with firm soles when being transferred.

   a. _____

   b. _____

3. What should you do if a patient begins to fall during a transfer?

   _____

4. How would right-sided paralysis affect a patient's transfer? _____

   _____

5. What is the purpose of a transfer belt? _____

   _____

6. Name two transfer techniques for which a transfer belt is used.

   a. _____

   b. _____

7. Why is a patient changed from a lying-down to a sitting position slowly?

   _____

8. State two criteria that may be used in evaluating the transfer of a patient.

   a. _____

   b. _____

9. The response of a patient to transfer might be documented by observing

   _____ , _____ , and _____ .

MODULE 24

Range-of-Motion Exercises

MODULE CONTENTS

PREREQUISITES

Successful completion of the following modules:

OVERALL OBJECTIVE

To perform range-of-motion exercises on patients' joints, using proper sequence and joint positioning.

SPECIFIC LEARNING OBJECTIVES

	Know Facts and Principles	Apply Facts and Principles	Demonstrate Ability	Evaluate Performance
1. Purposes of ROM	State two purposes of ROM	Given a patient situation, identify purpose of ROM	In the clinical setting, identify purpose of ROM for a specific patient	Evaluate with instructor
2. Contraindications to ROM	State two major contraindications to ROM	Given a patient situation, identify whether a contraindication to ROM is present	In the clinical setting, assess patient to determine presence of contraindications to ROM	Evaluate with instructor
3. Types of ROM	Know three types of ROM	State reasons for selecting a specific kind of ROM for a specific patient	In the clinical area, select correct kind of ROM for patient	Check decision with instructor

4. *Joints to be exercised*	State principles for deciding which joints need exercising	Given a patient situation, describe side of body or joints requiring ROM	In the clinical area, perform ROM on appropriate joints for particular patient	Evaluate own performance using Performance Checklist
5. *Sequence used for exercising various joints*	List order for exercising various joints		Use prescribed sequence, making adaptations for particular patients	
6. *Special attention to certain joints*	Explain rationale for exercise of particular functional joints	Determine mobility or lack of mobility of key joints	Emphasize functional joints when doing ROM	
7. *Performing ROM*	Give frequency of ROM for optimum benefit to patient	Determine frequency of ROM for particular patient	Do ROM at predetermined intervals	Evaluate frequency by checking joint flexibility
8. *Documentation*	List data needed for chart	Determine correct manner of recording data for facility	Record procedure correctly, adding pertinent data	Evaluate own performance with instructor

LEARNING ACTIVITIES	VOCABULARY

LEARNING ACTIVITIES

1. Review the Specific Learning Objectives.
2. Read the section on range-of-motion and active and passive exercises (in the chapter on activity and rest) in Ellis and Nowlis, *Nursing: A Human Needs Approach,* or comparable material in another textbook.
3. Review the anatomy of the skeletal and muscular systems.
4. Look up the module vocabulary terms in the Glossary.
5. Read through the module and study the figures.
6. In the practice setting:
   a. Standing, move the joints on one side of your body through range of motion. Begin with your neck. Use the Performance Checklist as a guide.
   b. Practice ROM, with a partner, for one side of the body.
   c. Change positions and have your partner perform ROM on one side of your body.
   d. Together, evaluate your performances of steps b and c.
7. In the clinical setting:
   a. Perform ROM on a patient with your instructor's supervision.
   b. Using the Performance Checklist, evaluate yourself with the help of your instructor.

VOCABULARY

abduction
adduction
circumduction
contracture
contraindicate
distal
dorsiflexion
eversion
extension
external rotation
flexion
hyperextension
internal rotation
inversion
opposition
plantar flexion
pronation
proximal
radial deviation
rotation
supination
ulnar deviation

RANGE-OF-MOTION EXERCISES

Rationale for the Use of This Skill

A joint that has not been moved can begin to stiffen within 24 hours and will eventually become inflexible. With longer periods of joint immobility, the tendons and muscles can be affected as well. The strong flexor muscles pull tight, causing a contraction of the extremity or a permanent position of flexion. This position is called a contracture. *Many people with an illness or injury become unable to move one or more of the body's joints themselves and have a nursing diagnosis of impaired physical mobility. The nurse must promptly take over this function. With skill in handling the various body parts and knowledge of their movements, the nurse can maintain joint and extremity function until the patient can move joints independently. Performing range-of-motion (ROM) exercises on patients can often save them a lengthy rehabilitation.*[1]

Range-of-Motion Exercises

Range-of-motion (ROM) exercises are ones in which a nurse or patient moves each joint through as full a range as is possible without causing pain. Most people move and exercise their joints through the normal activities of daily living. When any joint cannot be moved in this way, the patient or nurse must move it at regular intervals *to maintain muscle tone and joint mobility.*

Purposes of Range-of-Motion Exercises

The two purposes of range-of-motion exercises are the maintenance of current joint function and the restoration of joint function that has been lost through disease, injury, or lack of use. The restorative process requires the special skills and techniques of a physical therapist. Maintaining current function may be done by nurses, physical therapists, assistants, family members, and the patient.

[1]You will note that rationale for action is emphasized throughout the module by the use of italics.

Contraindications to Range-of-Motion Exercises

Range-of-motion exercises require energy and tend to increase circulation. Any illness or disorder in which increasing the level of energy expended or increasing the demand for circulation is potentially hazardous is a contraindication to routine range-of-motion exercises. This is seen particularly in those with heart and respiratory diseases. If these conditions are present, the nurse should consult with the physician to determine whether range-of-motion exercises are appropriate or are contraindicated by the individual's condition.

Range-of-motion exercises also put stress on the soft tissues of the joint and on the bony structures. These exercises should not be performed if the joints are swollen or inflamed or if there has been injury to the musculoskeletal system in the vicinity of the joint. Gentle exercises may be appropriate in some situations, but this requires consultation with the physician.

Types of ROM

Active

In active ROM, instruct the patient to perform the movements on a nonfunctioning joint. When patients are taught a planned ROM program, they feel more independent *because they are participating actively.* They can also carry out additional ROM *by participating in their own care.* Combing the hair exercises joints of the upper extremity; lifting the foot for bathing exercises joints of the lower extremity. Encourage other appropriate activities as well.

Active-Assistive

Active-Assistive ROM is carried out with both patient and nurse participating. Encourage the patient to carry out as much of each movement as possible, within the limitations of strength and mobility. You support or complete the desired movement.

Passive

Passive ROM is performed by a nurse on a patient's immobilized joints. Your assessment skills are needed *to determine which parts or joints must be ranged and with what frequency.*

Joints Needing Exercise

When an individual is weak and inactive, planned exercises of all joints may be needed because the ordinary activities of daily living may not provide sufficient exercise to maintain range of motion. Elderly individuals in particular may need assistance in planning for range-of-motion exercises when a sedentary lifestyle places them at risk of loss of joint function. Daily range-of-motion exercises are usually adequate to maintain full mobility for these individuals.

Any joint that is immobile as a result of paralysis is in particular need of range-of-motion exercises. When a patient is completely paralyzed on one side of the body, ideally the joints should be exercised four to five times daily *for full maintenance of joint flexibility.* In reality, however, the staff's time restrictions may limit the exercise to only one or two times a day. Of course, limited ranging does not lead to optimum joint mobility.

It is difficult to assess need when extremities or joints are just weak or partially affected. Through the use of assessment skills, *you should be able to determine which joints are not being moved adequately by the patient and must therefore receive ROM.* When a patient receives ROM for the first time, it is helpful to exercise both affected and unaffected joints *to establish a baseline of normal functioning for the patient.* With each ROM procedure, put each joint through the range six to eight times. If you are also bathing the patient, you will not have to range all the joints that many times *because several of the bathing movements are also ROM movements. Never* force a joint to the point of pain.

Sequence of Exercises

Joints are exercised sequentially, starting with the neck and moving down. Remember that joints move in different ways: the knee and elbow move in just one direction; the neck, wrist, and hip move in several directions. Several movements can be done together. For example, flexion of the knee and external rotation of the hip (see Figure 24.6) can be done simultaneously, as can abduction and external rotation of the shoulder (see Figure 24.2). Never grasp

joints directly. *It is more comfortable for the patient, and better for ROM*, if you grasp the extremities gently but firmly either distally or proximally to the joint. When it is necessary to support the joint itself, gently cup your hand under the joint and allow the joint to rest on the palm of the hand. *This prevents pressure on the joint.* Do not grasp the fingernails or toenails; *this can be very uncomfortable for the patient.* When exercising extremities, work from the proximal joints toward the distal joints.

Every joint should receive adequate exercise, but it is crucial that several particular joints remain functional. For example, flexion of the thumb must be maintained *so that there is opposition of the thumb to the other fingers—otherwise the patient's hand will be useless. Hip and knee extension allows the patient to walk successfully when he or she is again mobile, and maintaining ankle flexion helps to prevent footdrop.*

Time of Exercise

Bath time is one appropriate time to administer ROM. *The warm bath water relaxes the muscles and decreases spasticity of the joints. During the bath, also, areas are exposed so that the joints can be both moved and observed.* Other appropriate times might be when the patient is rested in the morning or before bedtime.

Evaluate the effectiveness of the ROM regime by observing the flexibility and range of the joints. Then adjust the regime to the individual needs of the patient.

General Procedure for Range-of-Motion Exercises

Note: After each movement, return the part to its correct anatomical position. Each joint movement is described separately here. Remember that it is possible to move two joints, such as the shoulder and the elbow, at the same time.

Assessment
1. Assess the patient's joint mobility and activity status to determine the need for range-of-motion exercises.
2. Assess the patient's general health status to determine whether any contraindications to range-of-motion exercises are present.

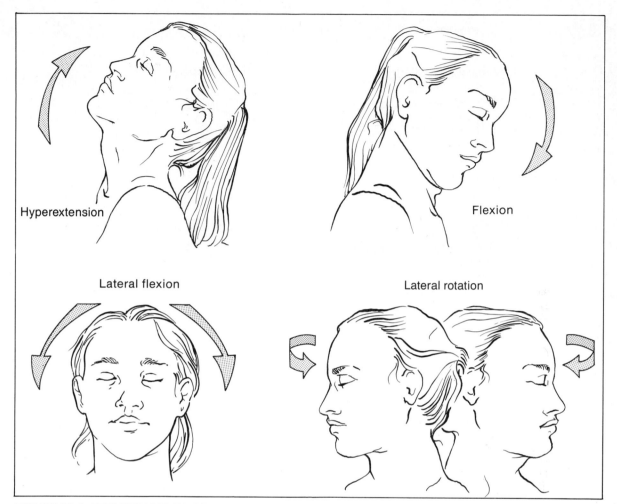

Hyperextension

Flexion

Lateral flexion

Lateral rotation

FIGURE 24.1 EXERCISING THE NECK

3. Assess the patient's ability and willingness to cooperate in range-of-motion exercises.

Planning

4. Plan when range-of-motion exercises should be done.
5. Plan whether exercises will be active, active-assistive, or passive.

Implementation

6. Wash your hands *for asepsis.*
7. Identify the patient *to be sure you are carrying out the procedure for the correct patient.*
8. Provide privacy by closing the door or pulling curtains around the bed.
9. Explain to the patient what you are about to do and ask for the patient's cooperation.

10. Lower the head of the bed *so that the patient is in the supine position.* Raise the entire bed to a comfortable working level for you. Remember to maintain your own proper body mechanics as you carry out the exercises for the patient *in order to avoid strain.*
11. Follow the procedure below in order to administer ROM to one side of the body.
    a. Neck (see Figure 24.1)
       (1) *Flexion* Position the head as if looking at the toes.
       (2) *Extension* Position the head as if looking straight ahead.
       (3) *Hyperextension* Position the head as if looking up at ceiling.
       (4) *Lateral flexion* While the head is positioned looking straight ahead,

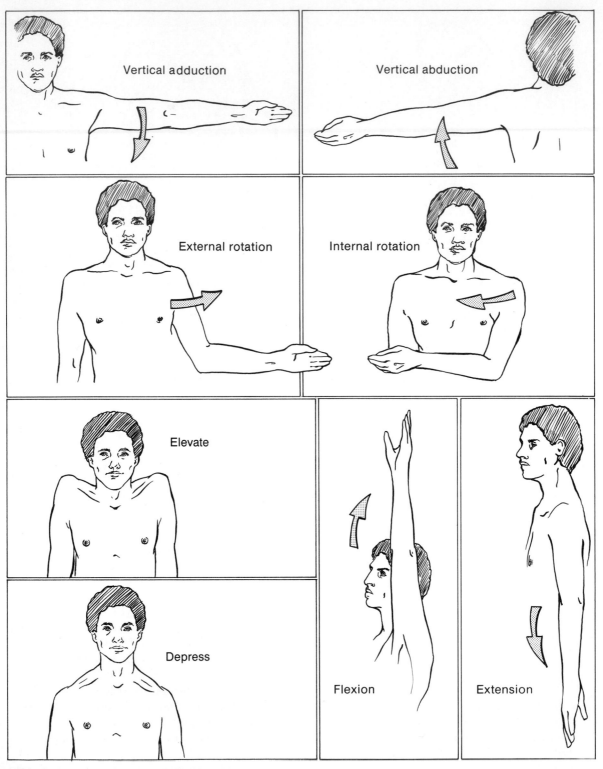

FIGURE 24.2 EXERCISING THE SHOULDER

tilt the head toward the shoulder, first to the left and then to the right.

    (5) *Lateral rotation*   Position the head so that the head is looking first toward the right and then toward the left.

b. Shoulder (see Figure 24.2)

    (1) *Flexion*   Raise the arm forward and overhead. The elbow may be bent *to avoid the head of the bed*.

    (2) *Extension*   Return the arm to the side of the body.

    (3) *Vertical abduction*   Swing the arm out from the side of the body and up.

    (4) *Vertical adduction*   Return the arm to the side of the body.

    (5) *Internal rotation*   Swing the arm up and across the body.

    (6) *External rotation*   Rotate the arm out and back, keeping the elbow at a right angle.

    (7) *Elevate shoulder*   Raise the shoulder in a shrug.

    (8) *Depress shoulder*   Lower the shoulder below the horizontal line.

c. Elbow (see Figure 24.3). These movements can be performed in conjunction with the shoulder movements.

    (1) *Flexion*   Bend the elbow.

    (2) *Extension*   Straighten the elbow.

d. Wrist (see Figure 24.4)

    (1) *Flexion*   Grasping the palm with one hand and supporting the arm with the other hand, bend the wrist forward.

    (2) *Extension*   Straighten the wrist.

    (3) *Radial deviation*   Bend the wrist toward the thumb.

    (4) *Ulnar deviation*   Bend the wrist toward the little finger.

    (5) *Circumduction*   Move the wrist in a circular motion.

e. Fingers and thumb (see Figure 24.5) *A hand can be partially functional* if a patient is able to place the thumb in opposition to the index finger or third finger. Therefore, you should take special care to range these joints

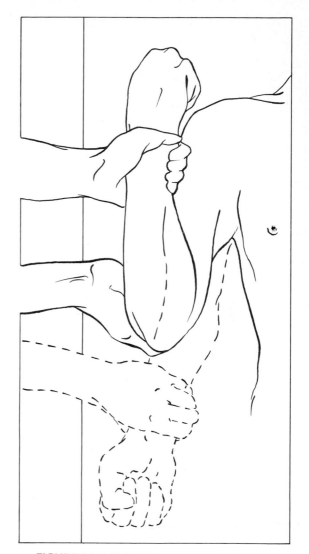

FIGURE 24.3 *EXERCISING THE ELBOW*

as thoroughly as possible. All three joints of each finger and the fingers and thumb can be moved through flexion and extension together

    (1) *Flexion*   Bend the fingers and thumb onto the palm.

    (2) *Extension*   Return them to their original position.

    (3) *Abduction*   Spread the fingers.

    (4) *Adduction*   Return the fingers to the closed position.

    (5) *Circumduction*   Move the thumb in a circular motion.

    (6) *Opposition*   Touch the thumb to each of the fingers in turn.

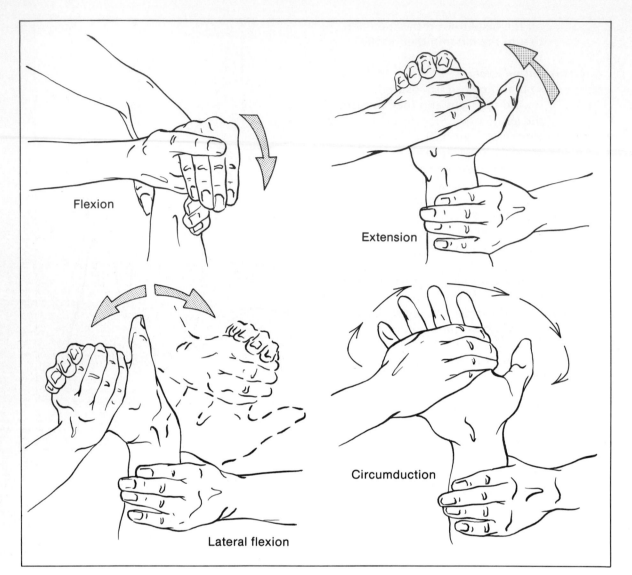

FIGURE 24.4 EXERCISING THE WRIST

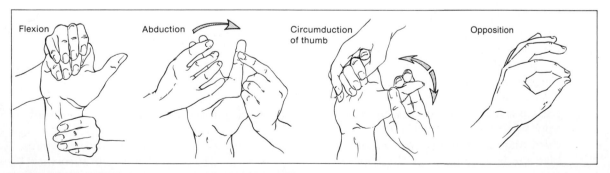

FIGURE 24.5 EXERCISING THE FINGERS AND THUMB

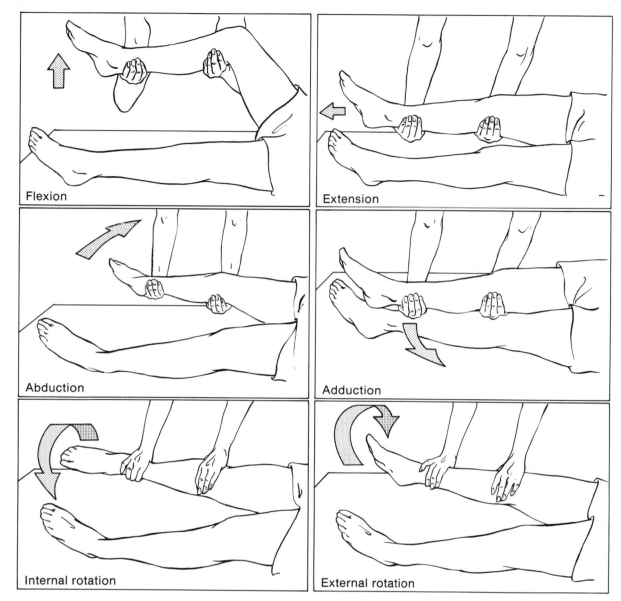

FIGURE 24.6 *EXERCISING THE HIP AND KNEE*

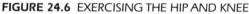

f. Hip and knee (see Figure 24.6). The hip and knee can be exercised together. Place one hand under the patient's knee, and, with the other hand, support the heel.

    (1) *Flexion* Lift the leg, bending the knee as far as possible toward the patient's head.

    (2) *Extension* Return the leg to the surface of the bed and straighten.

    (3) *Abduction* With the leg flat on the bed, move the entire leg out toward the edge of the bed.

    (4) *Adduction* Bring the leg back toward the midline or center of the bed.
    Note: Steps (3) and (4) can be performed with the knee bent. *This allows you to give better support to some patients and affords a greater range of movement.*

    (5) *Internal rotation* With the leg flat on the bed, roll the entire leg inward *so that the toes point in. This will rotate the hip joint internally.*

    (6) *External rotation* With the leg flat

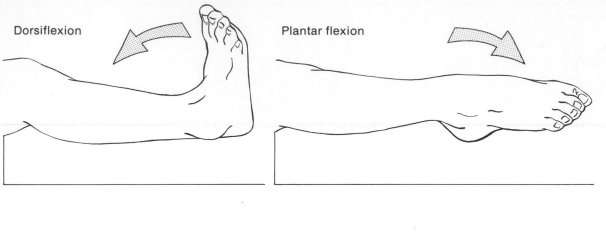

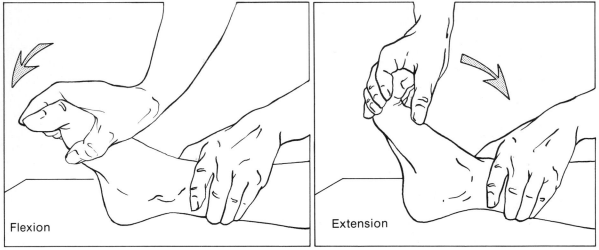

FIGURE 24.8 EXERCISING THE TOES

on the bed, roll the entire leg outward, *so that the toes point out. This will rotate the hip externally.*

g. Ankle (see Figure 24.7)

(1) *Dorsiflexion*   Cup the patient's heel with your hand and rest the sole of the foot against your forearm. Steady the leg just above the ankle with your other hand. Put pressure against the patient's toes with your arm to flex the ankle.

(2) *Plantar flexion*   Change your hand from above the ankle to the ball of the foot. Move the other arm away from the toes, keeping the hand cupped around the heel, and push the foot downward to point the toes.

(3) *Circumduction*   Rotate the foot on the ankle, moving it first in one direction and then in the other.

h. Toes (see Figure 24.8)

(1) *Flexion*   Bend the toes down. Avoid grasping the nails *because this can be uncomfortable for the patient.*

(2) *Extension*   Bend the toes up.

i. Spine (see Figure 24.9)

These exercises can be done only by the individual who is able to stand. The elderly person should be directed to hold the back of a chair or a railing for balance while doing these exercises.

(1) *Extension*   Stand straight.

(2) *Flexion*   Bend forward.

(3) *Hyperextension*   Bend backward.

500

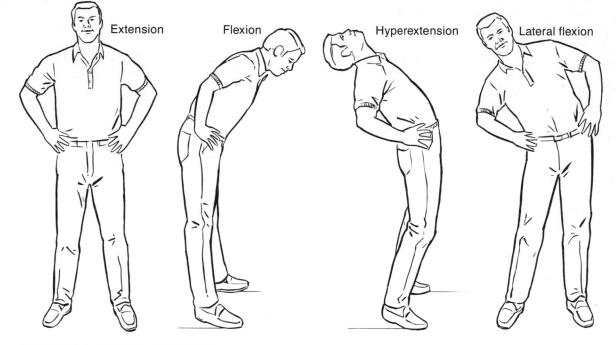

Extension Flexion Hyperextension Lateral flexion

FIGURE 24.9 EXERCISING THE SPINE

(4) *Lateral flexion*   Bend toward the side, first left, then right.
12. Wash your hands *for asepsis*.

☐ *Evaluation*
13. Evaluate the patient in terms of fatigue, joint discomfort, and joint mobility.

☐ *Documentation*
14. ROM is frequently placed on a flow sheet in order to facilitate record keeping. If no flow sheet is available, a narrative note may be used. If there is any adverse response, a narrative or SOAP note must be made in addition to a flow sheet recording. Notations about the extent to which joints can be moved are usually made in degrees.

Example of Charting   Narrative Style

12/3/88
1015   Passive ROM performed after bedbath. Left upper and lower extremities spastic with movement. Extension of leg at knee limited to approx. 120°.

        W. Dennis, R.N.

Example of Charting—Flow Sheet

Treatment	12/3	12/4	12/5	Date 12/6	12/7	12/8	12/9
ROM to left side	0800 RL 2000 MM						
Signature	R. Lot, R.N. M. May, R.N.						

PERFORMANCE CHECKLIST

General procedure for range-of-motion exercises	Unsatisfactory	Needs More Practice	Satisfactory	Comments
☐ *Assessment*				
1. Assess joint mobility and activity status.				
2. Assess general health status.				
3. Assess patient's ability to participate.				
☐ *Planning*				
4. Plan time for exercises.				
5. Plan type of exercises.				
☐ *Implementation*				
6. Wash your hands.				
7. Identify patient.				
8. Provide privacy.				
9. Explain to the patient what you are going to do and elicit the patient's help.				
10. Lower the head of the bed so that the patient is in the supine position.				
11. Follow the procedure below to administer ROM to one side of the body: a. Neck: (1) Flexion				
(2) Extension				
(3) Hyperextension				
(4) Lateral flexion				
(5) Lateral rotation				
b. Shoulder: (1) Flexion				
(2) Extension				
(3) Vertical abduction				
(4) Vertical adduction				
(5) Internal rotation				
(6) External rotation				
c. Elbow: (1) Flexion				

	Unsatisfactory	Needs More Practice	Satisfactory	Comments
(2) Extension				
d. Wrist:				
(1) Flexion				
(2) Extension				
(3) Radial deviation				
(4) Ulnar deviation				
(5) Circumduction				
e. Fingers and thumb: .				
(1) Flexion				
(2) Extension				
(3) Abduction				
(4) Adduction				
(5) Circumduction (thumb)				
(6) Opposition				
f. Hip and knee:				
(1) Flexion				
(2) Extension				
(3) Abduction				
(4) Adduction				
(5) Internal rotation				
(6) External rotation				
g. Ankle:				
(1) Dorsiflexion				
(2) Plantar flexion				
(3) Circumduction				
h. Toes:				
(1) Flexion				
(2) Extension				
i. Spine:				
(1) Extension				
(2) Flexion				
(3) Hyperextension				
(4) Lateral flexion				

	Unsatisfactory	Needs More Practice	Satisfactory	Comments
12. Wash your hands.				
☐ *Evaluation*				
13. Evaluate:				
a. Fatigue				
b. Joint discomfort				
c. Joint mobility				
☐ *Documentation*				
14. Record on flow sheet or narrative.				

QUIZ

Short-Answer Questions

1. List two purposes of ROM.

    a. _____

    b. _____

2. Identify two contraindications to ROM exercises.

    a. _____

    b. _____

3. Contractures occur when the stronger muscle group of an extremity
   shortens or pulls. These muscles are the _____ .

4. ROM that is performed by the patient is called _____ .

5. When the hand is held in an outward, upward position, it is called

   _____ .

6. To comb the hair, the shoulder assumes a position of _____ .

Multiple-Choice Questions

_____ 7. ROM should be performed

   a. every time a patient is repositioned.
   b. at bath time.
   c. when ordered by the physician.
   d. four to five times a day.

_____ 8. Joints of the body should be exercised sequentially; that is,

   a. alternately, from one side to the other.
   b. from distal to proximal.
   c. from proximal to distal.

_____ 9. "Scissoring" one leg over the other may bring about

   a. hip flexion.
   b. hip extension.
   c. adduction.
   d. circumduction.

U N I T V

Providing for Comfort, Elimination, and Nutrition

MODULE 25

Special Mattresses, Frames, and Beds

MODULE CONTENTS

PREREQUISITES

1. Successful completion of the following modules:

   VOLUME 1

   Module 1 / An Approach to Nursing Skills
   Module 2 / Medical Asepsis
   Module 3 / Safety
   Module 4 / Basic Body Mechanics
   Module 5 / Assessment
   Module 6 / Documentation
   Module 7 / Bedmaking
   Module 8 / Moving the Patient in Bed and
     Positioning

2. If the patient has traction in place, consult Module 31, Applying and Maintaining Traction.

OVERALL OBJECTIVE

To use special mattresses, frames, and beds effectively and safely with emphasis on both physical and psychological aspects of care.

SPECIFIC LEARNING OBJECTIVES

	Know Facts and Principles	Apply Facts and Principles	Demonstrate Ability	Evaluate Performance
1. *Rationale for use*	State two reasons for the use of special mattresses, frames, and beds	Given a specific situation, identify reason for use of specific device	In the clinical setting, identify reason for use of special device with specific patient	Evaluate with your instructor
2. *Special mattresses*	Name and describe three types of special mattresses	Identify one precaution common to all three types of mattresses	In the clinical setting, use special mattress correctly in specific situation	Evaluate with your instructor
3. *Special frames and beds*				
a. *Specific types*	Name and describe four special frames and beds. Name one unique feature of each device.	Identify two appropriate uses for each	In the clinical setting, identify which special frame or bed is appropriate for a specific situation	Evaluate with your instructor
b. *Manufacturer's instructions*	Locate and read manufacturer's instructions for any device used	Given a patient situation and a specific device, indicate how many people are needed to help	In the clinical setting, read manufacturer's instructions and secure adequate number of people for specific procedure	Evaluate using manufacturer's instructions

512

c. *Necessary equipment and accessories*	State equipment necessary and accessories available for each device	Given a patient situation and a specific device, list equipment necessary for a specific procedure	In the clinical setting, using manufacturer's instructions, gather necessary equipment for specific situation	Evaluate using manufacturer's instructions
d. *Explanation to the patient*	State reasons for use of each device	Given a patient situation and a specific device, describe what would appropriately be included in explanation to the patient	In the clinical setting, prepare a patient appropriately for a procedure involving a specific bed or frame	Evaluate with your instructor
e. *Privacy*	State ways to provide for privacy		In the clinical setting, provide for privacy of the patient about to undergo procedure on special frame or bed	Evaluate with your instructor
f. *Operating the device*	List steps in operation of device used for specific procedure	Given a specific device and procedure, describe how to proceed	In the clinical setting, perform procedure correctly for patient on special bed or frame	Evaluate with your instructor, using manufacturer's instructions
	List critical aspects of care of equipment as noted from manufacturer's instructions	Given a specific situation, describe appropriate care of equipment	In the clinical setting, care appropriately for equipment in use	Evaluate with your instructor, using manufacturer's instructions
g. *Evaluating the procedure*	State two appropriate observations to make in evaluating procedure	Given a specific situation, list observations and actions appropriate to procedure performed	In the clinical setting, evaluate in relation to short- and long-term goals	Evaluate with your instructor
4. *Documentation*	State at least two items of data to be included in record	Given a patient situation, record appropriately using chart form provided	In the clinical setting, record appropriately	Evaluate with instructor

LEARNING ACTIVITIES	VOCABULARY

LEARNING ACTIVITIES

1. Review the Specific Learning Objectives.
2. Read the section on special devices (in the chapter on activity and rest) in Ellis and Nowlis, *Nursing: A Human Needs Approach,* or comparable material in another textbook.
3. Look up the module vocabulary terms in the Glossary.
4. Read through the module.
5. In the practice setting:
   a. Find out what special mattresses, frames, or beds are available.
   b. Read the instruction manual for each device.
   c. Working in groups of three (one patient and two nurses), practice using each device, with particular attention to safety measures and to explanations to the "patient" and his or her family.
6. In the clinical setting:
   a. Find out what special mattresses, frames, or beds are available in the facility. Observe them in use if possible.
   b. Read the instruction manual and facility procedure for each device.
   c. Arrange with your clinical instructor for an opportunity to care for a patient using a special mattress, frame, or bed.

VOCABULARY

alternating pressure mattress
CircOlectric bed
Clinitron bed
decubitus ulcer
egg-crate mattress
Foster bed
hypostatic pneumonia
pulmonary embolus
quadriplegia
radiolucent
renal calculi
Roto-Rest bed
Stryker turning frame
Trendelenburg position
venous thrombosis
water bed

USING SPECIAL MATTRESSES, FRAMES, AND BEDS

Rationale for the Use of This Skill

Patients are placed on special mattresses, frames, and beds for a variety of reasons. One reason is to prevent and treat "pressure sores," or decubitus ulcers. Another is to keep the patient immobile to allow healing after disease, surgery, or fractures and to allow the patient to be turned without healing being disrupted. Patients who are immobile because of disease, injury, or other physical conditions may be placed on special devices. Frequent changes of position help to prevent the many complications of immobility (including hypostatic pneumonia, renal calculi, venous thrombosis, pulmonary emboli, and skin breakdown) and to promote physical and psychological comfort.

Patients suffering from multiple fractures, extensive burns, quadriplegia, acute arthritis, or dermatitis may be placed on one of a number of special mattresses, frames, or beds. The device selected varies with the problems of the patient and the availability of the device, which is usually ordered by the physician after consultation with appropriate members of the health care team.

To use these devices effectively and safely, you must know which mattress, frame, or bed is appropriate in a specific situation, the principles upon which it operates, and the details specific to its operation, such as the attachments that are available and the purpose of each attachment.[1]

Special Mattresses

Several types of special mattresses have been designed to assist in the prevention and treatment of decubitus ulcers (pressure sores). The primary goal of those that either inflate or operate on the principle of alternating pressure is to reduce the pressure on capillaries to below 32 mm Hg. Pressure above this level overcomes the internal blood pressure, and the capillaries collapse, increasing the risk of tissue damage and ulcer formation (Landis, 1983). This number is an average; the person with high blood pressure (hypertension) may be able to

tolerate more pressure before capillary collapse occurs, whereas the capillaries of those with lower blood pressure may collapse with much less pressure (Porth, 1982, p. 329). Some special mattresses have a motor attached to alternate the mattress pressure, and others have an attachment for inflation purposes.

All special pads and mattresses are most effective when there is only one layer of untucked linen between the patient and the mattress. This prevents the mattress from being confined by linen, so that it can inflate or provide the surface for which it was intended. If dampness due to excessive perspiration is a problem, a cotton blanket (or "sheet blanket") can be used for extra absorption.

With incontinent patients, using a single layer of linen may not be feasible. It may be necessary to use an incontinent pad under the patient's buttocks. If so, use as thin a layer of padding as possible and place it over the minimum area under the patient, so that the mattress continues to benefit most of the skin as usual, and benefits the coccyx and buttocks at least partially. Check the patient frequently and change the padding as needed to keep the patient dry.

Foam Rubber Mattress Pads

The foam rubber mattress pad (often called an egg-crate or egg-carton mattress) is placed over the regular mattress on the bed. Its surface of rounded projections allows air to circulate near the skin. The result is twofold: moisture is reduced, so that there is less danger of skin maceration, and pressure is distributed over a wider area, so that the pressure on any one spot is lower. These mattresses can be large enough to cover an entire bed or small enough to use with wheelchairs or other chairs. Again, only a single layer of linen should be used between the patient and the mattress to allow for optimum air circulation and pressure distribution.

Inflated Mattresses

A water-filled mattress is a special mattress that is placed on an ordinary bed; it is used to distribute pressure evenly over the entire body. It is similar in principle to the water bed, which has become popular in recent years as a piece of bedroom furniture. The rubber mattress is filled with water so that the body floats. The feeling of weightlessness can induce nausea, and hip and

---

[1]You will note that rationale for action is emphasized throughout the module by the use of italics.

knee contractures are common *because the pelvis tends to sink deeper than the trunk and lower extremities.* Although the outer covering is strong, take care with safety pins and other sharp articles *to avoid punctures and leaks.*

Sof-Care is the brand name for a commercial air-inflated mattress that is used over the regular mattress and secured by corner straps. This "bed cushion" consists of interlocking layers of air compartments that are inflated using a special device. This mattress can be individualized to the body weight and needs of each patient by varying the amount of air infused. Capillary pressure is reduced to below 32 mm Hg. The Sof-Care mattress is for single patient use and can be cleaned easily with soap and water if soiled. (See Figure 25.1.)

Alternating Pressure Mattress

The alternating pressure mattress is a plastic mattress that is placed on top of a standard mattress. *An attached motor alternately inflates and deflates tubular sections of the mattress, so that the pressure against any section of the patient's body changes continuously.* This constant motion can cause nausea, but the nausea usually disappears after the first few hours. You should warn the patient, family, and other staff to be careful with safety pins or other sharp objects *because punctures will cause the mattress to leak and be ineffective.* Use only a single layer of linen between the mattress and the patient *because multiple layers of linen tend to bunch up between the inflated tubes and mask the pressure variation.* The covering used can be a regular sheet, or a cotton blanket can be used *for greater absorption.* Take care not to pinch or bend off the tubing that connects the mattress to the motor, *since this will interfere with the action of the mattress.*

Special Frames

Stryker Frame

The Stryker Frame, like the very similar Foster bed, is used *to maintain immobilization and, at the same time, provide for turning.* The frame, which may be used as a surgical table as well as a rehabilitation bed, has a bottom mattress or support attached to a frame on wheels. When the patient is to be turned, a second frame is fas-

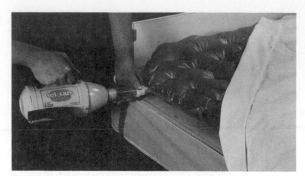

FIGURE 25.1 AIR-INFLATED MATTRESS
Courtesy Gaymar Industries, Inc.

tened into place above the patient, and safety straps are applied. The patient is then turned laterally either from back to abdomen or from abdomen to back. Nursing care is planned around the turning schedule. The Stryker Frame can be operated safely by one nurse if the Wedge turning frame is used. *The wedge design prevents the patient from falling, since the opening is uppermost when the turn is made* (see Figure 25.2). If the Wedge turning frame is not used, two nurses must be present. Some facilities require two nurses to be present even when the Wedge turning frame is used *to ensure safety.*

The Stryker Frame has an opening in the bottom mattress to accommodate a bedpan. A face support is used when the patient is turned face down *to facilitate eating and reading.* Many patients have a fear of falling, however, and are not comfortable in that position, although some do adjust after a period of time on the frame.

CircOlectric Bed

The CircOlectric bed is actually a frame designed for patients with severe injuries or other acute conditions where the objective, again, is immobilization with provision for turning. The difference is that the CircOlectric bed turns vertically, and the bed and patient can be placed in several positions, including standing, sitting, and Trendelenburg positions (see Figure 25.3). The patient is again placed between two mattresses or supports if the turn is to be a complete one, and the bed is rotated using an electric or manual control. This bed will rotate a full 210° and can also be used as a tilt table *to help a patient regain gradually the ability to tolerate an upright position.* Again, there is an opening in the bottom

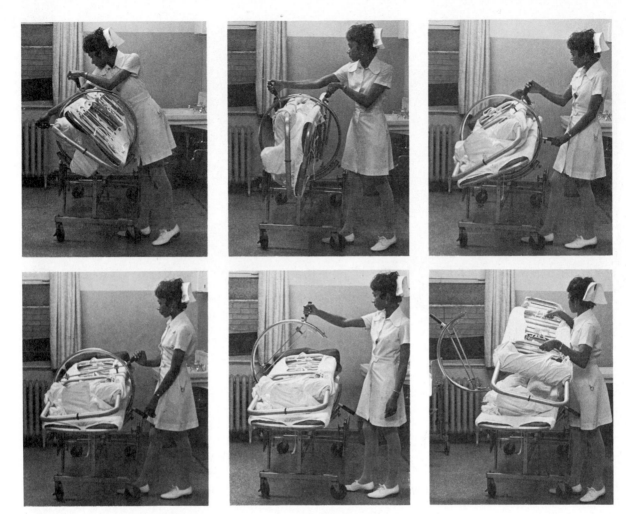

FIGURE 25.2 TURNING A PATIENT WITH THE STRYKER WEDGE TURNING FRAME
Courtesy Stryker Corporation, Kalamazoo, MI

mattress *to accommodate a bedpan,* and the patient can eat and read when in the face-down position. Turning can be a frightening experience for the patient, especially when going forward, and every effort should be made to make the turn as smooth as possible.

The patient can be transported to other areas of the facility on the CircOlectric bed, which makes transfer to a stretcher unnecessary.

Special Beds

There are a variety of special beds that can be obtained by hospitals and long-term care facilities. Many are similar in function. In general, the primary purpose of special beds is *to preserve*

the integrity of the skin by facilitating change in position and/or minimizing pressure on the capillaries of the skin.

One type of special bed is the Roto-Rest bed, which focuses on change of position; another type is the Clinitron Air-Fluidized bed, which is designed to minimize and equalize pressure on skin tissue. Several air support beds can also be obtained commercially. Among these are the Mediscus, the Kin-Air, and the Air Plus (Stat Medical, Inc.). The air support beds have the advantage of encouraging healing *by not drying wounds.*

Several other special beds are, in reality, bed-chair combinations that allow the care provider to adjust the device from a bed to a chair or a chair to a bed. *This action allows the patient*

517

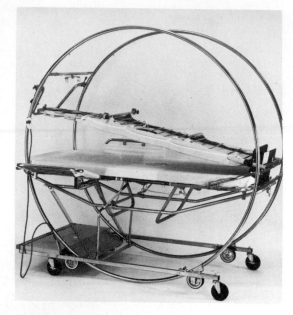

FIGURE 25.3 CIRCOLECTRIC BED
Courtesy Stryker Corporation, Kalamazoo, MI

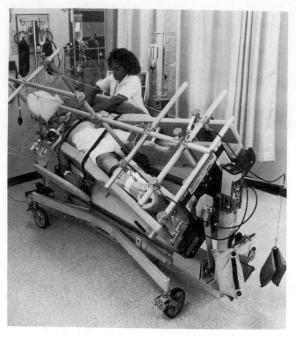

FIGURE 25.4 ROTO-REST KINETIC BED
Courtesy Kinetic Concepts, Inc.

convenient changes in position between lying and sitting.

Roto-Rest Kinetic Bed

This bed operates electrically and *offers continuous side-to-side turning*—180° in either direction. With the patient's body securely immobilized in place by bolsters, *postural drainage can be accomplished while the complications of immobility* are avoided. *Since the turning is continuous,* the patient's sleep pattern is not disturbed by a turning schedule. The Roto-Rest bed may be used as a surgical table, and it is radiolucent (x-rays may be taken through the table) as well (see Figure 25.4).

Clinitron Air-Fluidized Bed

This bed provides uniform support to all parts of the body, eliminating pressure and minimizing shear while decreasing pain. Shear occurs when tissue layers move relative to each other, and it can cause a reduction in the blood supply to the part involved. The 12-inch-thick mattress is filled with ceramic beads. When air is blown through them—a process known as "fluidizing"—the beads go into a state of constant motion. This

action results in pressure against the skin that is less than capillary filling pressure and thus improves blood flow to the skin (Lucke, 1985). Instant "defluidization" can be accomplished if a firm surface is needed, as in cardiac arrest (see Figure 25.5). If cardiac arrest occurs, be sure to unplug the bed at the wall socket *because if the bed is merely turned off, it will automatically restart after thirty minutes.*

An order is needed to initiate Clinitron Air-Fluidized therapy. These beds are very costly. If a hospital has these beds available, they may be obtained through the housekeeping or central supply department. They may also be rented. A special filter sheet that comes with the unit is spread over the surface of the bed and tucked under an elasticized band around the bed. These sheets are also expensive and should never be put with the usual soiled laundry. If the unit is rented, the supplier provides clean sheets on a return basis. If the unit belongs to the hospital, follow the facility's policy regarding cleaning. A hospital sheet is doubled and placed loosely on top of the filter sheet *for purposes of cleanliness and for turning the patient.*

Patients who may benefit from the Clinitron Air-Fluidized bed include those who have a very

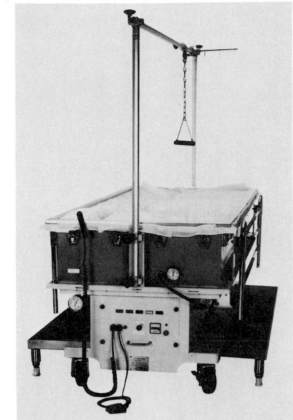

FIGURE 25.5 THE CLINITRON AIR-FLUIDIZED BED
Courtesy UHI Corporation, Los Angeles, California

limited number of possible positions, have potential or actual skin breakdown, and have extreme pain or discomfort that is exacerbated by movement. It is not appropriate for spinal cord-injured patients *because the surface of the bed is not firm enough to provide the spinal alignment that is essential for these persons. Because the head of the bed cannot be elevated,* a foam wedge is used if the patient's head needs to be raised. A wedge should always be used when you are tube feeding a patient *to prevent accidental aspiration.*

The nurse must take special precautions when caring for the patient in the Clinitron bed. Never use pins or clamps on the filter sheet *because these can cause damage to the special fabric. Because it may be possible for microscopic particles to escape through the filter sheet,* see that x-ray plates are put into pillowcases. The unit should also be turned off when x-rays are being taken *because the movement of the ceramic beads may obliterate or*

distort the image. It is best if you and the patient do not wear wrist watches around the Clinitron bed *because of the possible dispersion of microscopic particles.* It will be useful for you to carefully read the detailed booklet of instructions that accompanies the unit.

Air Support Bed

The air support bed sold under the brand name Mediscus consists of U-shaped sacs of a heavy nylon material that are arranged widthwise to form the bed. These sacs are attached to a blower system that inflates or deflates them independently *in order to meet the patient's specific needs for position change.* The desired capillary pressure is at a level *that allows the capillaries to maintain their function.* The unit is controlled through a large console that is placed by the bed. Hand controls allow the nurse to select six different patient positions and different pressure settings on various sections of the bed. In this way, the nurse can implement position changes easily. Temperature regulation can also be maintained for the patient *so that the person can be warmed or cooled as appropriate.* As with the Clinitron bed, these units can be instantly deactivated *for purposes of administering resuscitation (CPR) in the event of a cardiac arrest.* The Mediscus can be purchased or rented by the facility. Patients who will benefit from using the Mediscus bed are similar to those who will benefit from the Clinitron bed. In addition, this bed may be used for those with unstable spinal cord injuries. Knowledge of the accompanying instruction manual is essential for proper operation. (See Figure 25.6.)

Other Manual or Electric Positional Change Beds

There are several other types of beds which can be changed into the configuration of a chair to allow the patient to assume a sitting position. This is done with a manual crank or an electric control. These beds are most often used for patients who have difficulty getting out of bed but benefit from spending time in the sitting position. The Nelson bed and cardiac "stretcher" are only two of these beds. Check with your institution for the availability of these units.

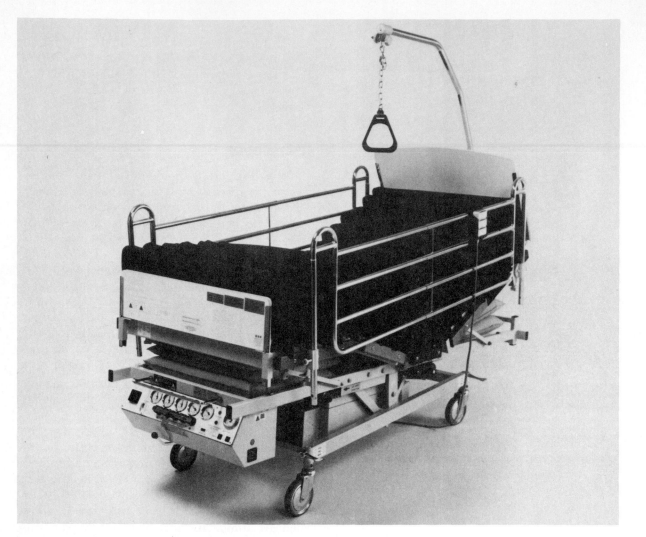

FIGURE 25.6 MEDISCUS AIR SUPPORT BED

Courtesy Mediscus Products, Inc. The Mediscus Air Support Therapy System is a relief system designed for prevention and treatment of pressure sores. The system delivers measurable therapeutic support pressures below capillary closures with operable pressure gauges. It reduces maceration, shear force, friction, and moisture.

Comparison of Special Frames and Beds

On the following pages is a comparison of the special frames and beds discussed above, using the nursing process as a framework. Appropriate points about each device are included with each step in the nursing process.

Example of Charting   Narrative Style

1/30/88

1015   Patient placed on Clinitron Air-Fluidized unit per order. Health teaching in the following areas completed:
1. Reason for bed
2. Operation of bed
3. Familiarize patient with bed
4. Demonstration of control system
5. Placement of the call signal
6. Reassure patient and answer questions
Patient to be assessed qlh for first eight hours.

                J. Buckwald, R.N.

COMPARISON OF SPECIAL FRAMES AND BEDS

Nursing Process	Stryker Frame	CircOlectric Bed	Roto-Rest Bed	Clinitron Bed	Mediscus Bed
Assessment					
1. Assess patient's need for special frame or bed	Used for cervical traction, spinal fusion, and laminectomy	Used for patients with multiple fractures, extensive burns, quadriplegia, acute arthritis, dermatitis, spinal fusion	Used for postural drainage of severely injured patients and for prevention of the complications of immobility (e.g., pressure sores, hypostatic pneumonia, deep vein thrombosis, pulmonary embolus)	Used for patients with limited movement, pain with movement or handling, and at risk for skin breakdown. Not for patients with unstable spinal cord injury.	Used for patients with limited movement, pain with movement or handling, and at risk of skin breakdown. Used for patients with orthopedic problems and spinal cord injury.
2. Check order	Confer with other members of health care team and suggest an order as appropriate. Check any special details of order.	Confer with other members of health care team and suggest an order as appropriate. Check any special details of order.	Confer with other members of health care team and suggest an order as appropriate. Check any special details of order.	Confer with other members of health care team and suggest an order as appropriate. Check any special details of order.	Confer with other members of health care team and suggest an order as appropriate. Check any special details of order.
3. Check the patient unit for supplies and equipment you will need to carry out procedure	To turn the patient, you will need: (a) Anterior or posterior frame, correctly padded and covered (b) Two safety belts, one for chest, the other for thighs	To turn the patient, you will need: (a) Anterior or posterior frame, correctly padded and covered (b) Accessories include: safety/restraining straps traction bars IV bottle holders overbed table	Bed is in constant motion. Posterior hatches open to allow care of cervical, thoracic, and rectal areas. Traction apparatus available.	(a) "Fluidized" temperature-controlled air flows constantly around patient (b) Standard equipment: foam wedge turn sheet IV holder side rails call signal	(a) Air sacs inflated to meet individual needs of patient (b) Standard equipment: turn sheet IV holder side rails call signal

COMPARISON OF SPECIAL FRAMES AND BEDS *continued*

Nursing Process	Stryker Frame	CircOlectric Bed	Roto-Rest Bed	Clinitron Bed	Mediscus Bed
	(c) Accessories include: footboard armrests tray table bedpan cervical traction				
Planning					
4. *Review manufacturer's instructions*	Be sure you are familiar with directions printed by manufacturer. One person may turn Stryker Wedge Frame alone—two are needed with other equipment. You may also need help handling anterior and posterior frames. Check recommended procedure for performance of CPR on this frame.	Be sure you are familiar with directions printed by manufacturer. This will ensure patient safety and maximum efficiency for you. One person can operate the bed, but you may need help handling the anterior and posterior frames. Check recommended procedure for performance of CPR on this bed.	Be sure you are familiar with directions printed by manufacturer. Since bed is in constant motion, it is not necessary to use extra people, except as a special nursing procedure (e.g., dressing change) might make necessary. Check recommended procedure for performance of CPR on this bed. In case of cardiac arrest, firm surface allows CPR to be done without special board.	Be sure you are familiar with directions printed by manufacturer. When bed is "fluidized," one person can turn the patient for procedures. Check recommended procedure for performance of CPR on this bed. In case of cardiac arrest, patient can be resuscitated without being removed from the bed by simply "defluidizing" the bed.	Be sure you are familiar with directions printed by manufacturer. When bed is inflated, procedures can be performed without returning to original pressure settings. Instant deflation is possible in cases of cardiac arrest.
5. *Wash your hands for asepsis*					

6. Gather needed equipment	Obtain any needed supplies and equipment that are not in patient unit	Obtain any needed supplies and equipment that are not in patient unit	Obtain any needed supplies and equipment that are not in patient unit	Obtain any needed supplies and equipment that are not in patient unit	Obtain any needed supplies and equipment that are not in patient unit
Implementation					
7. Identify patient to be sure you are carrying out the procedure on the correct patient					
8. Explain to the patient what you plan to do	Explain specifically why this particular piece of equipment is being used for this patient. Explain turning or other procedure planned.	Explain specifically why this particular piece of equipment is being used for this patient. Explain turning or other procedure planned.	Explain specifically why this particular piece of equipment is being used for this patient. Explain specific procedure planned.	Explain specifically why this particular piece of equipment is being used for this patient. Explain specific procedure planned.	Explain specifically why this particular piece of equipment is being used for this patient. Explain specific procedure planned.
9. Provide for privacy	Covers will need to be removed to turn the patient. Pull curtain around patient or close door. Be certain that gown covers patient.	Remove top covers and be certain that gown covers patient adequately. Pull curtain around patient or close door.	To change position of bolsters, top covers will be removed. Be certain that gown covers patient. Pull curtain around patient or close door.	Pull curtain around patient or close door. If procedure requires defluidization, position patient as necessary prior to defluidization.	Pull curtain around patient or close door. Cover patient before moving onto inflated bed.
10. Prepare the frame or bed for the procedure	Prepare the frame for turning or other procedure. Position any apparatus attached to the patient (e.g., IV line, catheter) to prevent dislodgement.	Prepare the bed for turning or other procedure. Position any apparatus attached to the patient (e.g., IV line, catheter) to prevent dislodgement.	Remove cushions or restraining straps as necessary. Position any apparatus attached to the patient (e.g., IV line, catheter) to prevent dislodgement.		

COMPARISON OF SPECIAL FRAMES AND BEDS *continued*

Nursing Process	Stryker Frame	CircOlectric Bed	Roto-Rest Bed	Clinitron Bed	Mediscus Bed
11 Carry out the procedure	Medicate patient if painful procedure is planned. When using Wedge frame, turn patient toward yourself *to promote a greater feeling of security*—patients often have a fear of falling, especially when first on the frame. Narrowness of mattress, as well as turning, contribute to fear. Attach anterior or posterior frame and fasten securely. Remove or adjust attachments as necessary. Secure safety belts (around both anterior and posterior frame and the patient)—one around chest, the other around thighs.	Medicate patient if painful procedure is planned. Stand facing patient and where patient can see you as you operate controls. Create calm and quiet environment *to make patient less fearful*—fear of falling is especially great when patients are turning face forward. Attach anterior or posterior frame and fasten securely. Remove or adjust attachments as necessary. Ask patient to hold onto frame if able. Otherwise restrain arms next to the body.	Medicate patient if painful procedure is planned. Bed can be placed in extreme lateral position. Care may be given and procedures performed through posterior hatches with bed in this position. Awake patient may benefit from presence of second person *for face-to-face contact and psychological comfort.*	Medicate patient if painful procedure is planned. Bed promotes relaxation, but the flotation sensation can have disorienting effect on patient. You may need to turn the unit off and on *several times to relieve patient's fear.*	Medicate patient if painful procedure is planned. Inflation may be altered in such a way as to accommodate a variety of positions for procedures. You may reassure patient during procedure by offering touch and comfort.
	Be sure patient knows which way frame is to be turned. Arrange signal so that patient will know when you will turn frame (e.g.,	Be sure patient knows which way frame is to be turned. Be sure patient is ready to be turned. Stand where you can	Perform procedures planned. You may need to remove cushions or restraining straps or perform procedure through one of the	Perform procedure planned. Rising airflow provides clean environment, and the special "filter sheet" is permeable both to rising flow of	Perform procedure planned. Protect surface of bed with folded sheets. Adjust airflow pressure for patient comfort and convenience of car-

	on count of three). Use smooth, uninterrupted motion and moderate speed. Remove frame that is now in uppermost position. If patient is now in prone position, use safety belts, since side rails cannot be used.	see patient's face if verbal communication is not possible. Remove frame that is now in uppermost position. If patient is now in prone position, use safety belts, since side rails cannot be used.	posterior hatches. Be certain to reposition patient and cushions carefully.	air and downward flow of fluids like plasma, blood, perspiration, and urine, thus removing them from contact with the patient.	rying out procedure. Return to preset pressure readings.
12. *Make the patient comfortable*	Position patient carefully. Check for proper position and support of face and shoulders. Arrange linen so that patient is not lying on wrinkles. Replace top covers and any attachments needed. Safety belt is necessary in prone position. Call light and personal items within reach.	Position patient carefully. Check for proper position and support of face and shoulders. Arrange linen so that patient is not lying on wrinkles. Replace top covers and any attachments needed. Safety belt is necessary in prone or standing position. Call light and personal items within reach.	Replace any cushions or restraining straps removed. Replace top covers. Call light and personal items within reach.	Position patient carefully. Replace any covers removed. Call light and personal items within reach.	Position patient carefully. Replace any covers removed. Call light and personal items within reach.
13. *Care for equipment*	Replace linen as necessary on anterior or posterior frame removed from bed. Store frame carefully where it will not get dirty or fall over and hurt someone.	Replace linen as necessary on anterior or posterior frame. Lock frame in place above patient.	Be sure to close any posterior hatches opened while caring for patient.	The Clinitron system should be cleaned every week and disinfected between patients.	The Mediscus bed should be cleaned every week and disinfected between patients.

COMPARISON OF SPECIAL FRAMES AND BEDS *continued*

Nursing Process	Stryker Frame	CircOlectric Bed	Roto-Rest Bed	Clinitron Bed	Mediscus Bed
Evaluation					
14. *Evaluate procedure*	Assess patient's response, both physical and psychological, to procedure	Assess patient's response, both physical and psychological, to procedure	Evaluate the results based on goals set before the procedure was performed. In some cases, the goals will be long-term. Complete evaluation will not be possible.	Evaluate the results based on goals set before the procedure was performed. In some cases, the goals will be long-term. Complete evaluation will not be possible.	Evaluate the results based on goals set before the procedure was performed. Goals may have to be long-term.
Documentation					
15. *Record Data*	Record turn on flow sheet or progress notes. Include any physical or psychological response of patient.	Record turn on flow sheet or progress notes. Include any physical or psychological response of patient.	Record procedure on flow sheet or progress notes. Include any physical or psychological response of patient.	Record procedure on flow sheet or progress notes. Include any physical or psychological response of patient.	Record procedure on flow sheet or progress notes. Include any physical or psychological response of patient.

Special Considerations

Should not be used if patient can be positioned on side, is broader than external frame, or is over 6 feet tall or 200 pounds.

Should not be used if patient has unstable spine, since feet bear weight during turn, causing pressure on spine.

Constant motion may exacerbate diarrhea. Bed should be protected, since it is hard to clean.

Patient does not need to be turned for skin care, but *should* be turned to maintain lung and kidney function. To turn, press down on bed beside patient while pulling patient toward you. Defluidize to provide firm surface for coughing. Constant circulation of warm, dry air may affect temperature and hydration status. Check patient closely.

Patient should be turned to check skin and maintain lung and kidney function. Patient is easily turned with a turn sheet. Change pressure settings to initiate changes in pressure on patient's tissues.

REFERENCES

"A Comparison of Static Pressure Sore Prevention Products." Orchard Park, N.Y.: Garmar Corporation, 1984.

Baier, R. E., R. W. King, and A. E. Meyer. "Pressure Relief Characteristics of Various Support Surfaces for Human Tissue." Buffalo, N.Y.: Arvin Calspan Corporation.

Brackett, Thomas O., and Nancy Condon. "A Comparison of the Wedge Turning Frame and Kinetic Treatment Table in the Acute Care of Spinal Cord Injury Patients." *Forum,* 4, No. 5 (September/October 1984).

Landis, E. M. "Micro-injection Studies of Capillary Blood Pressure in Human Skin." *Heart,* 15 (May 1930), 209.

Lucke, Kathleen, and Connie Jarlsberg. "How Is the Air-Fluidized Bed Best Used?" *American Journal of Nursing* (December 1985), 1338–1340.

Porth, Carol. *Pathophysiology: Concepts of Altered Health Status.* Philadelphia: J. B. Lippincott Co., 1982.

PERFORMANCE CHECKLIST				

General procedure for using special mattresses, frames, and beds	Unsatisfactory	Needs More Practice	Satisfactory	Comments
☐ *Assessment*				
1. Assess patient's need for special frame or bed.				
2. Check order.				
3. Check patient unit for supplies.				
☐ *Planning*				
4. Review manufacturer's instructions.				
5. Wash your hands.				
6. Gather needed equipment.				
☐ *Implementation*				
7. Identify patient.				
8. Explain procedure to patient.				
9. Provide for privacy.				
10. Prepare frame or bed for procedure.				
11. Carry out procedure.				
12. Make patient comfortable.				
13. Care for equipment.				
14. Wash your hands.				
☐ *Evaluation*				
15. Evaluate procedure.				
☐ *Documentation*				
16. Record data on flow sheet or progress notes.				

| QUIZ |

Short-Answer Questions

1. Give two reasons for the use of special mattresses, frames, and beds.

   a. _____

   b. _____

2. Describe the principle by which the egg-crate mattress helps protect the
   skin. _____

   _____

3. Compare the construction of the Stryker frame with that of the CircOlectric.

   _____

   _____

4. List two precautions that the nurse should take when caring for the
   patient using a Clinitron Air-Fluidized bed. _____

   _____

5. What provision is made for administering resuscitation (CPR) measures to
   patients on the Clinitron or Mediscus special beds? _____

   _____

Multiple-Choice Questions

_____ 6. Which of the following is not an inflatable device?

   a. The Mediscus bed
   b. An egg-crate mattress
   c. A water bed
   d. The alternating positive pressure mattress

_____ 7. Which of the following actions regarding x-rays is
   appropriate when caring for the patient on a Clinitron bed?

   a. X ray plates should be placed in pillow cases.
   b. The unit should be operating so that the x-ray plates
      stay in position.
   c. Always place a foam wedge beneath the patient's head.
   d. No x-rays should be taken.

_____ 8. Capillary collapse occurs when surface pressure levels rise
   above

   a. 20 mm Hg.
   b. 32 mm Hg.
   c. 42 mm Hg.
   d. 50 mm Hg.

_____ **9.** Bottom linen that covers a special mattress

    a. is tucked tightly so that the mechanism does not wrinkle it.

    b. is never tucked tightly because this interferes with the principle underlying the mattress.

    c. always consists of two sheets rather than one in order to protect the mattress.

    d. is always of special fabric and supplied by the manufacturer.

_____ **10.** Which of the following special beds can be used for the patient with an unstable spinal cord injury?

    a. Clinitron bed

    b. Sof-Care

    c. Mediscus bed

    d. Water-inflated bed

MODULE 30

Caring for Patients with Casts

OVERALL OBJECTIVE

To assist efficiently with the application of a cast, accurately assess the patient for complications related to the cast, and prevent problems related to the presence of a cast while providing psychological support.

SPECIFIC LEARNING OBJECTIVES

	Know Facts and Principles	Apply Facts and Principles	Demonstrate Ability	Evaluate Performance
Cast Application				
1. Casting materials	List common kinds of casting materials and describe characteristics of each	Give advantages and disadvantages of each material for specific cases	In clinical setting, observe type of cast being used	Share observation with instructor
2. Procedure	Explain steps of procedure for assisting with application of plaster of Paris cast	Apply steps to specific casting situation	If possible, assist with the application of a cast in clinical setting	Evaluate performance with instructor
3. Adaptations in cast application	State adaptations needed for application of fiberglass casts	Apply adaptations to specific situation	If possible, assist with fiberglass cast application	Evaluate performance with instructor
4. Types of casts	Briefly discuss the four types of commonly used casts	Given a patient situation, give rationale for type of cast applied	In the clinical setting, observe presence of different types of casts and know why each cast was used	Share with instructor
5. Adaptations to casts	Describe method and reason for bivalving or windowing a cast	Given a patient situation, explain when and where bivalving or windowing might be appropriate	In clinical setting, observe a bivalved or windowed cast and know why adaptation was done for specific patient	Evaluate with instructor

Giving Care

1. *Guidelines*	List steps to be taken when caring for the patient in a cast	Given a patient situation, give rationale for specific steps taken for care of patient	In the clinical setting, care for the patient in a cast	Evaluate performance with instructor
2. *Problems*	State potential problems related to being in a cast	Identify specific problems that may arise with a particular patient	In clinical setting, identify potential problems in nursing care plan	Evaluate with instructor
3. *Preventive measures*	List measures that can be taken to avoid problems	Identify preventive measures that could be taken with a particular patient	In clinical setting, incorporate preventive measures in nursing care plan	Evaluate with instructor
4. *Emotional support*	State why emotional support is important for the patient in a cast	Given a patient situation, show ways of offering emotional support	In clinical setting, include emotional support in nursing care plan	Share with instructor
5. *Documentation*	State information that should be recorded		In clinical setting, document on patient's record	Review notes with instructor

LEARNING ACTIVITIES

1. Review the Specific Learning Objectives.
2. Read the section on immobilization (in the chapter on activity and rest) in Ellis and Nowlis, *Nursing: A Human Needs Approach,* or comparable material in another text.
3. Look up the module vocabulary terms in the Glossary.
4. Read through the module.
5. In the practice setting, observe any available casts or casting materials.
6. In the clinical setting:
   a. Read the material in your facility's procedure book on assisting with the application of a cast and the care of the patient in a cast.
   b. Arrange with your instructor for an opportunity to observe or assist in the application of a cast.
   c. Review the care plan for a patient in a cast.
   d. Arrange with your instructor for an opportunity to care for a patient in a cast.

VOCABULARY

bivalving
cast padding
cure
epigastrium
fiberglass cast
"green" cast
isometric exercises
logrolling
malleable
petaling
plaster of Paris cast
stockinette
tepid
torso
trapeze
twist support
walking heel
windowing

CARING FOR PATIENTS WITH CASTS

Rationale for the Use of This Skill

The treatment of fractures by immobilizing a body part through the application of a cast is very old. Casts, to be effective and relatively problem-free, must be applied very carefully. Highly trained technicians usually apply a specific cast according to the physician's order. Some physicians apply their own casts to patients.

Casts are used to immobilize the trunk or a body part so that a fracture of a bone or an injury to soft tissue can heal. To be effective, casts must be contoured or molded carefully to the body surface being covered. Although padding is used, pressure from the hard casting material can produce complications in the covered area such as pain, decreased circulation, and skin breakdown.

Although nurses seldom apply casts, they do assist in their application and maintenance and should be competent and knowledgeable in order to recognize and prevent problems. Nurses should be able to gather the appropriate equipment and assist the person applying the cast and be available to provide the patient with emotional support. Because the area or part being treated is covered by the cast, it is often difficult to discern problems unless the nurse carries out frequent and careful assessment and intervention for problems.

The long-term immobilization caused by a hard cast can also lead to a variety of complications. These can, in large part, be prevented through conscientious nursing assessment and intervention. For problems that do arise, early intervention is essential. The nurse needs to be skillful both in caring for the patient immediately after a cast has been applied and in long-term care. Any cast, regardless of type or size, forces the patient to make some immediate and long-term adaptations.[1]

Nursing Diagnoses

Examples of some nursing diagnoses related to patients with casts include:

---

[1]You will note that rationale for action is emphasized throughout the module by the use of italics.

Alteration in Activity: impairment of physical mobility related to body cast.
Potential for Injury: skin breakdown related to leg cast.

Casting Materials

Many casting materials have been tried over the years, each of which has its own advantages and disadvantages for the patient. The physician orders the type of cast to be applied and the material to be used. The patient may be taken to a special "casting room" where all the casting equipment is available, or a "cast cart" with the materials may be brought to the unit. Two types of cast material are most often used today. The oldest, and still the most commonly used, material for casting is plaster of Paris. The second most frequently used material is fiberglass.

Padding and/or wrapping is used beneath both types of cast before the material is applied. It is said, "Cotton for plaster, synthetic for synthetic." This means that soft cotton material is the fabric of choice for the plaster of Paris cast because it absorbs perspiration, *thereby decreasing skin irritation.* Synthetic material is preferred for the fiberglass cast because cotton could fray under the hardness of the fiberglass surface, *causing skin-irritating particles to become embedded beneath the cast.*

Plaster of Paris Casts

Plaster of Paris, or calcium sulfate, when combined with water, forms gypsum, a hard but fairly light substance. After being wet in a waterbath, crinoline rolls impregnated with plaster of Paris can be molded to a body part and allowed to dry. The advantages of plaster of Paris casts are not only that they are hard but also that they are inexpensive and relatively nonallergenic to most patients. Disadvantages are that the larger casts are quite heavy and that the material has a tendency to become crumbly if worn over long periods or if it becomes damp or wet. Plaster of Paris is used *to immobilize fractures and damaged soft tissue parts and as a protective device for newly amputated limbs.*

Fiberglass Casts

A type of cast that has gained in popularity is the synthetic or fiberglass cast, sometimes re-

621

ferred to as a "light" cast. Casts made from fiberglass, like those made from plaster of Paris, have both advantages and disadvantages. *Fiberglass is easier to apply, more rigid, and durable.* For these reasons, fiberglass is commonly used for children with minor fractures and injuries, since they are more active and may damage a softer cast. Another advantage is that the drying time is only about twenty-four hours. Although these casts are more resistant to moisture and water than are plaster of Paris casts, the manufacturer does not recommend that the patient shower or swim in such a cast, mainly *because the padding underneath will become wet and can macerate the skin.*

There are several disadvantages to fiberglass. It is more expensive than plaster of Paris. The substance is not as "forgiving" as plaster, and so once the cast is "molded" to the part, *the rigidity may cause problems if even minimal swelling takes place.* When the cast is dry, *this rigidity may continue to cause problems for the underlying tissue.* For this reason, fiberglass is usually not used for the elderly patient.

General Procedure for Assisting with the Application of a Plaster of Paris Cast

Assessment

1. Review the patient's record to determine the kind of injury, and read the physician's notes about casting.
2. Find out what the physician has told the patient about the procedure *so that you can clarify, if necessary, any information that has been given.* The physician sometimes orders a sedative about 30 minutes before casting *to alleviate any anxiety or discomfort.*

Planning

3. Wash your hands *for asepsis.*
4. Gather equipment on a cart if a special "cast cart" is not available.
   a. Rolls of plaster of Paris. Assemble more than you think might be needed, and include various widths. The physician will often wish to reinforce certain areas or add more casting material than originally planned. It is frustrating not to have enough casting rolls at hand. Physicians usually elect to use the larger rolls, *since they produce a smoother cast with less chance of undue constriction.*
   b. A bucket or deep container for immersing the rolls.
   c. Stockinette. This soft, stretchy, ribbed tubular material comes in different circumferences. When pulled over a body part, it *provides a smooth surface and protection from the inner surface of the cast.* Choose an appropriate circumference and cut off a length 6 inches longer than the area to be casted.
   d. Large, heavy-duty scissors.
   e. Cast padding. This padding consists of soft, thin cotton layers between two outer layers of more closely woven cotton material. It comes pressed into a "waffled" configuration to prevent wadding underneath the cast. Gather several rolls of various widths.
   f. A cast knife for trimming.
   g. A cast saw in case "windowing" is needed (see Windowing, p. 625).
   h. Adhesive cloth tape.
   i. A plastic apron and gloves. These are used by the physician or technician applying the cast *to protect the clothing and hands.*

Implementation

5. Identify the patient *to be sure you are performing the procedure for the correct patient.*
6. Drape the patient *so that there is no unnecessary exposure.* Place a plastic-covered sheet or pillow under the part to be casted *to protect the linen from moisture and plaster.*
7. Offer the patient emotional support and reassurance.
8. Inspect the skin over which the cast is to be applied. Skin that has a rash or lesion of any kind should never be covered by cast material without the full knowledge of the physician. Surgical wounds are often exposed for inspection through a window—a small square cut—after the cast has been applied.

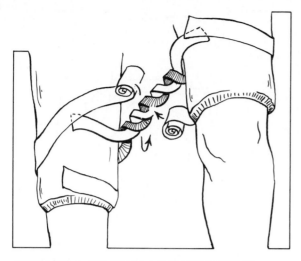

FIGURE 30.1 FORMING A "TWIST" SUPPORT

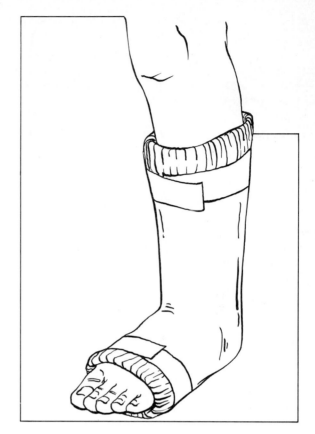

FIGURE 30.2 FOLDED STOCKINETTE OVER CAST EDGES

9. Fill the bucket with water that is warm but not hot. *Warm water facilitates the drying process.*

10. Stand a plaster roll on its end in the water *so that absorption is more uniform.*

11. As soon as the bubbles stop, remove the roll and gently squeeze (but do not twist) out the excessive water. "Free up" the end of the roll.

12. Hand the roll to the person applying the cast. The casting rolls are wrapped around the body part in an overlapping fashion.

13. Repeat steps 10, 11, and 12 until enough plaster rolls have been used.

14. Twist supports and walking heels can be incorporated into the cast during the wet or "green" stage or can be glued on later. Twists are made by twisting a plaster roll, wrapping the ends around the two sites of attachment, then rolling another plaster roll around the twist. When dry, this appears as a strong plaster bar between two extremities or between an extremity and the patient's body (see Figure 30.1).

15. The rough edges of the cast are trimmed with a cast knife and can be covered with either stockinette or, when dry, adhesive petals made by the nurse or the person applying the cast. Stockinette may simply be folded down over the outer surface of the cast and fastened with tape (see Figure 30.2). Adhesive petals can be made

by cutting small strips of adhesive tape into pointed or rounded ends. These strips are tucked smoothly vertically up and over the cast edges. Pointed petals wrinkle more readily than rounded ones. Moleskin cut into round sections *provides a smoother and softer surface and has less tendency to wrinkle up than tape* (see Figure 30.3).

16. Protect casts that surround the perineal or anal area from soiling by edging or covering them with plastic secured by tape (see Figure 30.4).

17. Clean excess plaster of Paris from the patient's skin *to prevent irritation.*

18. Reassure the patient again about the procedure.

19. Remove unused materials.

20. Clean the area. Water from the plaster application is disposed of in a special sink with a plaster trap. *Plaster will clog a regular sink.*

A

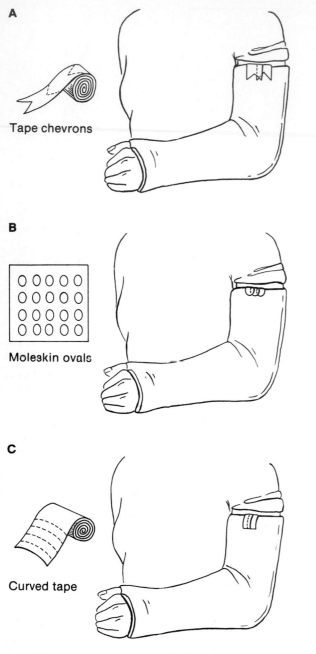

Tape chevrons

B

Moleskin ovals

C

Curved tape

FIGURE 30.3 MOLESKIN OR ADHESIVE USED AS "PETALING"

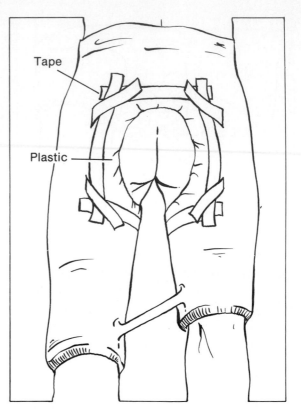

Tape

Plastic

FIGURE 30.4 PROTECTING CAST FROM SOILING

Evaluation

24. Check the patient for comfort and warmth, as well as for circulation, motion, and sensation of casted body parts.

Documentation

25. Chart the type of cast applied and any observations.

Assisting with the Application of Fiberglass Casts

Fiberglass casts are applied in basically the same way as plaster of Paris casts. However, the rolls of material come in sealed packages that are opened individually before application. The fiberglass remains flexible while it is being molded to the patient. Additional fiberglass material that comes in a can with a brush top is often used to smooth areas or to stick surfaces together.

21. Stay in attendance until the patient can be moved to a prepared bed.
22. Wash your hands.
23. Instruct the patient regarding length of drying time and the need to keep the extremity immobile.

Common Types of Casts

Figure 30.5 illustrates the various casts.

Short arm or leg casts extend from below the elbow to the fingers or from below the knee to the toes. The elbow or knee can still be flexed.

Long arm or hanging arm casts extend from under the axilla to the fingers. The elbow is maintained in flexion so that the arm can be supported by a sling or strap. Module 26, Applying Bandages and Binders, gives directions for tying a sling. *Long leg casts* extend from above the knee to the toes.

Shoulder spica casts immobilize the upper torso and one shoulder and arm. A support bar is used *for stability*, and a window is cut over the epigastrium *to allow comfort after eating.*

Hip spica casts can extend over the torso from just under the axilla or from the lower rib cage downward, enclosing both hips. One, one and one-half, or both legs may be casted, depending on need. A support bar is used if both legs are enclosed, and a window is again placed at the epigastrium.

There are many variations on these more commonly used casts.

Cast Changes and Adaptations

Cast Changes

Casts are changed for a variety of reasons. The cast may become too tight as a result of swelling or weight gain. The cast may no longer immobilize effectively. This may be a result of weight loss, a decrease in swelling, or a decrease in underlying muscle bulk related to disuse. In the infant or child requiring long-term casting, normal growth patterns can cause the original cast to become too snug, and a new one must be applied. Wrinkling of the padding under the cast can cause extreme discomfort and necessitate a change. The cast can also be changed because of fears that there is infection beneath it. The cast itself may soften, crumble, or become badly soiled or odoriferous. When this happens, a cast change may be needed.

Bivalving

A usable cast can be bivalved instead of being totally removed and discarded. An electric cast saw is used to cut the cast lengthwise in two pieces (see Figure 30.6). This usually is done *because of skin problems or for comfort* when a fracture is partially healed and, although support is still needed, an enclosed cast is unnecessary. An elastic bandage wrap can be used when the patient is moving *to keep the two halves together.* The top half can be lifted off when the patient is resting *to relieve constant pressure from the cast* (see Figure 30.6).

Windowing

Windowing involves cutting a square or diamond-shaped section from the cast *to allow for the observation and care of the skin underneath.* In some cases this is done to care for a surgical incision underneath the cast. In others, pins that have been used to hold bones together must be removed through a window in the cast. Windows are also cut *to relieve pressure* when the tissue below includes a bony prominence or an area that will expand or swell. The swelling might be due to injury or, more normally, to gastric enlargement caused by eating (see Figure 30.5). Edges of windows should be "petaled" *to prevent skin irritation* (see step 15 of the general procedure). Handle the windowed part of a cast carefully, *since it is the weakest point and cracking can occur.*

Caring for the Patient in a Cast

The patient in a cast is at risk for specific problems. These problems are more probable and more severe if a large proportion of the body or extremity is casted. There are many important nursing actions that can be taken to ensure the patient's comfort and safety. Consider the following guidelines carefully and, if appropriate, incorporate them into the plan of care.

Preparation

1. If the patient is to remain in bed for any length of time, use a firm mattress or place a board underneath the existing mattress. This firm surface *allows proper body alignment and supports a heavy cast.*
2. Obtain a trapeze or side rails *to help the patient to move more easily in bed.*

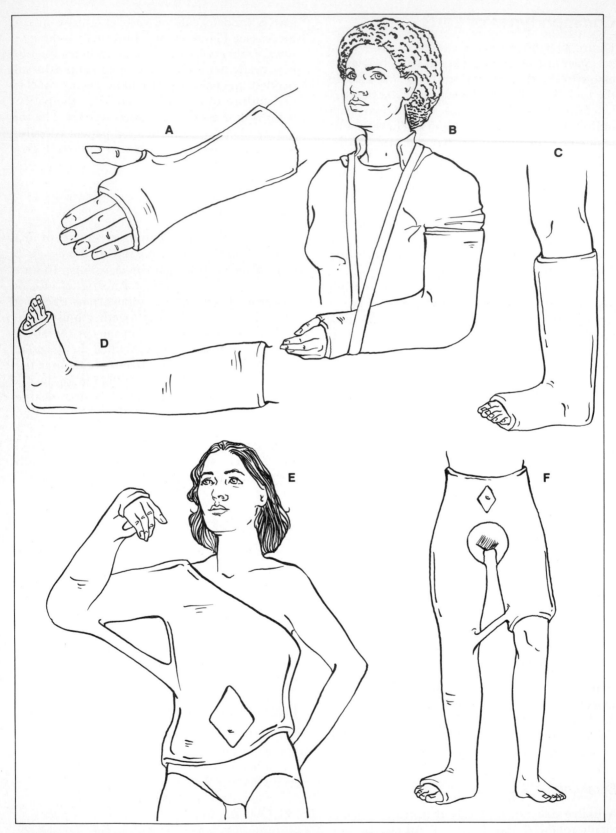

FIGURE 30.5 CAST TYPES *A:* short arm cast; *B:* hanging arm cast; *C:* short leg cast; *D:* long leg cast; *E:* shoulder spica cast; *F:* hip spica cast.

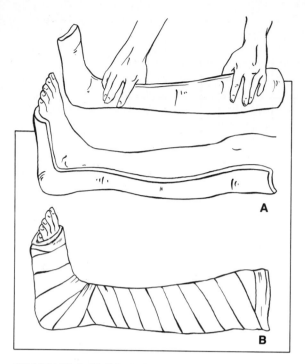

FIGURE 30.6 BIVALVING A CAST

Immediate Care after Casting

1. Get help when transferring the patient from a stretcher to the bed—the cast is heavy. One nurse can support the cast itself while a helper assists the patient. Supporting the cast well *prevents undue strain on muscle groups adjacent to it.*

2. Handle a plaster of Paris cast carefully until it is completely dry. Use the flat palms of the hands *so that your fingers do not place indentations in the wet or damp cast because this weakens the surface and causes uneven pressure on the skin.*

3. Place small plastic-covered pillows under and around the cast, leaving some air space at the sides until the cast is dry. Extending the pillows above and below the cast *will allow the cast to dry more evenly and also keep the cast from pulling on muscle groups.* Elevating an extremity slightly higher than the heart will help to prevent swelling of the tissues and excessive tightness of the cast *by improving venous return.*

4. During the drying period, leave the cast uncovered. A fan or a hair dryer on a cool setting can be used to hasten the drying process. Never apply heat, *for it tends to dry the surface of the cast too quickly, causing cracking.* Simple exposure to the air will dry a plaster cast in 10 to 20 hours time, depending on the size and thickness of the cast. The patient may feel cold as a result of evaporation from the cast. Keep the rest of the body covered *to prevent chilling and discomfort.*

5. While the cast is "green" or in the drying stage, check circulation, motion, and sensation carefully every hour. This is done *to detect any sign that the cast may be too tight.* Elevate the extremity above the level of the heart if possible *to improve venous return.*

    Circulation checks   Check first for warmth of the toes or fingers of the extremity. Do not rely on the patient's report that the fingers or toes do not feel cool. *When the circulation is restricted, the patient's sensitivity is reduced.* Feel the surface of the skin with your own hand. Also check for adequate circulation by observing the color of the nails. Nailbeds should be pink. Compare the pulse rates and quality of the two extremities. Any differences could indicate that circulation is compromised. Check for capillary filling by pressing on tissues. This causes blanching by emptying the capillary bed. Release the pressure and observe for the return of pink color. It should return immediately. *Delayed capillary filling indicates that arterial circulation is impaired. Swelling and darkened color indicate impairment of venous return.*

    Motion checks   Ask the patient to wiggle the fingers or toes. *Decreased ability to do this may indicate pressure on nerves or decreased circulation.*

    Sensation checks   Ask whether the patient can feel pressure when you press on the nails of the fingers or toes. Ask also about pain. Pain from the injury is expected, but *severe pain may result from decreased circulation or swelling of tissues. Numbness may indicate pressure on nerves from the cast or from swelling.* Some facilities use a convenient form for thorough assessment (see Figure 30.7).

	Admission/Pre-Op Assessment				Date	Extremity to be Assessed:												Frequency:													
	RUE	LUE	RLE	LLE	Time																											
Pain																																
Color																																
Temperature																																
Capillary Filling																																
Edema																																
Numbness/ Tingling																																
Pulse																																
Sensation																																
Motion																																
Comments																																

Pain: Severe, Moderate, Minimal
Color: Pink, Pale, Cynotic
Temperature: Cool, Increasingly warm
Capillary Filling: Rapid , Sluggish
Edema: Present (+), Absent (0) (specify degree)

Numbness Tingling: (+), (0)
Pulse: (+), (0) - Specify intensity
Sensation: Present, Decreased, Absent (if present, specify with, without stimuli)
Motion: Present, Decreased, Absent
WNL - Within Normal Limits

NORTHWEST HOSPITAL
SEATTLE, WASHINGTON 98133

NEUROVASCULAR ASSESSMENT

NWH M53 8/82

FIGURE 30.7 FORM FOR ASSESSING PATIENT IN A CAST

Long-Term Care of the Patient in a Cast

1. You should check casts every shift or more often for the following:
   a. *Tightness or looseness   Either of these conditions can cause complications.* You should be able to easily slip one finger between the cast and the patient's skin.
   b. *Circulation, motion, and sensation (CMS)* These checks are often recorded on a separate parameter sheet in the record. Assess the color of the toes or fingers, the patient's ability to move the tips of the extremities, and the patient's ability to feel (see above). Also note the temperature of the toes or fingers.
   c. *Drainage*   Observe for signs of drainage coming through the cast. Report, record, and describe the size of any area stained with drainage. Most facilities have a policy of outlining the area of drainage with a felt-tipped pen, noting date and time. This allows one to see any increase in drainage quickly. *Because some patients can become anxious over this procedure,* reassure the patient that this is a method of assessment so that he or she does not become unduly alarmed.
   d. *Odor*   Check the odor of the cast. *A musty, foul odor can signal infection and should be reported immediately.*
2. Try to keep water or moisture away from the plaster of Paris cast when the patient is bathing or being bathed *so that the cast will not be damaged.*
3. If the patient has a leg cast, protect the toes against cold with a heavy sock. Also prevent contact with sharp or dangerous objects, *since, because of the presence of the cast, the extremity cannot be flexed and hence cannot be withdrawn from danger.*
4. Discourage the patient from attempting to scratch beneath the cast with sharp objects. Sharp objects can, without its being detected, *damage or even puncture the underlying skin surfaces.* Itching is usually present to some degree and is especially likely when the cast is in place for a long time. Physically, little can be done about this problem except changing the cast. The best intervention for itching is distraction. Keeping the mind focused on something interesting will make other sensations recede. A cool environment also helps, *since perspiration under the cast increases itching.*
5. If the cast is an extensive one, perspiration and bacteria can cause unpleasant odors. These odors are different from the odor of infection. Commercial cast deodorants, which are sometimes mixed with the casting materials, are largely ineffective. A cast change is sometimes necessary if the odor becomes too unpleasant.
6. After the cast is completely dry, the patient will be allowed to turn more frequently and should be encouraged to do so. Turning *prevents respiratory complications and helps elimination, as does other exercise.* Teach the patient to move in one plane *so that muscle groups are not stretched.*
7. If the patient is on continuous bed rest, give instructions in performing isometric exercises. These exercises *can help prevent loss of muscle tone and strength.*
8. If the patient in a leg cast is ambulatory, the *weight of the cast can cause problems* in body balance, leading to unsteadiness and possible falls. The patient will accommodate more rapidly to this imbalance if the nurse or physical therapist gives instruction in safe ambulation. Assistive aids such as a cane, crutches, or a walker may be necessary. Consult Module 23, Ambulation.
9. Chart carefully on patients in casts. Whether your entry refers to a patient who has just been casted or to one who has been in a cast for some time, include specific findings relating to circulation, motion, and sensation as outlined above. Also record any relevant psychological data.

   Never ignore the patient's complaints. *They might be the first indication of a problem that could develop into serious complications.* You should offer emotional support to all patients in casts. *Being encased within a cast of any size imposes restrictions on activities of daily living that cause concern and inconvenience to the patient.*

Examples of Charting   Narrative

2/11/88
1520   Long leg cast applied to right leg
by Dr. Stone. Toes warm to touch,
pink, and easily moved. Returned
to room.

                     S. Thayer, R.N.

POMR Charting

2/13/88
1420   Nursing Diagnosis: Alteration in
comfort: Increasing pain in small
area of thigh under long leg cast.

S   "It's just that one spot that
keeps hurting."

O   Points to small area of cast and
grimaces.

A   Pressure under cast causing
tissue irritation.

P   Call physician, possible
bivalving of cast.

                     S. Thayer, R.N.

PERFORMANCE CHECKLIST				

Assisting with the application of a plaster of Paris cast

	Unsatisfactory	Needs More Practice	Satisfactory	Comments
Assessment				
1. Review patient's record and doctor's notes.				
2. Find out what information has been given to patient and whether clarification is needed. Determine whether sedative has been ordered.				
Planning				
3. Wash your hands.				
4. Gather equipment: a. Rolls of plaster of Paris				
b. Bucket or deep container				
c. Stockinette				
d. Scissors				
e. Cast padding				
f. Cast knife				
g. Cast saw				
h. Cloth adhesive tape				
i. Plastic apron and gloves				
Implementation				
5. Identify patient.				
6. Drape patient.				
7. Offer emotional support and reassurance.				
8. Inspect skin over which cast is to be applied.				
9. Fill bucket or container with warm water.				
10. Place first plaster of Paris roll in the water vertically.				
11. As soon as bubbles stop rising, remove roll and squeeze. "Free up" end of roll.				
12. Hand roll to person applying cast.				
13. Repeat steps 9, 10, and 11 until all rolls needed are used.				
14. If appropriate, assist with twists or walking heels.				

	Unsatisfactory	Needs More Practice	Satisfactory	Comments
15. Cover trimmed edges of cast using either stockinette or petals when dry.				
16. Protect cast area around perineum or anus with plastic.				
17. Clean excess plaster from patient's skin.				
18. Reassure patient.				
19. Remove unused material.				
20. Clean casting area.				
21. Stay until patient is moved.				
22. Wash your hands.				
☐ *Evaluation*				
23. Check patient for comfort and warmth, as well as for circulation, motion, and sensation of casted body part.				
☐ *Documentation*				
24. Chart type of cast applied and any observations.				

Caring for patients with casts

	Unsatisfactory	Needs More Practice	Satisfactory	Comments
☐ *Preparation*				
1. To provide a firm surface, obtain a firm mattress or place a board beneath mattress.				
2. Obtain trapeze or side rails as needed.				
☐ *Immediate Care*				
1. Obtain help when transferring patient from stretcher to bed.				
2. Handle cast only with palms of hands until completely dry.				
3. Place small plastic-covered pillows under and around cast as appropriate.				
4. Leave cast uncovered during drying process.				
5. While cast is "green," make hourly checks for circulation, motion, and sensation.				

	Unsatisfactory	Needs More Practice	Satisfactory	Comments
☐ *Long-term Care*				
1. Each shift, check cast for looseness or tightness and continue checks for impairment of circulation, motion, and sensation. Observe any drainage on cast or foul odor. Report any findings.				
2. Keep water or moisture away from plaster of Paris casts.				
3. Protect exposed toes from cold with a heavy sock.				
4. Discourage use of sharp objects for scratching underneath cast.				
5. Assess for unpleasant odors.				
6. Encourage patient to turn frequently after cast is dry.				
7. If patient is on bedrest, instruct in isometric exercises.				
8. If patient is ambulatory, instruct in safe walking with aids as needed.				
9. Chart any untoward observations and patient's responses. Never ignore patient's complaints. Continue to offer emotional support.				

QUIZ

Short-Answer Questions

1. The two kinds of casts are _____ and _____ .

2. Two advantages of a plaster of Paris cast are _____ and

 _____ .

3. Two advantages of a fiberglass cast are _____ and

 _____ .

4. The skin is inspected carefully before casting in order to prevent _____ .

5. The rough edges of a cast can be finished or covered by either of two methods,

 _____ or _____ .

6. The fingers and toes are checked for decreased circulation, which is

 identified by checking _____ , _____ ,

 and _____ .

Multiple-Choice Questions

_____ 7. Spica casts cover basically

 a. an arm or leg only.
 b. the body.
 c. the body and only one arm or leg.
 d. the body and one or more extremities.

_____ 8. Windowing is done to

 a. enlarge the cast.
 b. relieve pressure on underlying tissue.
 c. feel the fracture.
 d. do none of the above.

_____ 9. The toes or fingers of the patient in a green cast should be
 checked

 a. every 15 minutes.
 b. every hour.
 c. once per shift.
 d. once per day.

MODULE 31

Applying and Maintaining Traction

OVERALL OBJECTIVE

To apply skin traction to the patient and maintain commonly used skin and skeletal traction devices effectively and safely.

SPECIFIC LEARNING OBJECTIVES

	Know Facts and Principles	Apply Facts and Principles	Demonstrate Ability	Evaluate Performance
1. *Purposes*	State two or more basic purposes of traction. Explain how pull or tension is applied to the tissue.	Apply principles when setting up traction appliances. Explain purpose of a particular type of traction for specific patient.	In the clinical setting, identify the type of traction used for a particular patient	Evaluate with instructor
2. *Traction equipment*	Name various types of equipment used in setting up traction	Given a patient situation, explain use of each piece of equipment	In the clinical setting, locate equipment for traction	Evaluate with instructor
3. *Special problems*	List, by body system, special problems that may arise from the immobilization imposed by traction	Given a patient situation, assess patient and suggest intervention for problems	In the clinical setting, assess the patient for special problems, using previously learned theory	Evaluate with instructor
4. *Types of traction*	Explain the basic difference between skin and skeletal traction	Given a patient situation, identify type of traction suitable for patient	In the clinical setting, discuss the rationale for the type of traction being used to treat a particular patient	Evaluate with instructor

5. *Procedures* a. *Skin traction:* *Humerus (side-arm)* *Buck's* *Russell's* *Bryant's* *Pelvic* *Pelvic sling* *Cervical halter*	State position of bed and patient, equipment needed, direction of pull, and special potential problems with each	In the practice setting, correctly set up skin traction. With a patient in traction, determine purpose and effectiveness of treatment and assess for potential problems.	In the clinical setting, care for the patient requiring skin traction, performing either application or maintenance	Evaluate performance with instructor
b. *Skeletal traction:* *Balanced suspension* *Skull tongs*	State position of bed and patient, equipment applied to the patient, direction of pull, and potential problems of each	Given a patient in traction, determine purpose and effectiveness of treatment and identify potential problems	In the clinical setting, maintain skeletal traction under supervision	Evaluate performance with instructor
6. *Documentation*	State what information should be recorded regarding the type of traction being used and the patient's response	Given a patient situation, give an example of appropriate recording	In the clinical setting, record for a patient using either skin or skeletal traction	Evaluate performance with instructor

LEARNING ACTIVITIES	VOCABULARY

LEARNING ACTIVITIES

1. Review the Specific Learning Objectives.
2. Read the section on sensory disturbance in Ellis and Nowlis, *Nursing: A Human Needs Approach,* or comparable material in another textbook.
3. Look up the module vocabulary terms in the Glossary.
4. Read through the module.
5. In the practice setting:
   a. Inspect the bed trapeze, pulleys, and weights available.
   b. Practice tying a traction knot.
   c. When you feel proficient doing this, have a partner check your knot and check your partner's knot.
   d. With a partner, practice applying one type of skin traction in order to experience the "pulling" sensation. Use both tape and a boot, if possible.
   e. Together, evaluate the traction experience with attention to the feeling of immobility and psychosocial concerns.
   f. With a partner, practice applying Buck's traction and pelvic traction.
6. In the clinical setting:
   a. Arrange with your instructor for an opportunity to care for a patient in traction.
   b. Review the care plan for this patient, with particular attention to parts of the care plan relating to traction or problems with immobilization.
   c. Administer care to the patient in traction, based on what you have learned.
   d. Evaluate your performance with your instructor.

VOCABULARY

anorexia
cervical traction
countertraction
excoriate
footboard
footdrop
footrest
"hairline" fracture
humerus
iliac crest
integument
occiput
popliteal space
prism glasses
pulley
skull tongs
spreader bar
thrombophlebitis
traction
trapeze
weights
"whiplash"

APPLYING AND MAINTAINING TRACTION

Rationale for the Use of This Skill

Traction devices are used to treat many injuries and conditions of the musculoskeletal system. Nurses on the unit can safely and effectively apply the simpler, more commonly used traction devices to keep an injured body part in proper alignment by using the prescribed pull or tension. Some of the more complicated traction devices must be applied by nurses or technicians with special training. If reduction of a fracture requires surgery, the patient may return from the operating room to the unit with traction already in place. It is then your responsibility to maintain it properly. Traction and the immobility associated with it place the patient at risk for other complications, of which you should be aware.[1]

Nursing Diagnoses

Examples of some nursing diagnoses related to traction include:

Impairment of physical mobility related to traction

Sleep pattern disturbance: difficulty sleeping related to confinement by traction device

Potential impairment of skin integrity related to pin insertion sites

Diversional activity deficit: boredom related to confinement imposed by traction

General Information on Traction

Traction has several uses in the treatment of musculoskeletal conditions and injury. A pulling force on bones can be used to correct deformities. Immobilizing and aligning fractures with traction *allows healing and mending to take place.* When traction is applied to muscles by a pull on the skin, *pressure on nerves can be decreased, which provides relief from muscle spasm.* Traction is most commonly applied to the arms, legs, and spine—including the cervical spine, or neck.

[1]You will note that rationale for action is emphasized throughout the module by the use of italics.

The principles of traction vary with the type of traction used. Generally, each type of traction relies on one or several of these principles to produce "force" or pull. In traction, however, countertraction is imposed. This can be done by using the weight of the body, by applying external weights to the traction device, or by simply positioning the bed at an angle. Most traction is continuous.

The Traction Bed and Frame

The regular hospital bed can be easily converted to a traction bed by installing an overhead bar and a rod at the head and foot. A trapeze device can be added overhead *to assist the patient to move* (see Figure 31.1). All traction beds should have a bedboard *to provide a firm foundation.* A special egg-carton or alternating pressure mattress may be needed *to protect the patient against skin breakdown.*

Equipment and Setup

Ropes Inspect all ropes for kinking or fraying. Only clean ropes in good condition should be used. Ropes must hang freely without interference from bedding or bars. The ends of ropes near the patient's body should be wrapped with a pull tape. These tapes, which can easily be removed *prevent slipping and fraying.* They are made by covering the end of the rope with ad-

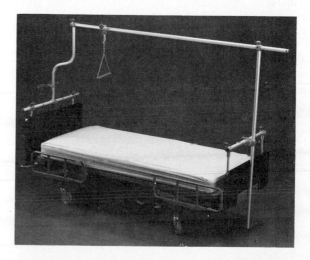

FIGURE 31.1 BED PREPARED FOR TRACTION APPLICATION
Courtesy Zimmer, Inc.

A

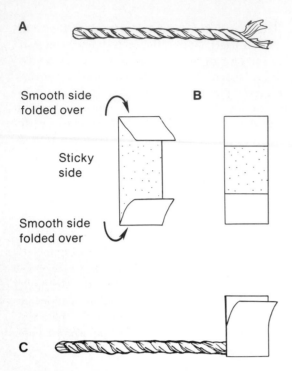

FIGURE 31.2 PULL-TAPE ON END OF ROPE *A:* rope with frayed ends; *B:* prepared tape with folded-over ends to make removal easy; *C:* tape folded over end of rope to prevent further fraying.

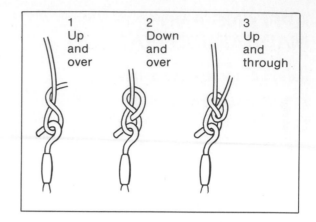

FIGURE 31.3 *HOW TO TIE A TRACTION KNOT*

hesive tape and folding the two free ends of the tape over on themselves to form two pull tabs that can easily be removed (see Figure 31.2). When tying ropes, use a traction knot, as shown in Figure 31.3. All knots are taped for safety.

Pulleys   Be sure all pulleys move freely and function properly. Initially lubricate all pulleys with an oiled cotton sponge or silicone spray.

Weights   The physician decides how much weight is to be applied. Metal blocks and sand bags, with hooks for attachment to the ropes, are used as weights. If weights are used intermittently, they should always be removed slowly and gently while support is simultaneously given to the affected body part *in order to avoid jarring the patient.* You may need assistance to do this properly. Weights must hang freely from the pulleys at all times.

Special Problems for the Patient in Traction

All patients in traction are immobilized to some degree, ranging from minimal restriction of ac-

tivity to complete immobilization. Because of this immobilization, many body systems are at risk.

The *integument* (skin) is prone to breakdown in any area where there is pressure, whether pressure caused by the traction devices or pressure from lying in bed. Frequent inspection, good hygiene, and massage are essential. You may need to adjust devices or place extra padding over bony prominences *to relieve pressure.*

The patient in traction may have a slow *respiratory* rate and shallow breathing. Breathing exercises and frequent repositioning (within the confines of the order) may be needed *to prevent pulmonary complications.*

Range-of-motion exercises, either active or passive, and other movements of the muscles and joints *can promote joint mobility, maintain muscle strength, and improve circulation in general.*

Gastrointestinal disorders may include anorexia (loss of appetite) and constipation. The diet should be made as appealing as possible and have increased fiber content *to aid bowel function.* Stool softeners may also be prescribed. Taking at least 3,000 ml of fluids per day also *helps to prevent constipation and maintain adequate urinary output.*

Pain can increase restlessness. Adequate pain management, therefore, is essential *for more effective traction and patient comfort.*

If the patient appears disoriented, you may have to apply restraints and should give frequent explanations and reassurance.

Boredom and sensory deprivation can also be problems for the immobilized traction patient. The room should be made as colorful and attractive as possible. Plan recreational activities for the patient. These might include music, television, crafts, or other activities suggested by the patient or family. These measures greatly *alleviate irritability, restlessness, and boredom.*

Patients may have secret fears of being trapped or abandoned in the event of a disaster. You should discuss these fears openly with the patient, and you should conscientiously deal with any concerns or complaints that he or she may have *in order to avoid more serious problems.*

Skin Traction

Skin traction applies traction to muscles or bones by pulling on the skin, using tapes or harnesses with protective padding. Skin traction has some limitations *because of the danger of skin irritation and breakdown.* It cannot be applied over skin that is broken or has poor blood supply *because of the danger of more serious tissue damage.* The weights are usually limited to less than 10 pounds and are left on for periods of less than three weeks.

Skin traction is generally used to treat fractures in children and minor fractures in adults, and to temporarily immobilize fractures in adults before permanent fixation. It is also commonly used for muscle strains or spasms.

Although the physician decides the type of skin traction to be used, the nurse or a specially trained technician can apply it. Whether or not it can be removed intermittently to facilitate hygiene, elimination, or exercise depends on the physician's order or the policy of the facility. The decision is usually guided by the purpose of the traction. For example, if the traction is being used to immobilize a fracture, it will generally not be removed. If the patient is being treated for muscle strain or spasm, the traction can usually be taken off for varying periods.

The skin should be clean before traction is applied. Follow the policies of the physician or facility regarding skin preparation. The area that is to be confined or taped is sometimes shaved. Tincture of benzoin is often applied to the skin *for protection.*

Types of Skin Traction

There are many variations of skin traction. In this module, we will discuss the following com-

monly-used types: humerus (side-arm), Buck's, Russell's, Bryant's, pelvic, pelvic sling, and cervical halter traction.

Humerus (Side-Arm) Traction

Humerus skin traction is used for stabilizing fractures of the upper arm and for dislocations of the shoulder. The patient is in the supine position. The head may be elevated *for comfort* as long as the forearm is in flexion and is extended 90 degrees from and in the same plane as the body.

Traction is applied in two directions by producing one pull on the elbow and another on the hand. Procedures vary with the preference of the physician, but generally the following steps are used. The skin is prepared by thorough cleansing. Strips of adhesive tape or special commercial adhesive (Skin-Trac) are attached to the

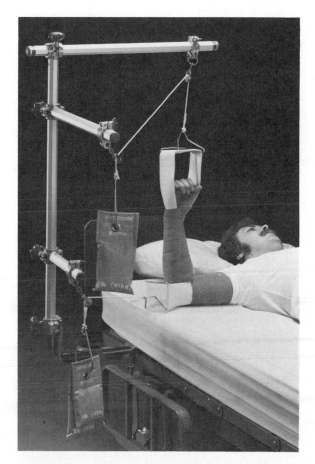

FIGURE 31.4 HUMERUS (SIDE-ARM) TRACTION
Courtesy Zimmer, Inc.

skin, with the ends of the tape protruding above the hand. The part is then wrapped with an elastic bandage. Refer to Module 26, Applying Bandages and Binders. Figure 31.4 shows the proper positioning of the ropes, pulleys, and weights. *To protect the skin over the bony prominence of the elbow,* moleskin or lamb's wool padding can be used.

Problems associated with this type of traction include skin breakdown, particularly over the elbow, and compromised circulation. Observe the patient's fingers closely for objective signs of coolness, pallor, or swelling, and ask about such subjective signs as numbness and tingling. These are most often caused by wrappings that are too tight and interfere with circulation. If any of these danger signs appear, rewrap the bandage *for comfort and safety.*

Buck's Traction

Buck's extension skin traction may be applied to one leg (unilateral) or both (bilateral). It is used primarily for immobilizing fractures of the femur, for lower-spine "hairline" or simple fractures and for temporary immobilization of a hip fracture. Muscle spasm of the lower back can also be treated with Buck's traction.

The patient in Buck's traction is placed in the supine position with the bed flat. The foot of the bed is sometimes placed on blocks *so that the weight of the patient's body will produce countertraction.*

Traction is applied in one direction on the leg or legs distally and with straight alignment. A foam and Velcro traction boot is often used to apply the traction and is the most convenient and comfortable means of doing so. An Ace bandage may be used instead of the boot to hold the footrest and sidestrips to the leg. If tape is used, wide strips are applied lengthwise to the inner and outer aspects of the calf. The calf is then padded and wrapped, and a footrest and spreader bar are put in place. The ropes, pulleys, and weights are positioned at the foot of the bed (see Figures 31.5 and 31.6).

Problems include possible skin breakdown at the ankle and over the heel. Wrappings that are too tight may compromise the circulation. The foot should be in dorsiflexion on the footrest and should be covered only by light linen *to prevent footdrop (permanent plantar flexion of the foot).*

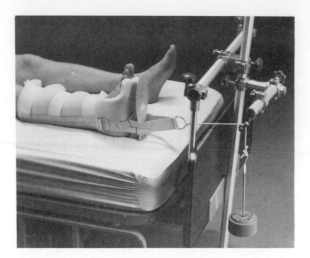

FIGURE 31.5 UNILATERAL BUCK'S EXTENSION TRACTION USING A FOAM BOOT WITH VELCRO STRAPS
Courtesy Zimmer, Inc.

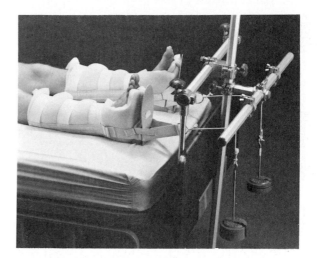

FIGURE 31.6 BILATERAL BUCK'S EXTENSION TRACTION
Courtesy Zimmer, Inc.

If the diagnosis permits, the boot and wrappings should be removed *for observation and skin care* and rewrapped. When traction is held in place by Ace bandages only, rewrapping every eight hours is usually essential.

Russell's Traction

Russell's traction combines, in principle, Buck's and balanced-suspension traction (see p. 649). With children, Russell's traction is used to re-

644

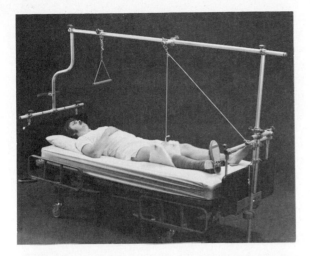

FIGURE 31.7 RUSSELL'S TRACTION USING A SINGLE WEIGHT
Courtesy Zimmer, Inc.

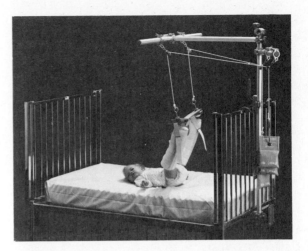

FIGURE 31.8 THE SMALL CHILD IN BRYANT'S TRACTION   Side rails are lowered to show traction clearly. In the clinical setting, side rails would be in place unless a nurse is at the crib side.
Courtesy Zimmer, Inc.

duce or align fractures of the femur and is applied as skin traction. With adults, Russell's traction is usually skeletal, with the pull being exerted on a pin or wire that has been surgically inserted through the proximal portion of the femur. Skeletal traction is used *because the pull required for the reduction of the fracture in an adult* could not be tolerated by the skin. Russell's traction is used for fractures of the femur and for knee injuries.

In general, with this type of traction the patient is supine and the bed is flat. If ordered, the head can be elevated *to a more comfortable level.* Russell's traction allows more mobility than Buck's or balanced-suspension traction, and the patient can be in high-Fowler's position and can move a little from side to side with care.

With this traction, two methods can be used to provide two-directional pull on the leg. In the first, two weights are used, one hung from an overhead bar lifting the knee and the second hung at the foot of the bed, exerting a proximal pull on the lower leg. In the second method, a single weight is added so that it exerts the two-directional pull used in the first method (see Figure 31.7).

Excessive pressure on the popliteal space behind the knee can impinge on nerves and constrict circulation. Pressure over the heel can irritate the skin and cause breakdown. Extra padding may have to be used. The foot must remain in flexion on the footrest *to prevent footdrop.*

A sock can be put on *for warmth.* The patient in Russell's traction should be continually assessed.

Bryant's Traction

Bryant's traction is a variation of bilateral Buck's traction and is used for children under the age of two who have an unstable hip joint or a fracture of the femur. The child is supine with the bed flat. Both legs, whether affected or not, are suspended so that the hips are flexed at 90 degrees to the bed surface. The traction must be applied to both legs *in order to maintain proper alignment of the affected leg.* The buttocks should be a few inches off the mattress *to ensure proper traction on the legs.* Traction boots are preferable to tape, particularly with children, *because the boots are less likely to cause skin breakdown.* Ropes are threaded from the footrests of the boot through pulleys on the overhead bar and onto the foot of the bed, where a weight is hung (see Figure 31.8).

Children adjust surprisingly well and quickly to such an apparently uncomfortable position but are at risk for a variety of problems. Both feet should be assessed frequently for decreased circulation, as evidenced by poor color, coolness, and decreased femoral, popliteal, or pedal pulses. There may also be a decrease in motion and sensation. The skin, including the back, should be inspected for excoriation. When Bryant's traction is first applied, the child may need to have the upper body restrained for a short time until he or she no longer attempts to roll the body or pull on the traction ropes or boots.

You should give the child in Bryant's traction additional support and comfort and should plan to spend extra time with the child. The family can also comfort and support the youngster and provide ideas for the amusement and diversion that are so important to the child's contentment.

Pelvic Traction

Pelvic traction is used to treat minor fractures of the lower spine, low back pain, and muscle spasm. A flannel or foam-lined canvas girdle or belt is placed snugly around the patient, often over pajama bottoms. The belt is placed somewhat lower than an abdominal binder—the lower portion ends just below the greater trochanter. It is secured with buckles or Velcro closures, and traction is applied through straps sewn into it. Traction is applied in the direction of the foot of the bed, either with two weights—one weight pulling to each side of the bed—or with only one weight, which is attached to a connector bar (see Figure 31.9).

Orders on the position of the patient vary. The most common is William's position, in which the patient is supine with the knees elevated. The patient's head is usually not elevated higher than the knees except for meals. *For countertraction,* the foot of the bed may be elevated. In certain cases, the traction is ordered as intermittent, meaning that it may be removed for elimination or hygiene. These cases usually involve patients with muscle spasm or minor pathology. For more serious conditions, such as minor aligned vertebral fractures, the traction is usually ordered as continuous so that the pull will remain constant. A fracture pan is used for elimination in these cases.

Take care to replace the pelvic belt when it becomes soiled. Inspect skin frequently, particularly over the iliac crests, *for irritation from the belt,* and provide any special skin care or padding needed. Measures to prevent or relieve constipation may also be needed. A footboard will keep the feet in flexion, *thereby preventing footdrop.* Foot and leg exercises and position changes *help to relieve cramping, maintain muscle tone, and prevent venous congestion, which could lead to thrombophlebitis.*

Pelvic Sling Traction

Pelvic sling traction is used to treat a fracture of the pelvis that has resulted in a spreading of the pelvic girdle. A flannel-lined sling provides compression on the pelvic region by suspending it slightly. Ropes are threaded through pulleys to a free-swinging weight at the foot of the bed. The patient is supine with the bed flat. Continuous traction is usually ordered, so problems of hygiene and elimination may arise. A footboard is needed, as in pelvic traction. Breathing exer-

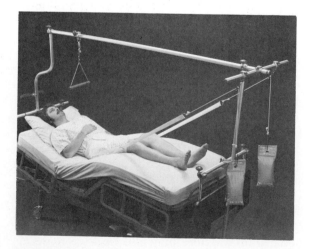

FIGURE 31.9 PELVIC TRACTION
Courtesy Zimmer, Inc.

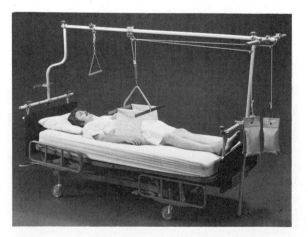

FIGURE 31.10 PELVIC SLING TRACTION
Courtesy Zimmer, Inc.

cises and exercises of the lower legs can help *prevent the complications of immobility.* (See Figure 31.10.)

Cervical Halter Traction

Cervical halter traction is used to treat a variety of conditions of the cervical spine (neck), including arthritis, "whiplash" injuries, spasms, and minor fractures.

A flannel-lined chin-head halter exerts pull on the cervical spine from the chin and occiput through a series of ropes and pulleys leading to a weight hanging freely over the head of the bed. Countertraction, if ordered, can be accomplished either by raising the head of the bed to a low-Fowler's position or by placing the head of the bed on blocks. A rolled piece of flannel or a small, flat pillow under the neck *increases extension and adds to patient comfort. A footboard prevents footdrop* (see Figure 31.11).

The occipital area (back of the head) can develop a decubitus ulcer from pressure and should be routinely inspected. The chin and cheeks are also susceptible to skin breakdown. The patient's diet may have to be modified if chewing becomes a problem. Prism glasses that direct vision upward and then horizontally can

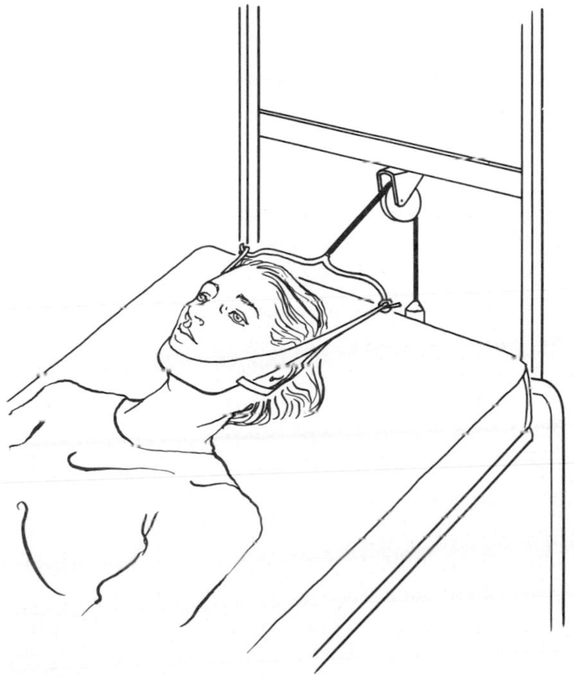

FIGURE 31.11 CERVICAL HALTER TRACTION

be obtained *so that the patient can enjoy television and books while in the supine position and thus relieve boredom.*

Procedure for Applying Skin Traction

Assessment
1. Check the order. The order for traction is written by the physician and should be followed accurately by the nurse. The order will state the type of traction to be used, the weight to be applied, and allowances for or restrictions on the activity of the patient.
2. Assess the patient for possible complications of traction. *To prevent the complications of immobilization that have already been discussed,* it is essential to make a careful assessment of the patient initially, and at regular intervals thereafter. The assessment should include all systems. If circulation, for example, is less than adequate, special padding over bony prominences may have to be added *to prevent skin breakdown.*

Planning
3. Wash your hands *for asepsis.*
4. Ensure that any assistance you might need will be available.
5. Gather the equipment you need. Skin traction will make use of several of the following: solutions, tapes, boots, bandages, harnesses, halters, ropes, pulleys, weights, padding, trapeze, spreader bars, footrests, footboard.

Implementation
6. Identify the patient *to be sure you are carrying out the procedure for the correct patient.*
7. Explain the procedure. Find out what the physician has told the patient and explain further, if necessary. Explain the purpose of the traction, whether weights are to be used intermittently or continuously, and how much the patient will be allowed to turn or move. Some patients in traction, particularly those in continuous skeletal traction, cannot move as much as those in intermittent skin traction.

8. Provide for privacy and drape the patient as appropriate.

9. Place the bed in proper position. *The degree of pull or tension required for effective traction often depends upon the level of the bed and the relative position of the patient. With some types of skin traction, the patient's body weight serves as a counterbalance, necessitating elevation of the foot or the head of the bed.*

10. Cleanse and prepare the skin according to the procedure of the facility. If tape is to be applied, the skin is often shaved beforehand *so that pain and irritation when the tape is being removed will be lessened.* Tincture of benzoin solution may be applied *to protect the skin* before any type of skin traction is initiated. (This is not done with cervical traction, *where the close proximity of the face* makes it inadvisable.)

11. To secure the traction, apply the tape, boots, slings, or halters that are appropriate to the specific procedure. Make sure all appliances are the right size for the particular patient.

12. Thread and knot ropes through lubricated pulleys. Check that both are aligned properly for the traction you are carrying out.

13. Using the hooks provided, attach ropes to the patient's appliance. Check for the security of the tapes, boot, or wrappings by gently tugging on the attached rope.

14. If more than one weight is to be applied, add one at a time with a gentle motion *to avoid jerking the body part.*

15. Tape the end of the rope *to prevent fraying.*

16. Carefully check that all appliances are functioning effectively.

17. Place the call signal, all personal possessions, and items needed for self-care within easy reach of the patient. *Having to reach for objects or call signals could not only misalign the traction but cause a fall.*

Evaluation

18. Ask the patient about comfort. Assess the unconscious patient very carefully, *since feelings of discomfort cannot be expressed.*

19. Make any necessary adjustments. You may need to add padding to bony prominences. Take care not to exert any additional pressure when adding padding. Ropes and pulleys may also need some adjustments *to correct alignment.*

20. Wash your hands *for asepsis.*

Documentation

21. Chart the type of traction applied, any observations or concerns, and the patient's tolerance of the procedure.

Skeletal Traction

Skeletal traction is accomplished by applying traction to wires or pins that have been surgically attached to or placed through bones. This type of traction, which exerts direct pull upon the bones, allows up to 30 pounds of weight to be applied for continuous periods of traction of up to four months. Although the skin is not covered or pulled upon, it is still at risk for breakdown, particularly in the elderly.

Skeletal traction is used for more serious fractures of the bones than is skin traction and more often in adults than in children. *This is because with adults, more weight must be applied to effectively align and reduce fractures.*

Although the principles of care for the patient in skin and skeletal traction are similar, the nurse who cares for the skeletal traction patient has added responsibilities.

Skeletal traction is constant and must never be discontinued or interrupted without a specific order. The state of immobility is more complete, and frequent and conscientious assessment for potential problems is required. One important potential problem is that of infection, *since the skin barrier is broken.* Bone infections are very difficult to treat successfully.

Patients in skeletal traction may understandably fear that they could not be moved or transferred quickly or easily in the event of a fire or natural disaster. It is sometimes well to explore these feelings and assure the patient that in such an event they would be given special attention. Having the call bell constantly within reach of these patients *greatly allays fears.* Answer any questions the patient may have.

Because skeletal traction devices are usually applied in surgery, the nurse's responsibilities center on maintenance and safety.

Types of Skeletal Traction

In this module, two of the more common types of skeletal traction will be discussed: balanced suspension traction and skull tongs traction.

Balanced Suspension Traction

Balanced suspension traction is used to stabilize fractures of the femur. It can be of either the skin or the skeletal type. If it is skeletal, a pin or wire is surgically placed through the distal end of the femur. If it is skin traction, tape and wrapping or a traction boot of the kind described under Buck's traction is used.

The patient is in the supine position, with the head of the bed elevated for comfort. As the name suggests, the affected leg is suspended by the ropes, pulleys, and weights in such a way that traction remains constant, even when the patient moves the upper body.

Two important components of balanced suspension traction are the Thomas splint and the Pearson attachment. The Thomas splint consists of a ring, often lined with foam, that circles and supports the thigh. Two parallel rods are attached to the splint and extend beyond the foot. A Pearson attachment consists of a canvas sling that supports the calf. A footrest completes the set-up (see Figure 31.12).

Parallel rods lead from the pin sites to the attachment for the rope. Traction to the femur is applied through a series of ropes, pulleys, and weights. These weights hang freely at the foot of the bed.

The skin should be inspected frequently *to identify problems early*. The ring of the Thomas splint can excoriate the skin of the groin. Special padding may have to be used. Again, the foot should always be in flexion on the footrest *to prevent footdrop*. If pins are used for fixation, aseptic technique must be used around pin sites until healing has taken place. From then on, clean technique can be used. The pin sites are cleansed carefully with soap and water and rinsed thoroughly, unless this varies from policy. Then an antiseptic such as povidone iodine solution may be applied. Dressings are usually not

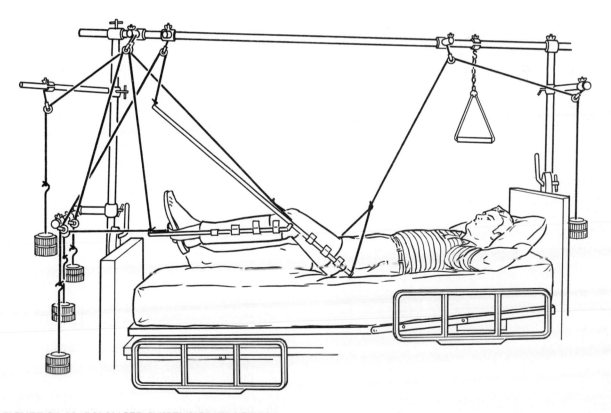

FIGURE 31.12 *BALANCED SUSPENSION TRACTION*

required. You should, however, constantly assess for infection at the pin sites. Indications include redness, heat, drainage, pain, or fever. Review your facility's policy on pin care.

Skull Tongs Traction

Skull tongs are used to immobilize the cervical spine in the treatment of unstable fractures or dislocation of the cervical spine. Although *Crutchfield tongs* have been used almost exclusively in the past, *Gardner-Wells skull tongs* are also now in wide use. These, some feel, are less likely to pull out than the Crutchfield tongs. The patient is prepared for either type with a local anesthetic to the scalp. The tongs are surgically inserted into the bony cranium, and a connector half-halo bar is attached to a hook from which traction can be applied (see Figure 31.13).

The patient is supine and is usually on a special frame instead of the regular hospital bed. See Module 25, Special Mattresses, Frames, and Beds. If a hospital bed is used, two or more people are required to assist the patient with any turning movements. The head of the bed may be elevated *to provide countertraction.*

Since patients remain in this type of traction for an extended period, the precautions taken for the patient in other types of skeletal traction must be observed here also. Difficulties with the performance of ADLs, infection at the tong sites, and restlessness and boredom are common concerns. It is useful to teach the patient range-of-

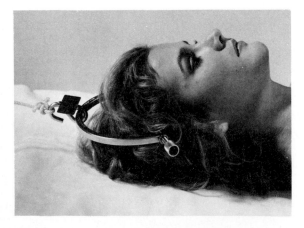

FIGURE 31.13 SKULL TONGS TRACTION
Courtesy Zimmer, Inc.

motion exercises, provide good nutrition, and suggest recreational or occupational activities.

Procedure for Maintaining Skeletal Traction

Assessment

1. Check the physician's order. Since the patient has usually returned to the unit from the operating room, the order will be contained in a list of post-op orders. It will state the weights to be used, any special restrictions on activity, and, often, the position of the heat or foot of the bed.
2. Patients just returning to the unit from surgery must be carefully assessed for signs of general discomfort or pain. See Module 47, Postoperative Care, for a more detailed discussion of this topic. For other patients being maintained in skeletal traction, carry out a complete systems assessment, with particular attention to skin, respiratory, gastrointestinal, musculoskeletal, and psychosocial systems.

Planning

3. Wash your hands *for asepsis.*
4. Ensure that any assistance you might need will be available.
5. Gather any equipment that assessment suggests you might need, such as pillows or padding.
6. If pain medication is ordered, be sure to give it long enough before the procedure for the patient to receive its full effect.

Implementation

7. Identify the patient *to be sure you are carrying out the procedure for the correct patient.*
8. Inspect the traction devices for effectiveness. Are all ropes and pulleys in proper alignment? Are ropes hanging freely? Are weights of the prescribed poundage?
9. Inspect all operative sites, such as pin or tong insertions. Is there any excessive bleeding? If there are dressings, are they clean and dry?
10. Carry out any nursing interventions

appropriate to the problems identified in assessment.

11. Place the call signal and any personal items within reach of the patient.
12. Teach the patient methods for moving in bed and any exercises that are appropriate.

Evaluation

13. Ask the patient about comfort.
14. Make any necessary adjustments, such as correcting alignment or adding extra padding.
15. Wash your hands *for asepsis.*

Documentation

16. Chart any observations you have made and all nursing actions taken.

Example of Narrative Charting

3/21/88

1630   Pelvic traction with 10 lbs. applied per order. C/o fatigue and discomfort after 2 hrs. Off 1 hour and reapplied. No skin redness.

                        A. Hartford, R.N.

Example of Narrative Charting

3/16/88

1230   Arrived on unit in balanced suspension traction. Right leg in good alignment. 10 lb. wt. hanging freely. Moderate discomfort at fracture site. Medicated × 1 with relief. Less restless, stated pain only mild and intermittent.

                        S. Adams, R.N.

PERFORMANCE CHECKLIST

Procedure for applying skin traction

	Unsatisfactory	Needs More Practice	Satisfactory	Comments
Assessment				
1. Check the physician's order regarding type of traction and weights.				
2. Carry out systems assessment.				
Planning				
3. Wash your hands.				
4. Plan for any assistance you may need.				
5. Gather equipment appropriate to the type of traction ordered.				
Implementation				
6. Identify patient.				
7. Explain procedure. Clarify any questions.				
8. Provide privacy and drape patient.				
9. Place bed in most effective position for type of traction being used.				
10. Cleanse and prepare skin according to facility policy.				
11. Apply appropriate tapes, boots, or halters.				
12. Thread and knot ropes, checking alignment.				
13. Attach ropes to patient's appliance and check security.				
14. Add weights ordered gently, one at a time.				
15. Tape loose ends of ropes.				
16. Place call signal and all personal items within reach of patient.				
Evaluation				
17. Ask patient about comfort.				
18. Make any necessary adjustments, such as correcting alignment or adding padding.				
19. Wash your hands.				

	Unsatisfactory	Needs More Practice	Satisfactory	Comments
☐ *Documentation*				
20. Chart type of traction applied, any observations you have made, and all nursing actions taken.				

Procedure for maintaining skeletal traction

	Unsatisfactory	Needs More Practice	Satisfactory	Comments
☐ *Assessment*				
1. Check the physician's order on the post-op order sheet.				
2. Carry out systems assessment, including level of discomfort or pain.				
☐ *Planning*				
3. Wash your hands.				
4. Plan for any assistance you may need.				
5. Gather any additional equipment you need based on assessment.				
6. Obtain any medication ordered.				
☐ *Implementation*				
7. Identify patient.				
8. Inspect all traction devices, ropes, pulleys, and weights.				
9. Inspect pin or operative sites.				
10. Carry out nursing interventions as identified in assessment.				
11. Place call signal and personal items within reach of patient.				
12. Teach methods for moving in bed and any appropriate exercises.				
☐ *Evaluation*				
13. Ask patient about comfort.				
14. Make any necessary adjustments, such as correcting alignment or adding padding.				

	Unsatisfactory	Needs More Practice	Satisfactory	Comments
15. Wash your hands.				
☐ *Documentation*				
16. Chart any observations you have made and all nursing actions taken.				

| QUIZ |

Short-Answer Questions

1. The primary difference between skin and skeletal traction is _____

_____ .

2. To prevent footdrop in patients in traction who must remain supine and

immobile, a(n) _____ can be used to keep the feet in _____ .

3. List four common patient problems that may result from the
immobilization associated with traction.

    a. _____

    b. _____

    c. _____

    d. _____

Matching Question

4. Match the most likely area for potential skin breakdown with the type of
traction listed below (more than one choice may be used):

    (1) ____ Humerus   **a.** elbow

    (2) ____ Buck's   **b.** groin

    (3) ____ Russell's   **c.** iliac crest

    (4) ____ Bryant's   **d.** heel

    (5) ____ Pelvic   **e.** occipital

    (6) ____ Cervical halter   **f.** ankle

    (7) ____ Cervical tongs   **g.** chin

                                h. back

Emergency Resuscitation Procedures

PREREQUISITES

Successful completion of the following modules:

VOLUME 1

OVERALL OBJECTIVE

To recognize the need for and to perform emergency resuscitation procedures on individuals of all ages.[1]

SPECIFIC LEARNING OBJECTIVES

	Know Facts and Principles	Apply Facts and Principles	Demonstrate Ability	Evaluate Performance
1. Cardiopulmonary resuscitation				
a. Airway	State usual method for opening airway. State method used in case of cervical injury.	Given a patient situation, identify appropriate method for opening airway	Open airway on mannequin, using both methods described	Evaluate with instructor and lab partner
b. Breathing	Describe usual method for rescue breathing. Describe alternative methods used in special situations.	Given a patient situation, identify appropriate method of rescue breathing	Demonstrate mouth-to-mouth and mouth-to-nose breathing	Evaluate effectiveness by checking chest for movement
c. Circulation	State where to palpate carotid pulse. State where to apply compression on adults and children. State distance sternum must be moved for effective compression.		Apply compression in appropriate location. Move sternum appropriate distance when doing cardiac compression.	Evaluate by checking for adequate compression on mannequin gauge, if available.
d. One rescuer	State ratio of breaths to compression for one rescuer		Perform CPR alone on mannequin	Evaluate with instructor using Performance Checklist
e. Two rescuers	State ratio of breaths to compression for two rescuers		Perform two-person CPR with partner on mannequin	Evaluate with instructor using Performance Checklist

f. *Age considerations*	State differences in procedure for adults, small children, and infants		Perform CPR on infant mannequin, incorporating techniques that differ from adult procedure	Evaluate with instructor using Performance Checklist
g. *Documentation*	State two items of particular importance to be observed and documented when CPR is carried out		Observe and document accurately during real or simulated CPR	Evaluate own performance with instructor
2. *Foreign-body airway obstruction*				
a. *Recognition*	Describe the universal distress signal for choking	Given a patient situation, state whether or not you would intervene	In a simulated situation, demonstrate how to determine that airway obstruction is present	
b. *Management*	Describe two aspects of attempting to dislodge a foreign-body airway obstruction	Given a situation (victim conscious or unconscious), state how procedure would be carried out	Using a mannequin, demonstrate correct procedure for dislodgment of foreign body in both upright and supine positions	Evaluate with your instructor
c. *Age considerations*	State differences in procedure for infants and small children		Using an infant mannequin, demonstrate correct procedure for dislodgment of foreign body	Evaluate with your instructor

[1]Material in this module, including Figures 32.1 through 32.14, conforms to the American Heart Association recommendations as of April 1986.

LEARNING ACTIVITIES

1. Review the Specific Learning Objectives.
2. Read the section on basic life support (in the chapter on circulation) in Ellis and Nowlis, *Nursing: A Human Needs Approach,* or comparable material in another textbook.
3. Look up the module vocabulary terms in the Glossary.
4. Read through the module.
5. In the laboratory, practice with a Resusci-Annie or similar mannequin under your instructor's supervision.
   a. Establish an airway on the adult mannequin.
   b. Breathe 12 times per minute into the adult mannequin, watching for the rise and fall of the chest wall and allowing for "exhalation."
   c. Practice closed-chest massage on the adult mannequin at a rate of 80–100 compressions per minute, compressing the sternum 1½ to 2 inches each time.
   d. Establish an airway on an infant mannequin.
   e. Breathe 20 times per minute into the infant mannequi.., using only the amount of air needed to cause the chest to rise.
   f. Practice closed-chest massage on the infant mannequin at a rate of 100 compressions per minute, using only the tips of your index and middle fingers to compress the sternum ½ to 1 inch each time.
6. With a partner, practice CPR on both adult and infant mannequins, using the Performance Checklist as a guide. Take turns doing the breathing and the closed-chest massage. Have your instructor evaluate your performances.
7. With your partner as observer and evaluator, practice CPR alone on both the adult and infant mannequins, using the Performance Checklist as a guide. When you are satisfied with your performance, trade places and have your partner demonstrate CPR on the adult and infant mannequins with you observing and evaluating. When you are both satisfied with your performances, have your instructor evaluate them.
8. Working as a pair, simulate the recognition and management of foreign-body airway obstruction on each other or on an adult mannequin, using the Performance Checklist as a guide. Practice management of foreign-body airway obstruction on the infant mannequin as well. When you are satisfied with your performance, have your instructor evaluate you.

VOCABULARY

airway
cardiac arrest
carotid pulse
Heimlich maneuver
respiratory arrest
sternum
trachea
tracheostomy
xiphoid process

EMERGENCY RESUSCITATION PROCEDURES

Rationale for the Use of This Skill

The nurse is expected to carry out emergency resuscitation procedures efficiently, whether on the street or in a health care facility. The nurse must be able to perform these lifesaving procedures as a member of a team or alone on individuals of all ages. At least once a year a refresher course must be taken to maintain expertise.[2]

Introduction

Although these procedures could have been written in such a way as to clearly show the nursing process approach, we chose not to do so for these reasons:

1. Rote memorization is necessary so that you can respond automatically in an emergency situation.
2. National organizations that teach these procedures do not use this format, and it may confuse those who have already been exposed to such courses.

When reviewing the procedures, you may wish to identify for yourself which steps constitute assessment, which planning, which implementation, and which evaluation.

Cardiopulmonary Resuscitation

Cardiopulmonary resuscitation (CPR) is a process of rescue breathing and chest compression that is provided to a person whose heart has stopped beating and who has stopped breathing. No matter where this person is, he or she needs immediate assistance *to restore breathing and circulation. If the delay is longer than four minutes, the potential for permanent brain damage is great.* CPR may be needed anywhere—in the home, on the street, in the health care facility. Eventually, you may be involved not only in performing the skill, but in teaching it to other professionals and lay people as well.

[2]You will note that rationale for action is emphasized throughout the module by the use of italics.

Basic CPR is as easy to remember as ABC: Airway, Breathing, and Circulation.

Airway

1. Determine unresponsiveness. When you find a person in a state of collapse, grasp the shoulder firmly, shake, and shout, "Are you all right?" If you get no response, call out for help, and when someone responds, send that person to activate the emergency medical system in the health care facility or, if you are outside the health care facility, in your community.
2. Position the person flat on the back on a firm, flat surface. If you must roll the person over, try to move the entire body at once, as a single unit, to avoid worsening any injury to the neck, back, or long bones.
3. Tilt the patient's head back by placing the palm of one hand on the forehead and applying firm backward pressure. Place the fingers of the other hand under the bony part of the lower jaw near the chin, and lift to bring the chin forward. *This will clear the tongue out of the airway.* (This is the chin-lift method of opening the airway.)

Breathing

1. Determine breathlessness. Place your ear close to the patient's mouth and do three things:
   a. *Look* at the chest and the stomach for movement.
   b. *Listen* for breathing sounds.
   c. *Feel* for air against your cheek (Figure 32.1).
   Sometimes a person begins to breathe spontaneously after an airway has been established. But if you cannot see chest movement, hear breathing sounds, or feel air on your cheek, the patient is not breathing, and you must provide rescue breathing.
2. Keeping the airway open by using the head-tilt/chin-lift maneuver, gently pinch the nose closed using the thumb and index finger of the hand on the forehead (see Figure 32.2). *This will prevent air from escaping through the patient's nose.*
3. Place your mouth over the patient's mouth,

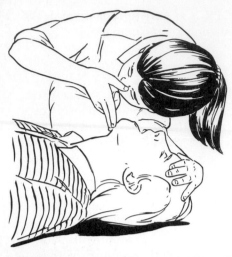

FIGURE 32.1 CHECKING FOR BREATHING Note that the patient's head is tilted back.

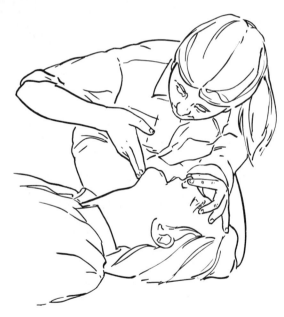

FIGURE 32.2 OCCLUDING THE NOSTRILS

make an airtight seal, and give two initial breaths of 1 to 1.5 seconds each. Be sure to allow time for deflation of the patient's lungs between breaths. If the patient's chest rises and falls, showing that air has entered, proceed to step 1 under "Circulation." If mouth-to-mouth breathing is not desirable or possible (for example, in the presence of vomiting or injury to the mouth or jaw), mouth-to-nose breathing can be done by closing the mouth with one palm and breathing into the nose. The position of the head is the same as for mouth-to-mouth breathing. Mouth-to-stoma breathing is possible if the patient has a permanent tracheostomy. In such a case it would not be necessary to tilt the head back to open the airway as you would for mouth-to-mouth and mouth-to-nose breathing.

4. If you feel resistance when you try to breathe into the patient's mouth and the patient's chest wall does not rise and fall as you breathe, reposition the head and attempt to breathe again. If you still feel resistance, proceed with foreign-body airway obstruction maneuvers, pp. 667–669.

Circulation

1. Determine pulselessness. Feel for the carotid pulse by locating the larynx (voice box) and sliding your fingers off into the groove beside it. You should feel for the pulse on your side of the patient (Figure 32.3) *to avoid compressing the other carotid artery with your thumb.* Adequate time (5 to 10 seconds) should be allowed, *since the pulse may be slow, irregular, or very weak and rapid. If you locate a pulse,* perform rescue breathing at a rate of 12 breaths per minute, rechecking the pulse after each 12 breaths. *If you cannot locate a pulse,* you will have to provide artificial circulation in addition to rescue breathing. Ask someone to call for help before beginning compression.

2. Kneel at the level of the patient's shoulders. *You will then be in a position to perform both rescue breathing and chest compression without moving your knees.* The patient should be on a hard surface to achieve best results. In a health care facility, slip a cardiac board under the patient.

3. Locate the lower margin of the patient's rib cage on the side nearest you. Run the fingers of the hand nearest the patient's legs up along the rib cage to the indentation where the ribs meet the sternum. Keeping one finger on the indentation, place another immediately above it, on the lower end of the sternum (Figure 32.4).

4. Place the heel of your other hand just

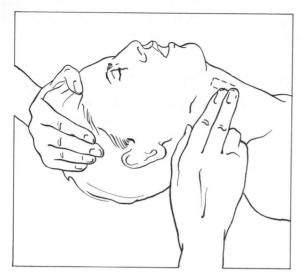

FIGURE 32.3 FEELING FOR THE CAROTID PULSE

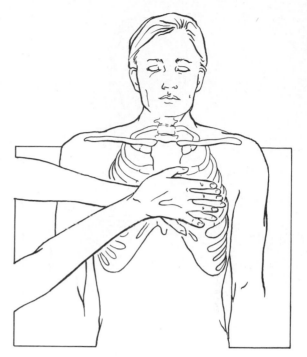

FIGURE 32.5 HANDS IN PLACE FOR CHEST COMPRESSION

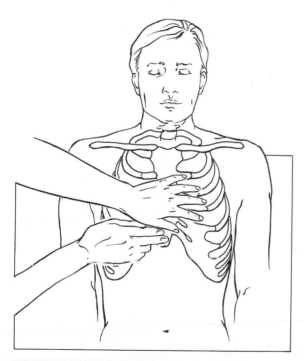

FIGURE 32.4 LOCATING THE LOWER MARGIN OF THE RIB CAGE

above that finger, at right angles to the sternum. *This will keep the main force of compression on the sternum and decrease the chance of rib fracture.*

5. Remove your fingers from the indentation and place that hand on top of the one already in position. Your hands should be parallel and directed away from you (Figure 32.5). Your fingers may be either extended or interlaced, but they must be kept off the chest *to avoid fracturing a rib* (Figure 32.6).

6. With your shoulders directly above the patient's chest, compress downward, keeping your arms straight. You should move the sternum of an adult 1½ to 2 inches with each compression (Figure 32.7). You must release compression pressure after each compression *to allow blood to flow into the heart.* The time allowed for release should equal the time required for compression. Therefore, your motion should be a rhythmical 50 percent down and 50 percent back up. Avoid quick, ineffective jabs to the chest *that can increase the possibility of injury and may decrease the amount of blood circulated by each compression.* Your hands should not be lifted from the chest or their position changed in any way *so that you do not lose correct hand position.*

One-Rescuer CPR

If you are the only rescuer present, you are responsible for both rescue breathing and cardiac

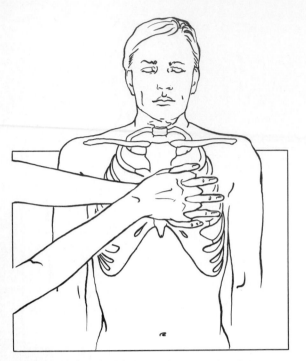

FIGURE 32.6 *HANDS IN PLACE WITH FINGERS INTERLACED*

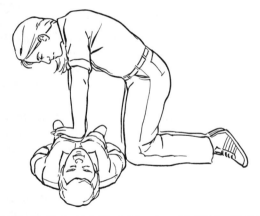

FIGURE 32.7 *PROPER POSITION OF RESCUER FOR AN ADULT*

compression. The proper ratio is 15 compressions to two breaths at a rate of 80–100 compressions per minute. You must maintain this rate to compensate for the compressions lost when you take time out to do the breathing. Move smoothly from one function to the other, keeping a steady rhythm. Say, "One and two and . . ." to yourself to maintain the correct rate. If there is no one in the immediate area to assist you, you should administer CPR for a full minute, after

which you may quickly phone for help and then resume CPR.

Two-Rescuer CPR

If two rescuers are present, it is best to position yourselves on opposite sides of the patient. Rescuer 1 should be positioned at the patient's side and compress the sternum at a rate of 80–100 compressions per minute. Rescuer 2, positioned at the patient's head, maintains an open airway, monitors the carotid pulse *for adequacy of chest compressions,* and ventilates the patient after every fifth compression. A pause should be allowed for the ventilation (1 to 1.5 seconds per breath). Rescuer 1 (the compressor) says, "One and two and three and four and five and . . ." (or any helpful mnemonic) aloud *to help both rescuers maintain the rate and ratio.*

When either of the rescuers tires, rescuer 1 calls for a change of tasks and completes the ongoing series of five compressions. Rescuer 2 breathes after the fifth compression as rescuer 1 moves up and checks the carotid pulse for five seconds. Rescuer 2 gets in position to compress the sternum and waits. If the carotid pulse is absent, rescuer 1 says, "No pulse," and ventilates once. Rescuer 2 restarts the compressions immediately after the breath.

Monitoring the Patient

Rescuer 2 assumes the responsibility for monitoring the pulse and breathing. The carotid pulse is checked during compressions *to assess the effectiveness of rescuer 1's external chest compressions. To determine whether the patient has resumed spontaneous breathing and circulation,* chest compressions must be stopped for five seconds at about the end of the first minute and every few minutes thereafter.

Terminating CPR

CPR is terminated when one of the following occurs:

1. Breathing and a spontaneous heartbeat are detected.
2. An advanced life-support team arrives to take over the patient's care.
3. A physician pronounces the patient dead and states that CPR can be discontinued.

4. The rescuer(s) becomes physically exhausted and no replacement(s) is available. This is the most difficult reality for a rescuer to face, but there are limits to one's physical endurance. Fortunately, this does not happen often.

Cervical Neck Fracture

If a patient has been in an accident (an automobile crash, a fall) and you suspect that he or she may have a cervical (neck) fracture, do not open the airway using the chin-lift method. Instead, keep the head in a flat position. Grasp the jaw at the angle, and pull the lower jaw forward so that it is higher than the upper jaw. (This is called *displacement of the mandible.*)

Infants and Small Children

Basically, the procedure used with infants and small children is similar to that used with adults. However, there are some important differences to keep in mind when you administer CPR to an infant or small child.

Airway   Some believe that overextension of the head closes the trachea in small babies. Although there is no proof of this, overextension is best avoided, *since it is unnecessary.*

Breathing   Cover both the mouth and the nose of the infant with your mouth (Figure 32.8). If the patient is a larger child, occlude the nostrils with the fingers of the hand that is maintaining head tilt, and make a mouth-to-mouth seal. Give two slow breaths (1 to 1.5 seconds per breath), pausing between to breathe yourself. *Since the volume of air in an infant's lungs is smaller than that in an adult's,* you should use only the amount of air needed to cause the chest to rise. Watch carefully—as soon as you see the chest rise and fall, you are using the right volume of air. For an infant, breathe once every 3 seconds, or 20 times a minute; for a child, breathe once every 4 seconds, or 15 times a minute.

Circulation   *Because the carotid artery is difficult to locate in an infant's short, chubby neck,* the brachial artery is recommended instead. Locate the brachial pulse on the inside of the upper arm, between the elbow and shoulder, by placing your thumb on the outside of the arm and press-

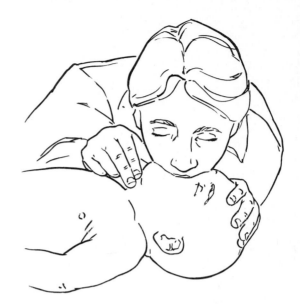

FIGURE 32.8 BREATHING FOR AN INFANT

ing gently with your index and middle fingers (Figure 32.9).

Position the child in a horizontal supine position on a hard surface, as you would an adult. For an infant, the hard surface can be the palm of the hand not performing the compressions. The weight of the infant's head and a slight lift of the shoulders then provide head-tilt.

In the infant, locate an imaginary line between the nipples over the sternum. Place the index finger of the hand farthest from the infant's head just under that line where it intersects with the sternum. The correct area for compression is one finger's width below this intersection, where your middle and ring fingers are located. Using two or three fingers, compress the sternum 0.5 to 1 inch at a rate of at least 100 times per minute (Figure 32.10).

In the child, the correct area for compressions is located the same way it is for an adult. Compress the chest with the heel of *one* hand 1 to 1.5 inches at a rate of 80 to 100 times per minute (Figure 32.11).

For both infants and small children, breathe after every fifth chest compression.

CPR in the Health Care Facility

Acute health care facilities follow a specific procedure whenever resuscitation is necessary.

1. The person who discovers the victim's collapse is expected to call for assistance,

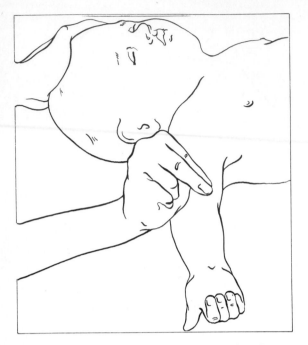

FIGURE 32.9 LOCATING AND PALPATING THE BRACHIAL PULSE

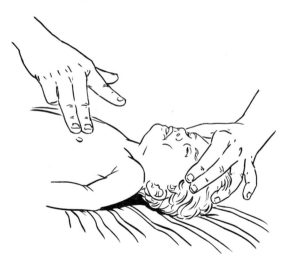

FIGURE 32.10 CORRECT COMPRESSION FOR AN INFANT

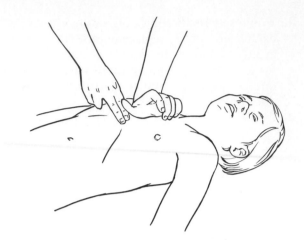

FIGURE 32.11 CORRECT HAND POSITION FOR CHEST COMPRESSIONS IN A CHILD

3. The person who responds to the call for help gathers the emergency equipment (cardiac board, breathing bag, oxygen setup, emergency meds, and the like) and brings it to the location of the victim's collapse.

4. The second person then assists as necessary. This might include placing the cardiac board and participating in two-person CPR.

5. Most facilities designate a team of specially trained personnel (including a physician) to respond to all codes. When the team arrives with special life-support equipment, such as a defibrillator and emergency drugs, it takes over care completely. The first persons with the victim relinquish care to the team. They can stay to assist if that is part of the facility's procedure, or they may return to their other duties.

6. If sufficient personnel are available, someone should reassure any family members and any patients in the immediate area.

Documentation

Certainly, the initiation of CPR is of primary importance, but the nurse's responsibility to maintain a record of all activities is also important. Whenever you find yourself an "extra" during CPR, you can fulfill an essential function by observing and recording, in particular the times of CPR initiation and discontinuation.

either by telephone or by actually calling to someone at the desk. *To simplify matters and to avoid alarming other patients,* the call is made with a designated code. The code number differs from facility to facility, but code 99 and code 199 are used in many places.

2. The discoverer initiates CPR following the above procedures.

666

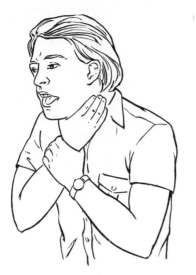

FIGURE 32.12 UNIVERSAL DISTRESS SIGNAL FOR CHOKING

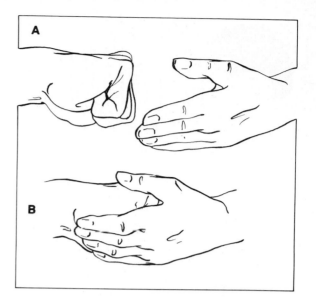

FIGURE 32.13 CORRECT HAND POSITION FOR MANUAL THRUSTS

Management of Foreign-Body Airway Obstruction

Foreign-body obstruction of the airway usually occurs during eating. Meat is frequently the cause of an obstruction in adults. Other foods and foreign bodies may be the cause in children and some adults. Choking on food may result from elevated blood alcohol level, poorly fitting dentures, or large, inadequately chewed pieces of food.

Recognition

A foreign body can cause partial or complete airway obstruction. If the victim's airway is only partially obstructed, some degree of air exchange may be possible. If the air exchange is good, the victim may be able to cough forcefully. You should not interfere in this situation. Encourage the victim to attempt to cough and breathe spontaneously

Initial poor air exchange or good air exchange that has deteriorated to poor air exchange (ineffective cough, crowing noises when inhaling, bluish color) should be managed as though it were complete airway obstruction.

Establish that the airway is obstructed. The victim may know the universal distress signal for choking—clutching the neck with his or her hand(s) (see Figure 32.12). Ask the victim, "Are you choking?" If the answer is an affirmative shake of the head, intervene immediately.

Management

1. The Heimlich maneuver (subdiaphragmatic abdominal thrusts) is recommended by the American Heart Association for relieving foreign-body airway obstruction. You may need to repeat the thrust six to ten times to clear the airway. Your hands should not be placed on the xiphoid process of the sternum or on the lower margins of the rib cage *in order to prevent possible damage to internal organs.* Your hands should be below this area but above the navel in the midline.

2. If the victim is sitting or standing (conscious), stand behind the victim and wrap your arms around his or her waist. Then grasp one fist with your other hand, and place the thumb side of that fist against the victim's abdomen in the midline slightly above the navel as described (Figure 32.13). Next, press into the victim's abdomen with a quick upward thrust (Figure 32.14a). Each thrust should be a separate and distinct movement. Continue until the foreign body is expelled or the victim loses consciousness.

3. If the victim is lying down (unconscious), position him or her on the back and kneel astride the victim's thighs. Place the heel of

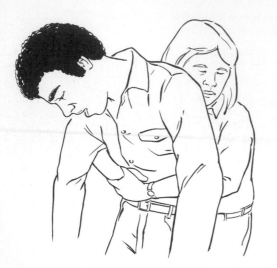

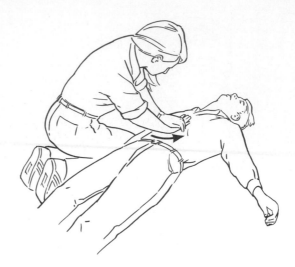

FIGURE 32.14 *HEIMLICH MANEUVER   A:* Conscious victim; *B:* Unconscious victim.

one hand against the victim's abdomen (as described) with the second hand directly on top of the first. Press into the abdomen with a quick upward thrust (Figure 32.14b). Do six to ten abdominal thrusts.

4. Chest thrusts are recommended *only* when the victim is in the late stages of pregnancy or when the Heimlich maneuver cannot be used effectively on the unconscious, very obese victim. In such cases, you should place the victim in the supine position and kneel at the victim's side. Using the same hand position as for external cardiac compression, deliver each thrust slowly and distinctly.

5. Use the finger sweep only in the unconscious patient to attempt to grasp the foreign body and remove it.

   a. With the victim face up, use one hand to open the mouth by grasping the lower jaw and tongue between your thumb and fingers and lifting. This draws the tongue away from the back of the throat and away from any foreign body lodged there.

   b. Insert the index finger of your other hand along the inside of the victim's cheek, using a hooking action to dislodge any foreign body so it can be removed. Be careful not to push the foreign body further into the airway.

6. If a victim who was initially conscious loses consciousness, the muscles may become

more relaxed, and techniques that were previously unsuccessful may be successful.

Infants and Small Children

In infants and small children, airway obstruction may be caused by an object, such as a small toy or a peanut, or by an infection that results in swelling of the airway. It is important to differentiate between the two. The procedure presented here is not effective in the case of infection and will only delay necessary treatment.

Although the procedure for relieving foreign-body airway obstruction in infants and small children is similar to that used for adults, there are some important differences to keep in mind.

Position   Straddle an infant over your arm, with the head lower than the trunk. Support the head by placing a hand around the jaw and chest (see Figure 32.15). After delivering four back blows between the infant's shoulder blades, place your free hand on the infant's back so that he or she is "sandwiched" between your two hands (one supports the neck, jaw, and chest while the other supports the back). Turn the infant and place him or her on your thigh, with the head lower than the trunk, then deliver four thrusts in the same way as for external chest compressions. If the infant is too large for this positioning, kneel on the floor and place him or

668

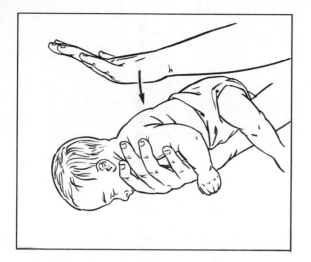

FIGURE 32.15 INFANT BACK BLOWS

her across your thighs, keeping the head lower than the trunk. Now deliver four back blows. Then, supporting the head and back, roll the infant over onto the floor and deliver four chest thrusts (as for external chest compression).

A child should be positioned face up, and you should kneel at the child's feet (or stand if the child is on a table). The "astride" position used for adults is not recommended for small children but may be used for a large child. Deliver the abdominal thrust as you would for an adult, but more gently in a small child.

Finger Sweep Because a foreign body can easily be pushed further back in the airway and cause increased obstruction, avoid blind finger sweeps in infants and children. If the victim is unconscious, open the mouth by lifting the lower jaw and tongue forward. If you can see the foreign body, remove it with your finger.

REFERENCES

American Heart Association, "Standards and Guidelines for Cardiopulmonary Resuscitation and Emergency Cardiac Care." *JAMA,* 255 (June 6, 1986), 2843–2984.

American Heart Association. *Interim Teaching Guidelines for Revisions in Basic Life Support.* Dallas: American Heart Association National Center, 1986.

"New CPR Guidelines: Bicarb Now a Last Resort." *AJN,* 86 (August 1986), 889.

PERFORMANCE CHECKLIST				

	Unsatisfactory	Needs More Practice	Satisfactory	Comments
One-rescuer CPR				
1. a. Shake and shout, "Are you all right?";				
b. Call out for help.				
2. Turn patient on back.				
3. Establish airway using head-tilt/chin-lift maneuver; look, listen, and feel.				
4. If patient does not begin to breath, occlude nostrils and give two full breaths, using mouth-to-mouth breathing. a. If chest rises and falls, continue with step 5.				
b. If chest does not move, clear the obstruction and then continue.				
5. Palpate carotid pulse. If absent, begin chest compression.				
6. Kneel beside patient's shoulders.				
7. Position hands correctly on patient's chest.				
8. Compress downward, keeping arms straight and moving sternum 1½ to 2 inches.				
9. After each 15 chest compressions at a rate of 80–100 compressions per minute, breathe twice (1 to 1.5 seconds per breath).				
Two-rescuer CPR				
1. Follow Checklist steps 1–6 for one-rescuer CPR.				
2. Have one rescuer breathe while the other compresses chest.				
3. Breather should give one breath between each five chest compressions at a rate of 80–100 compressions per minute.				
4. Rescuer 1 calls for change and completes ongoing series of five compressions.				
5. Rescuer 2 breathes after the fifth compression.				
6. Rescuer 1 moves up and checks carotid pulse for five seconds.				
7. Rescuer 2 gets in position to compress and waits.				

	Unsatisfactory	Needs More Practice	Satisfactory	Comments
8. If carotid pulse is absent, rescuer 1 says, "No pulse," and ventilates once. Rescuer 2 restarts compressions immediately after the breath.				

CPR for infants and small children

	Unsatisfactory	Needs More Practice	Satisfactory	Comments
1. Airway a. Avoid overextension of the head in infants.				
2. Breathing a. Cover both mouth and nose of infant with your mouth.				
b. Breathe once every three seconds for an infant. Breathe once every four seconds for a child.				
c. For infants, use only the amount of air needed to cause the chest to rise.				

3. Circulation
   a. Infants
     (1) Position 2 or 3 fingers one finger's width below an imaginary line between the nipples.				

(2) Compress at a rate of at least 100 times per minute.				
(3) Move sternum ½ to 1 inch.				
b. Small children (1) Use heel of one hand.				
(2) Position as for adult, using one hand only.				
(3) Compress at a rate of 80 to 100 times per minute.				
(4) Move sternum 1 to 1½ inches, depending on size of child.				

Foreign-body airway obstruction

	Unsatisfactory	Needs More Practice	Satisfactory	Comments
1. Recognition a. If victim has good air exchange, encourage attempts to cough and breathe spontaneously.				
b. If victim has poor air exchange, manage as complete airway obstruction.				
c. Ask victim, "Are you choking?" If answer is affirmative, intervene immediately.				

	Unsatisfactory	Needs More Practice	Satisfactory	Comments
2. Management				
a. Conscious victim				
(1) Stand behind victim and wrap your arms around waist.				
(2) Deliver six to ten abdominal thrusts.				
(3) Continue until foreign body expelled or victim loses consciousness.				
b. Unconscious victim				
(1) Position on back.				
(2) Kneel astride victim's thighs.				
(3) Deliver six to ten abdominal thrusts.				
(4) Use finger sweep to attempt to remove foreign body.				
(5) Continue management techniques.				

QUIZ

Short-Answer Questions

1. What is the *first* step you should take when you see a person collapse?

   _____

2. How do you position the victim's head if a cervical (neck) injury is suspected? _____

3. How can you quickly locate the carotid pulse? _____

4. How is the brachial pulse located in an infant? _____

5. Where should the chest of an adult be compressed? _____

6. How many chest compressions per minute should be performed in the following situations?

   a. One-rescuer CPR _____

   b. Two-rescuer CPR _____

   c. CPR for an infant _____

   d. CPR for a small child _____

7. What is the ratio of breaths to chest compressions in one-person CPR?

   _____

8. What is the ratio of breaths to chest compressions in two-person CPR?

   _____

9. What is the universal distress signal for choking? _____

10. Where is the Heimlich maneuver correctly delivered? _____

11. Under what circumstances is the finger sweep maneuver used? _____

abduction   The act of drawing away from the median line or center of the body.

accommodation   The adaptation or adjustment of the lens of the eye to permit the retina to focus on images or objects at different distances.

Ace bandage   A brand name that is commonly used as a synonym for a heavy, elastic roller bandage.

acetone   A colorless volatile solvent; commonly used as a synonym of ketone body; see *ketone body*.

acid   A substance that ionizes in solution to free the hydrogen ion; turns litmus paper pink.

acute care   Health care provided for a person who has a current problem that is expected to be resolved within a limited period of time.

adduction   The act of drawing toward the median line or center of the body.

ADLs   Activities of daily living.

adventitious sounds   Abnormal sounds, as in the lungs.

advocate   A person who speaks on behalf of another.

affected   Involved, such as the part of the body involved with pain or disease.

agility   The state of being nimble or of moving with ease.

AIDS (Acquired Immune Deficiency Syndrome)   A disease of the immune system that can be transmitted through the blood of infected persons.

airway   (1) The passageway by which air circulates in and out of the lungs. (2) A device used, generally when a patient is not fully alert, to prevent the tongue from slipping back and occluding the throat.

alkaline   Having characteristics of a base; neutralizes an acid.

alignment   Arrangement of position in a straight line. Used to refer to body parts being positioned so that they are in correct relationship, with no twisting.

alternating pressure mattress   A plastic mattress attached to a motor that alternately inflates and deflates the tubular sections of the mattress, so that the pressure against any one section of the patient's body changes constantly. It is placed over the regular mattress on the bed.

alveoli   Air sacs of the lungs, at the termination of a bronchiole.

A.M.A.   "Against medical advice."

ambulate   To walk from place to place.

amoeba   Any of various protozoans of the genus *Amoeba* and related genera, occurring in water, soil, and as internal animal parasites, characteristically having an indefinite, changeable form and moving by means of pseudopodia.

ampule   A small, sterile glass container that usually holds a parenteral medication.

anal sphincter   The two ringlike muscles that close the anal orifice. One is called the *external anal sphincter*; the other, the *internal anal sphincter*. The actions of both sphincters control the evacuation of feces.

anatomical position   A body position in which body parts are in correct relationship to one another and in which correct function is possible.

aneroid manometer   An air pressure gauge that indicates blood pressure by a pointer on a dial.

anorexia   Loss of appetite.

antecubital fossa   A depression in the contour of the inner aspect of the elbow; also called *antecubital space*.

antiemetic   An agent used to prevent vomiting.

antineoplastic   An agent which inhibits the growth of abnormal cell tissues or neoplasms.

antipyretic   A medication which lowers body temperature.

apex   The narrow or cone-shaped portion of an organ. In the heart, the point located in the area of the midclavicular line near the fifth left intercostal space; in the lung, the narrower, more pointed, upper end.

apical   Pertaining to the apex.

apical pulse   The heartbeat heard through a stethoscope held over the apex of the heart.

apnea   The absence of respiration.

arrhythmia   Any irregularity in the force or rhythm of the heartbeat.

ascending colon   The portion of the colon on the right side of the abdomen that extends from the junction of the small and large intestine to the first major flexion near the liver.

ascitic fluid   An abnormal accumulation of serous fluid in the abdominal cavity; also called *ascites*.

asepto syringe   A medical instrument that is used to aspirate and instill a fluid. The tip is graduated in size so that it fits into tubings of various sizes; the rounded bulb is used to create suction to fill the barrel and pressure to expel the fluid.

aspirate   To remove gases or fluids by suction.

aspiration   Removal of gases or fluids by suction.

assessment   The process of gathering data and analyzing it to identify patients' problems; the first step in the nursing process.

asymmetry   Different in form or function on opposite sides of the body.

auscultation   Listening with a stethoscope to the sounds produced by the body.

auscultatory gap   During the measurement of blood pressure, the disappearance of the usual sounds heard over the brachial artery when cuff pressure is high, and their reap-

pearance at a lower level as the pressure is reduced.

autopsy   An examination of the body after death to determine the cause of death and to further scientific investigation.

axilla   The armpit.

bacteria   Single-celled plantlike microorganisms that can cause disease.

bandage   A strip of fabric or other material that is used as a protective covering for a wound or to wrap a part of the body.

barrier   (1) Anything that acts to obstruct or prevent passage. (2) A boundary or limit.

base   The broad or wide end of an organ. In the heart, the area located at the second left and right intercostal spaces at the sternal borders; in the lungs, the wide lower end.

base of support   That which makes up the foundation of an object or person and supports the weight.

bath blanket   An absorbent, light-weight cotton blanket used for draping during the bath.

bedboard   A thin board, often hinged for easy use and storage, that is placed underneath a mattress when a firmer sleeping surface is wanted.

bedpan   A metal or plastic receptacle for the excreta of bedridden persons.

bell   On the stethoscope, the cone-shaped head that is most often used for listening to heart sounds.

bilirubin   A yellowish pigment that is derived from the normal or pathological destruction of hemoglobin.

binder   A type of bandage, worn snugly around the trunk or body part, that provides support.

bivalving   The process of using a cast saw to cut a cast in half lengthwise when the cast causes skin problems or undue pressure. The two parts of the cast are then held together by an elastic bandage when the patient is moving.

body language   Conveying thoughts or meanings through the posturing or positioning of the body.

body mechanics   The analysis of the action of forces on the body parts during activity.

body substances   A general term that includes saliva, sputum, vomitus, urine, feces, blood, genital secretions, wound drainage, pus, and the like.

bone marrow   Soft material that fills the cavities of bones.

bounding pulse   A body pulse that strikes the fingers with excessive strength.

brachial artery   An artery that supplies blood to the shoulder, arm, forearm, and hand.

bradycardia   An abnormally slow heartbeat, usually defined as below 60 beats per minute.

bronchi   The branches of the trachea that lead directly to the lungs.

bruit   An abnormal sound that results from circulatory turbulence.

burp   To cause to belch, especially a baby after feeding.

cane   A rehabilitative device used as an aid in walking.

canthus   The corner at either side of the eye, formed by the meeting of the upper and lower eyelids. *Inner canthus* is the corner next to the nose; *outer canthus* is the corner to the outside of the face.

cardiac arrest   The cessation of heart action.

cardiac sphincter   A circular muscle between the esophagus and the stomach that opens at the approach of food. The food then moves into the stomach as a result of peristalsis.

caries   The decay of bone or tooth.

cariogenic   That which contributes to the formation of dental caries.

carotid artery   Either of the two major arteries in the neck that carry blood to the head.

carotid pulse   The wave of blood felt as it passes through the carotid artery.

cast padding   A "waffled" padding, consisting of soft, thin cotton layers between two outer layers of closely woven cotton, used to provide cushioning between the patient's skin and a cast.

catheter   A slender flexible tube, of metal, rubber, or plastic, that is inserted into a body channel or cavity to distend or maintain an opening; often used to drain or to instill fluids.

caustic   Having the ability to burn, corrode, or dissolve by chemical action.

Celsius   A temperature scale, devised by Anders Celsius, that registers the freezing point of water at 0° C and the boiling point at 100° C, under normal atmospheric pressure; also called *centigrade*.

center of gravity   A point in an object or person at which gravitational pull functions as if the entire weight of the object or person were at that single point.

centigrade   See *Celsius*.

cerebrospinal fluid (CSF)   The serumlike fluid that bathes the lateral ventricles of the brain and the cavity of the spinal cord.

cerumen   A yellowish waxy secretion of the external ear; earwax.

cervical traction   Traction applied to the cervical spine by the use of weights attached by ropes to either skull tongs or a chin harness.

chart   The official, legal record of health care.

Cheyne-Stokes   A cyclic pattern of respirations that gradually increase in depth followed by respirations that gradually decrease in depth, with a short period of apnea between cycles.

circadian rhythm   The approximately twenty-four hour cyclic pattern of rest and activity in humans.

CircOlectric bed   A special bed designed to maintain immobilization and provide for turning. The patient is placed between two mattresses on frames and the turn is vertical.

circular bandage   A bandage that is wrapped in circular fashion around a body part.

circumcise   To surgically remove the prepuce (foreskin) of the penis.

695

circumduction   A circular movement of the eye or of a body part.

Clinitron bed   A special bed with a mattress filled with ceramic beads that move constantly when air is blown through them. This eliminates continuous pressure on any one point and minimizes shear while decreasing pain.

clove hitch   A knot that consists of two turns, with the second held under the first.

colic   Severe paroxysmal abdominal pain in infants, that usually results from the accumulation of gas in the alimentary canal.

comatose   Unconscious.

concurrent   Happening at the same time or place.

condiments   Seasonings for food.

confidentiality   The right to have personal matters kept private.

consensual   When both pupils move and focus together.

consent   The right of a competent adult to make his or her own decisions regarding health care.

constriction   A feeling of pressure or tightness.

contaminate   To introduce microorganisms to an object or person.

contracture   A shortening of a muscle that causes distortion or deformity of a joint.

contraindicate   To indicate the inadvisability of an action—for example, in treatment.

convergence   Two objects moving toward one another. When both pupils follow a point as it moves closer to the nose and both move medially (toward the nose).

coroner   A public officer whose primary function is to investigate by inquest any death thought to be of other than natural causes.

countertraction   Exerting pull in opposition to a traction system.

cradle   A frame shaped like an inverted baby's cradle that is used to protect the lower extremities from the pressure of bed linen or to supply electrical heat.

cradle cap   Yellowish oily scales on the scalp of an infant that result from the accumulation of sebaceous secretions.

cranium   The portion of the skull that encloses the brain.

critical care   Health care provided for acute, life-threatening illness.

crutch   A staff or support that is used by the disabled as an aid in walking; usually has a crosspiece that fits under the armpit and often is used in pairs.

crutch palsy   A weakness or paralysis of the hands caused by damage to the brachial nerve plexus through leaning on the crosspiece of crutches.

culture and sensitivity (C&S)   A laboratory test in which a swab or smear is placed in a nutrient medium to observe for growth of microorganisms. If microorganisms do grow, the culture is then tested with various antibiotics to determine whether the microorganisms are sensitive to the effects of these antibiotics. If the microorganism is destroyed, it is termed *sensitive* to the antibiotic. If the microorganism is not destroyed, it is termed *resistant*.

cure   A term used to describe the hardening stage of a cast.

cytology   A laboratory test in which cells are examined microscopically.

data   Information, especially material that is organized for analysis or used as a basis for decision making.

decubitus ulcer   An open sore or lesion of superficial tissue caused by pressure.

defecation   The act of expelling the contents of the bowel.

dependent edema   See *edema.*

descending colon   The portion of the colon on the left side of the abdomen that extends from the major flexion at the spleen to the point where the colon again flexes into the sigmoid portion.

dexterity   Skill in the use of the hands or body.

dialysis cannula   A surgically inserted tube

that provides access to the circulatory system for hemodialysis.

diaphoresis Perspiration, especially copious or medically induced perspiration.

diaphragm (1) A muscular membranous partition that separates the abdominal and thoracic cavities and that functions in respiration. (2) On a stethoscope, the flat, drumlike head that is used most often for listening to blood pressure, the lungs, and bowel sounds.

diarrhea Pathologically excessive evacuation of watery feces.

diastole The normal rhythmically recurring relaxation and dilatation of the heart cavities during which the cavities are filled with blood.

diastolic blood pressure The lowest pressure reached in the arteries during the heart's resting phase.

digestion The process by which food is broken down by enzymes into simpler substances which can be used by the body.

digital Pertaining to a finger. A digital examination is one carried out with a finger.

dignity Inherent worth.

dilation The condition of being enlarged or stretched.

displacement The act whereby a substance is replaced by another either in weight or in volume.

distal In anatomy, located far from the origin or line of attachment.

distention Bloat and turgidity from pressure within; usually refers to the stomach, bowel, or bladder.

diuresis The increased production and output of urine.

diuretic A drug that increases the production and output of urine.

dorsalis pedis artery An artery located on the top of the foot, used for palpating the pedal pulse.

dorsal recumbent position A position in which the person lies on back with knees bent.

dorsiflexion Bending or moving a part in a backward direction.

double T-binder A binder with two tails that is used to hold a dressing in place on the perineum of a male patient, so that the testicles are not restricted.

droplet nuclei Microscopic particles that, when surrounded by moisture, become airborne.

dullness In percussion, not sharp or intense.

dysphagia Difficulty in swallowing.

dyspnea Difficulty in breathing.

edema An excessive accumulation of serous fluid in the tissues. *Dependent edema* is fluid that has accumulated in the lower areas of the body due to gravity, *periorbital edema* is fluid that has accumulated in the soft tissue around the eyes, and *pretibial edema* is fluid that has accumulated over the tibia.

"egg crate" mattress A foam mattress which has rounded projections and indentations resembling an egg crate. Used to diminish pressure on tissues.

electroencephalogram A record of brain waves measured on the electroencephalograph.

electrolyte A substance that dissociates into ions in solution; in the body, electrolytes are critically important chemicals.

epigastrium The upper middle region of the abdomen.

ethical Pertaining to or dealing with principles of right and wrong.

ethnic Characteristic of a religious, racial, national, or cultural group.

evaluation The process of determining the outcomes of a course of action.

eversion Turned in an outward direction.

excoriate To chafe or wear off the skin.

excretion The process of eliminating waste matter, such as feces, urine, or sweat.

expectorate To eject from the mouth; spit.

extension The act of straightening or extending a limb.

external disaster   A disaster occurring in the community which may affect the medical facility.

external rotation   Moving a body part outward on an axis.

exudate   Fluid drainage from cells.

Fahrenheit   A temperature scale that registers the freezing point of water at 32° F and the boiling point at 212° F, under normal atmospheric pressure.

fan-fold   To fold or gather in accordion fashion; for example, the top linen of a bed toward the bottom or one side.

febrile   Having an elevated body temperature.

feces   Waste excreted from the bowels.

fetal   Pertaining to the unborn.

femoral artery   Either of the two large arteries that carry blood to the lower abdomen, the pelvis, and the lower extremities.

fever   Abnormally high body temperature.

fiberglass cast   A "light" cast, made of fiberglass, that is impermeable to water.

figure-8 bandage   A bandage that is wrapped around a body part in a figure-8 configuration.

flaccid   Lacking firmness; soft and limp; flabby.

flatness   A short, high-pitched sound without resonance or vibration.

flatus   Gas generated in the stomach or intestines and expelled through the anus.

flexion   Bending of a joint.

flow sheet   A schematic representation of a sequence of operations or events.

fontanel   Any of the soft membranous intervals between the incompletely ossified cranial bones of fetuses and infants.

footboard   A board or small raised platform against which the feet are supported or rested.

footdrop   The abnormal permanent extension of the foot that results from paralysis or injury to the flexor muscles.

footrest   A canvas sling or padded bar at the distal end of a leg cast used to support the foot.

forensic medicine   The legal aspects of medical practice.

foreskin   The loose fold of skin that covers the glans of the penis; the prepuce.

Foster bed   A special frame used to maintain immobilization and provide for turning. The patient is placed between two mattresses on frames and the turn is lateral.

Fowler's position   A position in which the patient is in bed on his or her back with the head elevated approximately 60° (also called *mid-Fowler's position*). Traditionally, knees were also elevated, but this is seldom done today. The degree of elevation of the head can vary: in *semi-Fowler's position (low-Fowler's position)* the head is at a 30° angle from the horizontal; in *high-Fowler's position*, the head is as close to 90° as possible.

fracture pan   A container of metal or plastic with a lower edge, or lip, than a conventional bedpan; used for purposes of excretion by bedridden patients, often with fractured hips or in casts.

friction   The rubbing of one object or surface against another.

funeral director   A licensed person who is responsible for a body from the time of death until ultimate disposition; *mortician*.

gait   A way of moving on foot; a particular fashion of walking, running, or the like.

gastric gavage   Introducing a feeding by tube into the stomach.

gastrocolic reflex   The emptying of the colon resulting from the filling of the stomach.

gastrostomy   A surgical opening into the stomach; usually for feeding by tube.

genital   Pertaining to the reproductive organs.

genital area   The body area that contains the reproductive organs.

glucose   A dextrose sugar.

gooseneck lamp   An adjustable lamp with a slender flexible shaft.

graphic   Represented by a graph; often used to refer to the record of temperature, pulse, and respiration.

gravida   A pregnant woman; used with numerals to designate the number of pregnancies a woman has had regardless of outcome.

gravity   The force exerted by the earth on any object, tending to pull the object toward the center of the earth.

"green" cast   A cast that is still damp or not thoroughly hardened.

guaiac   A natural resin that is used as a reagent to test for blood in specimens.

hairline fracture   A simple fracture of a bone that is not displaced. Shows on x-rays as a "hairline" image.

Harris flush   A term used to refer to a return-flow enema.

health care system   All those individuals, organizations, and agencies which provide health services and/or health financing considered as a whole.

health status   A person's level of ability in meeting his or her own needs.

Heimlich maneuver   An emergency procedure (also called subdiaphragmatic abdominal thrusts) devised for relieving foreign body airway obstruction.

Hematest   A brand name for a product that is used to test for the presence of blood in fecal specimens; commonly used to refer to the test itself.

Homan's sign   A pain in the dorsal calf when the foot is forcibly flexed that can indicate thrombophlebitis.

horizontal   Parallel to or in the plane of the horizon.

humerus   The long bone of the upper part of the arm, extending from the shoulder to the elbow.

hydraulic   Moved or operated by a fluid, especially water under pressure.

hydrometer   An instrument that is used to determine specific gravity.

hyperalimentation   The intravenous introduction of nutrients into a large vein, usually the subclavian.

hyperextension   Extension of the joint beyond the straight position.

hypertonic   Having a higher osmotic pressure than body fluid.

hypostatic pneumonia   Pneumonia due to lack of movement.

hypotonic   Having a lower osmotic pressure than body fluid.

hypovolemic shock   A state of shock that is caused by an abnormally low volume of body plasma.

iliac crest   The highest portion of the broad rim of the hipbone.

immunosuppression   The suppression of the body's natural immune system by drugs or disease.

impaction   Compressed material in a confined space; for example, hardened feces in the bowel.

implementation   The carrying out of a plan of action.

incubate   To warm (eggs), as by bodily heat, so as to promote embryonic development and the hatching of young; to brood.

inflammation   Localized heat, redness, swelling, and pain as a result of irritation, injury, or infection.

infused   Put into or introduced.

infusion   The introduction of a solution into a vessel; commonly, the introduction of a solution into a vein.

ingested   See *ingestion*.

ingestion   The taking in of food by swallowing.

inspection   A careful, critical visual examination.

instillation   The process of pouring in drop by drop; commonly used to indicate a slow process of introducing fluid.

integument   Skin.

interdigital   Between the fingers (digits).

intermittent   Stopping and starting at intervals.

internal disaster   A disaster occurring within the medical facility.

internal girdle   Those muscles of the abdomen, back, and hips that provide support to the abdominal contents and the pelvis.

internal rotation   Moving a body part inward on an axis.

intravenous infusion   The introduction of a solution into a vein.

invasive   Any procedure that involves the insertion or placement of a device through the skin or into a body orifice or cavity.

inversion   Turning in an inward direction.

isometric exercises   Contracting and relaxing the muscles voluntarily without obvious movement of the part.

isolation   To set apart from the environment so that organisms cannot be readily transferred from one person to another.

isotope   A radioactive substance used for diagnosis and treatment.

ketone body   A substance synthesized by the liver as a step in the combustion of fats. May be present in increased amounts in abnormal situations, such as uncontrolled diabetes mellitus.

Kling bandage   A brand name that is commonly used as a synonym for a loosely knit, lightweight, stretch roller bandage.

Korotkoff sounds   The characteristic sounds, produced by the pressure of blood entering the artery during systole, that are heard on auscultation of an artery after it has been occluded.

Kussmaul's respirations   Deep rapid respirations, often seen in states of acidosis or renal failure.

labia   The lips or folds of tissue that surround the female perineum.

lactase   An enzyme secreted by the intestine which is necessary for the digestion of lactose (sugar found in milk).

legibility   Able to be read or deciphered.

lesion   A wound or injury in which tissue is damaged.

Levin tube   A slender rubber or plastic tube that is usually used for decompression of the stomach.

lithotomy position   A position in which a person lies on back with legs flexed and spread apart.

litmus paper   White paper that is impregnated with litmus and is used as an acid-base indicator.

liver biopsy   The excision of microscopic liver tissue for examination.

logrolling   Turning a patient so that the entire body turns at one time with no twisting.

lumbar puncture (LP)   The insertion of a needle into the spinal canal for purposes of withdrawing spinal fluid or instilling contrast-dye materials; also called a *spinal tap*.

lumbrosacral   Pertaining to the lumbar and sacral regions of the spinal column.

lumen   The inner, open space of a needle, tube, or vessel.

macerate   To soften by prolonged contact with moisture.

macular   A skin rash consisting of separate, circular flat reddened spots.

malleable   Capable of being shaped or formed.

manometer   An instrument that measures the pressure of liquids and gases.

medical asepsis   The technique designed to prevent the spread of microorganisms from one person (or area) to another.

medical examiner   An appointed public official, usually a forensic pathologist, whose function it is to investigate deaths that result from traumatic causes (homicide, suicide, accident) and sudden natural deaths in the absence of medical attention.

meniscus   The curved upper surface of a liquid column.

metabolism   The complex of physical and chemical processes concerned with the disposition of the nutrients absorbed into the blood following digestion.

microorganism An animal or plant of microscopic size, especially a bacterium or protozoa.

midclavicular line An imaginary line running vertically through the midway point of the clavicle or collarbone.

military (24-hour) clock A system for noting time in which time is recorded as part of a 24-hour cycle, beginning at midnight. Hours before 10:00 a.m. are noted with a zero before the hour; minutes after the hour are noted immediately after the numbers for the hour. For example, fifteen minutes after 1:00 a.m. would be recorded as 0115; the hours after noon are numbered 13, 14, and so on, so 15 minutes after 1:00 p.m. would be 1315.

minibottle A small container for intravenous infusion solutions.

mitered corner A method of folding a sheet or blanket to achieve a smooth squared covering over the corner of the mattress.

morgue A place in a health care facility where the bodies of deceased patients are temporarily detained pending release to a mortician, coroner (medical examiner), or other authorized person.

mortician A funeral director and embalmer who is responsible for the care and disposition of a deceased person.

nares The openings in the nasal cavities; the nostrils.

narrative charting The traditional style of recording data on a patient's chart in a time-sequenced story-like form.

nasal mucosa The mucous membrane lining of the nose.

nasal speculum An instrument that is used to dilate the nostrils for purposes of inspecting or treating the nasal passages.

nasogastric tube A long, slender rubber or plastic tube that is introduced through the nose and esophagus into the stomach, for purposes of feeding or aspiration.

net binder A tube made of netlike material that is used to secure dressings to the body.

nosocomial An infection considered to have been hospital-acquired.

NPO Nothing by mouth.

nursing diagnosis The intellectual processes of sorting and classifying data collected, recognizing patterns and discrepancies, comparing these with norms, and identifying patient responses to health problems that are amenable to nursing intervention.

nursing history The initial data gathered through interview by the nurse.

nursing process A thoughtful, deliberate use of a problem-solving approach to nursing. Also the end statement of this process, which includes a statement of the problem and its etiology.

objective Based on observable phenomena.

occiput The posterior, inferior portion of the cranium.

occult Hidden.

ombudsman An official designated to act as an advocate for a member of the public in disputes with a health care agency.

ophthalmoscope An instrument that consists of a light and a disc with an opening through which the interior of the eye is examined.

opposition Positioned opposite one another; for example, the thumb to the fingers.

organ donor A deceased person who donates organs for transplantation through a personal pre-death bequest or through the bequest of the family after death.

organization The quality of order, structure, or system.

orthopnea A state in which a person has difficulty breathing in the recumbent position and is relieved by sitting upright or standing.

orthopneic Pertaining to difficulty breathing in the recumbent position. Also pertaining to a position in which the patient's head and arms rest on a table over the bed to relieve orthopnea.

osmolarity The number of osmotically active particles in a unit of fluid.

otoscope An instrument, for inspecting the ears, consisting of a light and a cone.

ova The female reproductive cells of animals; eggs. Microscopic examination of stool is often done to identify the ova of intestinal parasites.

oxygenation   Treating, combining, or infusing with oxygen.

palpation   Examining or exploring by touch.

para   Used with numerals to designate the number of pregnancies a woman has had in which a viable fetus (over 20 weeks gestation or 500 grams weight) is produced.

paracentesis   The insertion of a trocar into the abdominal cavity for the removal of excess fluid.

paralysis   Loss or impairment of the ability to move or have sensation in a bodily part as a result of injury to or disease of its nerve supply.

parasite   Any organism that grows, feeds, and is sheltered on or in a host organism while contributing nothing to the host's survival.

parenteral fluid   Fluid given directly into tissues or blood vessels.

patellar tendon   A continuation of the quadriceps tendon that leads from the patella to the tibia.

patent   Open.

pathogenic organism   A microorganism that causes disease.

pavilion   Related buildings forming a complex.

pectoralis muscles   Four muscles of the chest.

pedal pulse   A pulse wave that can be felt over the arteries of the feet.

penis   The male organ of copulation and urinary excretion.

percussion   (1) A process of striking a finger held against the body surface with a fingertip of the opposite hand and listening to the resulting sound as part of assessment. (2) The striking of a hand on the chest wall to produce a vibration or shock that loosens secretions retained in the lungs.

perineum   The portion of the body in the pelvic area that is occupied by urogenital passages and the rectum.

periorbital edema   Edema around the eyes or the orbits.

periphery   The outermost part or region.

peristalsis   Wavelike muscular contractions that propel contained matter along the alimentary canal.

petaling   Forming adhesive or moleskin "petals" by cutting strips into pointed or rounded ends and tucking around the rough edges of a cast in such a way that the skin is protected.

pH   A measure of the acidity or alkalinity of a solution; 7.0 is neutral, and numbers below that indicate an acid solution and numbers above it indicate an alkaline solution, in a range of 1 to 14.

piggyback   An intravenous infusion setup in which a second container is attached to the tubing of the primary container through a short tubing.

pinwheel   A wheel-like instrument with sharp points that is used to test peripheral sensation of the body.

planning   The second step in the nursing process, in which information is reviewed and synthesized in order to form goals and a plan of action.

plantar flexion   Bending the foot so that the toes point downward.

plaster of Paris cast   A cast made of calcium sulfate, which, when combined with water, forms gypsum producing a light but rigid and durable structure.

popliteal artery   The major artery that extends from the femoral artery down behind the knee.

popliteal space   The hollow area behind the knee joint.

postmortem examination   See *autopsy*.

postural hypotension   A sudden drop in blood pressure that is caused by a change in position, from lying to sitting or standing; may cause dizziness, fainting, and falling; also called *orthostatic hypotension*.

preformed water   The water content of ingested foods.

pretibial edema   Serous fluid over the tibia.

prism glasses   Glasses that direct the vision upward and then horizontally so that a patient in the supine position can make use of television and books.

privacy   The right to have matters of a personal nature not shared with anyone who does not have a need to know them.

problem-oriented medical record (POR or POMR)   A system of keeping medical records that is organized according to patients' problems.

proctoscope   An instrument that dilates the anus to allow inspection or treatment of the lower intestine.

profuse   Plentiful, overflowing, copious.

pronation   Turning the palm or inner surface of the hand or forearm downward.

protein   An organic compound that contains amino acids as its basic structural unit.

proximal   Near the center part of the body or a point of attachment, or origin.

ptosis   Paralytic drooping of the upper eyelid caused by nerve failure.

pulley   A grooved wheel that allows free movement of a rope.

pulmonary embolus   Obstruction of the pulmonary artery or one of its branches by an embolus.

pulse deficit   The difference in rate between apical and radial pulses.

pulse pressure   The difference between systolic and diastolic blood pressure readings.

pureed   Strained, as in food.

pyrexia   Fever.

quad cane   A cane with a 4-legged base for stability.

quadriplegia   Paralysis of all four extremities.

radial artery   The artery that descends from the brachial artery along the radius of the arm.

radial deviation   Bending the hand on the wrist in the direction of the thumb (toward the radius).

radiolucent   A surface through which x-rays can be taken.

rales   Abnormal or pathological respiratory sounds heard on auscultation.

reagent   A substance that is used in a chemical reaction to detect, measure, examine, or produce other substances.

rebound tenderness   The pain or discomfort that is experienced when pressure is quickly withdrawn from an area.

recurrent bandage   A bandage that is wrapped in such a way that it recurs, or folds over, on itself.

referral   A specific plan for directing a patient or client to other health care resources.

reflex contraction   An involuntary response of muscle contraction.

reflex hammer   A small rubber-headed hammer that is used to test body reflexes; also called a *percussion hammer.*

regurgitate   To vomit.

remittent   Increasing and decreasing in measurement.

renal calculi   Kidney stones.

repose   A body position that appears peaceful.

reservoir   A container used to hold a fluid for continuous administration, such as in tube feeding.

resonance   In percussion, a vibrating sound that is produced in the normal chest.

respiratory arrest   The sudden cessation of breathing.

respite   An interval of rest or relief.

resuscitate   To revive or restore to life.

retraction   An abnormal pulling in of soft tissue of the chest on inspiration; commonly seen in the supraclavicular, intercostal, and substernal areas.

reverse spiral   A bandage that is applied, usually on a limb, in a circular fashion with a reverse fold.

rhonchi   Coarse rattling sounds that are produced by secretions in the bronchial tubes; a type of rale.

rhythm   A variation of energy occurring in a regular pattern.

rigor mortis   Muscle stiffening after death.

roller bandage   Bandaging material that has been rolled to provide for easier application; commonly used to refer to rolls of gauze.

rotation   A circular movement around a fixed axis.

Roto-Rest bed   An electrically operated special bed that turns side to side continuously. Cervical, thoracic, and rectal areas can be cared for through posterior hatches.

sanction   Authoritative permission or approval.

scalpel   A sharp surgical knife.

scultetus binder   A heavy fabric binder that is held to the body by the interwrapping of cloth tails in an oblique fashion across the abdomen.

self-care   The ability to manage one's own life in such a way as to meet one's own needs.

self-determination   See *consent.*

semi-Fowler's position   See *Fowler's position.*

shock   A generally temporary state of massive physiological reaction to bodily trauma, usually characterized by marked loss of blood pressure and the depression of vital processes.

sigmoid flexure   The distal portion of the colon, which appears as an S-shaped curve preceding the rectum.

sigmoidoscope   A tubular instrument with a light that is used to dilate the anus for inspection and treatment of the sigmoid.

Sims's position   A side-lying position with the top leg flexed forward.

skull tongs   Device inserted into each side of patient's cranium as an attachment for the application of traction.

sling   A device that suspends and supports a body part.

smegma   A thick whitish substance, composed of epithelial cells and mucus, which is found around external genitalia.

Snellen chart   A chart printed with black letters in gradually decreasing sizes, used in testing vision.

sordes   Accumulation of dried secretions and bacteria in the mouth caused by not eating, mouth-breathing, and inadequate oral hygiene.

specific gravity   A measurement of the concentration of urine. Overhydration leads to a low specific-gravity figure; dehydration results in a high figure.

sphincter   A circular muscle that controls an internal or external orifice.

sphygmomanometer   An instrument that measures blood pressure in the arteries.

spiral bandage   A bandage that is applied, usually on a limb, in a circular ascending fashion.

spreader bar   A bar that extends from one side of the traction frame surrounding an extremity to the opposite side.

stab wound   A direct scalpel puncture into skin or membrane.

stereotype   A presumed form or pattern that is attributed to a group and generalized to an individual.

sternum   A long flat bone that forms the midventral support of most of the ribs; the breastbone.

stertorous   Respirations having a heavy snoring sound.

stethoscope   An instrument that is used for listening to sounds produced in the body; also see *bell* and *diaphragm.*

stockinette   A soft, stretchy, ribbed material that comes in a tube shape of different circumferences. When pulled over a body part, it provides a smooth surface and protection from the inner surface of a cast.

stopcock   A valve that regulates a flow of liquid through a tube.

straight abdominal binder   A large cloth that

is placed snugly around the lower part of the trunk to give support or to secure a dressing.

Stryker turning frame   A special frame used to maintain immobilization and provide for turning. The patient is placed between two mattresses on frames and the turn is lateral.

stylet   A slender pointed instrument; a surgical probe.

subjective   Personal; in assessment, refers to information from the patient's viewpoint.

subungual   Beneath the fingernails.

supine   Position in which the person is lying flat on the back.

supination   Turning or placing the hand and forearm so that the palm is upward.

suppuration   The formation or discharge of pus.

sutures   The thread, gut, or wire used to stitch tissues.

symmetry   The equal configuration of opposite sides.

symphysis pubis   The area at the front center of the pelvis, where the pubic bones from either side fuse into one bone.

systole   The rhythmic contraction of the heart, especially of the ventricles, by which blood is driven through the aorta and pulmonary artery after each dilation, or diastole.

systolic blood pressure   The highest pressure reached in the arteries, created by the contraction of the ventricles of the heart.

tachycardia   An abnormally rapid heartbeat, usually defined as above 100 beats per minute, in the adult.

T-binder   A binder with a single tail that is used to hold a dressing in place on the perineum of a female patient.

technical proficiency   Skill in the performance of tasks.

temporal artery   One of the two three-branched arteries that lie at the temple of the head.

tepid   Lukewarm.

thoracentesis   The insertion of a trocar into the pleural space of the chest for the removal of abnormal fluid.

thready pulse   A weak, faint pulse.

thrombophlebitis   Inflammation of the veins.

toe pleat   A method of folding top bed linen to provide extra room for the feet.

tolerance   In activity, the capacity to endure.

torsion   The act or condition of being twisted or turned; the stress caused when one end of an object is twisted in one direction and the other end is held motionless or twisted in the opposite direction.

torso   The trunk of the human body.

trachea   A thin-walled tube of cartilaginous and membranous tissue that descends from the larynx to the bronchi, carrying air to the lungs.

tracheostomy   A surgically devised opening into the trachea from the surface of the neck.

traction   Applying a pulling force to bones. Usually used to reduce bone fractures.

transverse colon   The portion of the colon across the top of the abdomen from the hepatic flexure to the splenic flexure.

trapeze   A short, horizontal bar suspended from a frame over the top of a bed. It is used by the patient to facilitate moving in bed and transfer.

tremor   An involuntary trembling motion of the body.

Trendelenburg position   A position in which the head is lower than the feet with the body on an inclined plane.

triage   A process for assessing the level of care needed for a group of patients, often in an emergency situation.

trocar   A sharp-pointed surgical instrument that is used with a cannula to puncture a body cavity for fluid aspiration.

trochanter   The bony processes below the head of the femur; often used to refer to the greater trochanter, which is on the lateral aspect of the femur.

tuning fork   A small two-pronged instrument that, when struck, produces a sound of fixed pitch; used to test auditory acuity.

turgor   Normal tissue fullness in relationship to superficial body fluids.

twist support   A strong plaster bar between two casted extremities or between a casted extremity and the body cast, formed by twisting a wetted plaster roll during the application of a cast.

tympany   In percussion, a low-pitched, drum-like sound.

ulnar deviation   Bending the hand on the wrist in the direction of the fifth, or small finger.

umbilicus   The navel.

urethral meatus   The opening of the urethra onto the surface of the body through which urine is passed.

urinal   A receptacle for urine that is used by bedridden patients.

urinalysis   The chemical analysis of urine, which commonly includes color, clarity, pH, specific gravity, and checks for the presence of glucose, RBCs, casts, and WBCs.

urination   The act of excreting urine.

urine refractometer   A microscopelike instrument that refracts a beam of light through a drop of urine to give a reading of glucose content. Often used by nurses on the nursing unit.

urinometer   An instrument that is used to determine the specific gravity of urine.

uvula   The small, conical fleshy mass of tissue that is suspended from the center of the soft palate above the back of the tongue.

vaginal speculum   An instrument that is used to dilate the vagina for purposes of inspecting or treating the vaginal passages or to obtain a specimen for a culture or smear.

venous   Of or pertaining to a vein or veins.

venous pressure   The pressure of blood in the veins; often measured in the superior vena cava. This measurement, called *central venous pressure* (CVP) is normally between 4 and 10 cm water.

venous thrombosis   Formation of a blood clot inside of a vein.

vesicant   Any agent which can cause blistering or necrosis, the sloughing of tissue.

void   The emptying of urine from the bladder through the urethra; to urinate.

vulva   The external female genitalia, including the labia majora, the labia minora, the clitoris, and the vestibule of the vagina.

walker   A rehabilitative device that is used by a disabled person for support while standing or walking.

walking heel   A metal or plastic implant embedded in the heel of a plaster or fiberglass leg cast to facilitate walking.

water balance   A state of the body in which the fluid intake is in equilibrium with the fluid output.

water bed   A special water-filled mattress used to distribute pressure evenly over the body.

weight-bearing   The side on which the weight of the body can be placed while standing; *partial weight-bearing* indicates that an individual cannot stand solely on the affected limb and must have other means of support also.

weights   Substances having bulk or mass, able to produce gravitational pull.

wheezes   Hoarse whistling sounds, produced by breathing, that are considered abnormal.

"whiplash"   Spasms, fracture, or other injury of the neck or cervical spine due to a sudden whiplike motion of the body.

windowing   The procedure of cutting an opening in a cast to allow for observation, care of the skin underneath, and relief of pressure.

xiphoid process   The lower tip of the sternum.

ANSWERS TO QUIZZES

Module 1 / An Approach to Nursing Skills

1. a. Right to self determination/consent
   b. Right to information upon which to base decisions
   c. Right to privacy/confidentiality
   d. Right to safe care
   e. Right to personal dignity
   f. Right to individualized care
   g. Right to assistance toward independence
   h. Right to complain and obtain changes in care
2. Any one of the following: calling patient by preferred name; helping person to be physically clean and attractive; always pulling drapes and closing doors for privacy
3. a. Assessment
      (1) Data Gathering
      (2) Nursing Diagnosis
   b. Planning
   c. Implementation
   d. Evaluation
4. Gathering data, analyzing data, and identifying the problems present
5. a. Correct technique
   b. Organization
   c. Dexterity
   d. Speed
6. Past practice and sound deductive reasoning from known facts
7. To identify the outcomes of nursing action

Module 2 / Medical Asepsis

1. d
2. d
3. d
4. b
5. a. Microorganisms move through space on air currents.
   b. Microorganisms are transferred from one surface to another whenever objects touch.
   c. Microorganisms are transferred by gravity whenever one item is held above another.
   d. Microorganisms move slowly on dry surfaces but very quickly through moisture.

Module 3 / Safety

1. a. The facility is complex and unfamiliar.
   b. Space is often limited.
   c. A variety of equipment is used.
2. a. Good body mechanics
   b. Walking, not running
   c. Keeping to the right in hallways
   d. Turning corners and opening doors carefully
   e. Using stretchers properly
   f. Using brakes on beds, wheelchairs, and stretchers
   g. Using elevators correctly
3. Smooth, in good repair, and free of spills and foreign materials
4. Government codes must be observed and all electrical cords and plugs must be in good repair.
5. Most needle sticks occur when nurses attempt to recap needles. All needles, syringes, and other sharp objects should ideally be disposed of in the room receptacle designed for this purpose.
6. Side rails or restraints used cautiously; bed in low position; patient positioned so extremities are free; protection from sharp objects, with special attention to eyes and air passages
7. Prevention of aspiration of materials or fumes
8. Cigarettes not for sale in facilities; designated smoking areas; placing patients in rooms according to smoking habits
9. a. Be familiar with code procedure.
   b. Remove patients from immediate vicinity of fire.
   c. Initiate code.
   d. Return to unit if you did not call code.
   e. Never use elevators.

    f. Return patients to rooms and close doors.

    g. Calm patients.

    h. Follow directions of person in charge.

    i. Stand in hallway.

    j. Evacuate according to procedure if necessary.

    k. Remain calm.

    l. Wait for directions at all clear signal.

10. To be knowledgeable of plans, to report as designated in plan, to perform skills as predetermined by plans

11. a. To document an event

    b. To serve as a record for insurance and legal purposes

    c. To identify need to modify or rectify a procedure or policy

Module 4 / Basic Body Mechanics

1. T

2. T

3. F

4. F

5. T

6. F

7. These muscles may become tired or injury to the back may occur.

8. It is easier to move an object on a level surface than to move it up a slanted surface against the force of gravity.

9. Enlarging the base of support in the direction of the force to be applied increases the amount of force that can be applied.

10. It takes less energy to hold an object close to the body than at a distance from the body; it is also easier to move an object that is close.

Module 5 / Assessment

1. a. Oxygenation

    b. Respiratory

2. a. Regulation and sensation/Comfort

    b. Neural

3. a. Oxygenation and possibly Rest and Sleep

    b. Respiratory and possibly Neural

4. a

5. c

6. b

7. e

8. S

9. O

10. S

11. O

12. O

Module 6 / Documentation

1. b

2. c

3. a

4. a. Source-oriented method

    b. Problem-oriented record

5. a. Narrative

    b. SOAP format

6. So that others may check the original data and make their own inferences

7. Upset

8. Error 175 ml   SJ

    or

    wrong amount   SJ
    clear yellow urine 175 ml

9. The hospital

10. Patients have a right to the information contained in the record. Usually there is a procedure to follow in the facility.

Module 7 / Bedmaking

1. clean and wrinkle-free; provides comfort

2. conserves energy

3. the post-op bed is in high position for easy transfer and the linen is fan-folded so the patient can be easily covered to prevent chilling

4. use siderails appropriately to protect the patient from falling

5. decreases the effectiveness of the mattress

6. b

7. d

8. a

9. c

10. b

11. 6, 8, 5, 2, 1, 4, 7, 3

708

Module 8 / Moving the Patient in Bed and Positioning

1. So as not to be working against the gravitational pull
2. **a.** Promotes physical progress
   b. Adds to patient's self-esteem
3. dislocation of the shoulder
4. The patient's trunk
5. **a.** For patients' comfort and safety
   b. To make sure there is no pressure on parts
6. **a.** To prevent pressure sores
   b. To prevent joint contractures
   c. To improve muscle tone and circulation
7. trochanter or ankle roll
8. flexed
9. **a.** Feet in space between mattress and footboard
   b. Roll placed under ankles
10. b
11. b

Module 9 / Feeding Adult Patients

1. **a.** Environment
   b. Emotions
   c. Physical disability
   d. Dentures
2. c
3. b
4. a
5. a
6. c
7. F
8. F
9. T
10. F

Module 10 / Assisting with Elimination and Perineal Care

1. **a.** Medical asepsis principles
   b. Psychological comfort principles
   c. Principles related to normal bowel function
2. **a.** Bedpan
   b. Urinal
   c. Fracture pan

   d. Emesis basin
3. **a.** Pad the pan.
   b. Warm it.
4. **a.** Lifting the buttocks
   b. Rolling onto the pan
5. Any five of the following: amount; color; consistency; odor; blood; mucus; foreign matter
6. **a.** Postpartum patients
   b. Surgical patients
   c. Patients with catheters in place
7. Refer to Performance Checklist.
8. For aesthetic purposes
9. On the nursing care plan
10. To prevent contamination of the urinary meatus with microbes from the rectal area

Module 11 / Hygiene

1. c
2. b
3. d
4. Sterile saline or special soaking solution
5. **a.** Place a drop of saline or lens solution in the eye.
   b. Place one finger on the upper lid and one on the lower lid.
   c. Raise the upper lid and gently push in on the lower lid at the lower margin of the lens to pop it out.
6. To avoid scratching the lenses
7. Remove the battery and place in a safe, dry place
8. F
9. F
10. T
11. F
12. T
13. F
14. T
15. T
16. F

Module 12 / Basic Infant Care

1. The thickest part is placed where the greatest absorbency is needed, and the infant has free movement of legs.

2. Urine or feces on the skin contributes to a variety of skin problems.
3. Close them and put them out of reach of the infant.
4. Diaper rash is a reddened rash throughout the diaper area. Scald is a solid red, burn-type area.
5. Place a small amount in your hand and smooth it over the infant's skin rather than "sprinkling" it on, because it acts as an irritant to the respiratory tract.
6. Shake some on the inner aspect of your wrist.
7. Hold the bottle so that the nipple is filled with fluid, not air.
8. Because once infants have tasted the naturally sweet fruit, they will prefer to continue eating it and will not want to finish the plain food
9. It will not slip and become tighter, cutting off circulation.
10. Any three of the following: avoid chilling; keep one hand on the infant; check water for correct temperature; place basin on a safe surface; put side rail or crib net in place when finished

Module 13 / Inspection, Palpation, Auscultation, and Percussion

1. Any five of the following: color, odor, size, shape, symmetry, movement
2. a. Size
   b. Shape
   c. Equality of pupils
3. In a position above 45 degrees
4. 4 and 10 centimeters
5. a. What is being done
   b. Why it is being done
   c. What the patient can do to make it easier for himself or herself and the nurse
6. Around the eyes
7. Because the breasts may be particularly sensitive at the time of menstruation
8. Because palpation and percussion can change the bowel sounds that might be heard
9. Fifth intercostal space near the nipple line (the apex)

10. Any one of the following: bronchial obstruction; chronic lung disease; shallow breathing

Module 14 / Admission, Transfer, and Discharge

1. b
2. a
3. c
4. c
5. d
6. d
7. d
8. d
9. b
10. a discharge planner
11. elevated temperature

Module 15 / Intake and Output

1. a
2. c
3. c
4. b
5. a
6. c
7. b
8. a
9. b
10. b
11. a
12. d

Module 16 / Temperature, Pulse, and Respiration

1. 37° C; 98.6° F
2. Any four of the following: time of day; age; presence of infection; environment; exercise; emotions; metabolism
3. prevent injury to the mucosa
4. 8 minutes; 3 minutes; 9 minutes; only seconds
5. 3, 2, 1
6. 50, 100
7. Any four of the following: exercise;

application of heat or cold; medications; emotions; blood loss

8. a. Radial
b. Carotid
c. Temporal
9. 16; 20
10. Any four of those listed in answer 7, as well as disorders of the respiratory tract

Module 17 / Blood Pressure

1. c
2. c
3. b
4. d
5. a
6. b
7. 140 / 80 / 70
8. Because low-pitched sounds are more easily heard with the bell head than with the diaphragm
9. a. The disappearance of the usual sounds heard over the brachial artery when cuff pressure is high and their reappearance at a lower level when the cuff pressure is reduced
b. By pumping the hand bulb on the blood pressure cuff to a point 30 mm of mercury beyond the point at which you last felt a pulse

Module 18 / Collecting Specimens

1. a. Equipment with which to obtain the specimen
b. Equipment in which to place the specimen
c. Equipment with which to observe the patient's response
2. a. Privacy
b. Lighting
c. Positioning
d. Draping
3. a. Right amount
b. Right container
c. Right time
d. Right patient
4. Any five of the following: patient's name;

identification number; age; room number; physician's name; date
5. 7/15/88 Coughed up approximately 15 ml in thick, blood-tinged sputum, which was sent to lab for C&S. c/o fatigue after coughing. Resting in bed.
S. Penobscot, NS
6. F
7. T
8. F
9. T
10. F

Module 19 / Assisting with Examinations and Procedures

1. a. Meeting the physical and psychological needs of the patient
b. Gathering necessary equipment and assisting the physician
2. Sitting on the edge of the bed, facing the physician
3. eyes
4. ears
5. supine
6. dyspnea, pallor, sudden pain, cough, or diaphoresis
7. reduce bleeding at the site
8. c
9. c
10. a

Module 20 / Performing Common Laboratory Tests

1. Urinometer
2. A measurement of the concentration of a liquid
3. The measurement of hydrogen ions (acidity)
4. Far fewer drugs interfere with testing
5. Percentages of glucose
6. Testape
7. If the patient has eaten red meat within the past three days
8. Because the material may dry out or change in character if left standing
9. b
10. d

11. b
12. c

Module 21 / Applying Restraints

1. a. To protect the patient
    b. To protect the staff
2. wrist; mitt
3. belt; vest
4. a. For hygiene
    b. For exercise
5. Injury, potential for, related to confusion
6. d

Module 22 / Transfer

1. Any four of the following: maintains and restores muscle tone; stimulates respiration; stimulates circulation; improves elimination; improves psychological well-being
2. a. They give the patient a sense of security.
    b. They prevent slipping.
3. Ease patient back onto bed or chair of origin
4. Chair must be placed on left side; extra support may be needed; right leg must be braced with nurse's leg or knee while pivoting
5. To provide a firm handhold and support for the nurse transferring the patient
6. a. Bed to chair: one-person maximal assist
    b. Bed to chair: two-person maximal assist
7. To prevent dizziness
8. Any two of the following: patient's body alignment; patient's comfort; safety for the patient; safety and proper body mechanics for the nurse(s) involved
9. Any three of the following: pain; fatigue; pulse and respiration rate; blood pressure changes; dizziness

Module 23 / Ambulation: Simple Assisted and Using Cane, Crutches, or Walker

1. Any four of the following: maintains muscle tone; restores muscle tone;

stimulates respiratory system; stimulates circulatory system; improves psychological well-being; facilitates elimination
2. Falls
3. They give better support, are less likely to slip, and usually stay on better.
4. A transfer and ambulation belt; a cane; a walker; or crutches
5. Crutches should extend from the floor, about 6 inches out from the foot, to the side of the chest 2 inches under the axilla.
6. When the patient needs balance and support but can use both legs and both arms
7. The arms of the chair (or the bed), not the walker
8. Opposite the weak leg
9. Hold both in one hand.
10. Three-point gait

Module 24 / Range-of-Motion Exercises

1. a. To maintain joint mobility
    b. To prevent lengthy rehabilitation
2. a. When increasing the level of energy expended or the level of circulation is potentially hazardous
    b. When joints are swollen or inflamed or there is injury near the joint
3. flexors
4. active
5. supination
6. abduction
7. b
8. c
9. c

Module 25 / Special Mattresses, Frames, and Beds

1. a. To prevent or treat pressure sores
    b. To keep patient immobile so healing can take place
2. Circulation of air
3. The Stryker frame turns laterally while the CircOlectric turns vertically.
4. Do not put the special sheets in with the general laundry; do not use pins which can puncture the mattress covering; remove

watches because they can be damaged by
the dispersement of microscopic particles
5. Unplug the bed to provide a firm surface.
6. b
7. a
8. b
9. b
10. c

Module 26 / Applying Bandages and Binders

1. a. To provide support
   b. To protect wounds
   c. To protect and hold underlying
      dressings
2. a. Circular
   b. Spiral
   c. Reverse spiral
   d. Figure-8
   e. Recurrent fold
3. a joint
4. distal; proximal
5. a. To hold layer dressings in place
   b. For support
6. male; female
7. d
8. c

Module 27 / Applying Heat and Cold

1. b
2. b
3. c
4. c
5. d
6. b
7. b
8. c
9. c

Module 28 / Administering Enemas

1. Any four of the following: *cleansing*—to
   remove fecal material and clean the bowel;
   medicated—to allow medication to be
   absorbed; *oil-retention*—to soften fecal
   material; *cooling*—for extremely elevated
   temperature; *return-flow*—to remove gas

2. a. Embarrassment
   b. Modesty
   c. Fear of discomfort
3. a. Color
   b. Respiratory rate
   c. Pulse
   d. Signs of excess fatigue
4. By lowering the fluid container below the
   level of the bowel
5. Slow the flow rate of fluid. If cramping
   still continues, stop the procedure until
   cramps subside.
6. Size 10 French
7. 300 ml

Module 29 / Tube Feeding

1. a
2. c
3. b
4. b
5. a
6. c
7. a
8. Silicone rubber
9. One
10. High osmolarity; lactose content; too rapid
    feeding; too cold a formula

Module 30 / Caring for Patients with Casts

1. plaster of Paris; plastic
2. hard; inexpensive
3. easy to apply; rigid and durable
4. serious skin breakdown or infection after
   casting
5. folded down stockinette; petaling
6. motion; sensation; pain
7. d
8. b
9. b

Module 31 / Applying and Maintaining Traction

1. Skin traction is applied to the muscles or
   skin through the use of tapes, belts, or
   halters. Skeletal traction is applied to the

skeletal frame or bones through wires, pins, or tongs that are surgically inserted through or into the bone.
2. footboard; plantar flexion
3. Any four of the following: constipation; respiratory complications; boredom; anorexia; skin breakdown; thrombophlebitis
4. (1) a
   (2) d, f
   (3) d
   (4) h
   (5) c
   (6) e, g
   (7) e

Module 32 / Emergency Resuscitation Procedures

1. Shake the person and say loudly, "Are you all right?"
2. Flat, with the neck straight
3. Locate the larynx (voice box), and slide your fingers to the hollow beside it.
4. By placing your thumb on the outside of the infant's upper arm and pressing gently with your index and middle fingers on the inside of the upper arm
5. 1½ inches above the xiphoid process
6. a. 80–100 per minute
   b. 80–100 per minute
   c. At least 100 per minute
   d. 80–100 per minute
7. 2 breaths to each 15 chest compressions
8. 1 breath to each 5 chest compressions
9. Clutching the neck in the area of the larynx between the thumb and index finger

10. In the midline, below the xiphoid process of the sternum but above the navel
11. Only in the unconscious patient to attempt to grasp a foreign body and remove it

Module 33 / Postmortem Care

1. c
2. the realization of offering an extension of life to another
3. kidneys, hearts, skin, corneas, pituitaries, and bones
4. viability and usefulness of tissues
5. Coroner is elected or appointed, not necessarily a physician. Medical examiner is an appointed physician, usually holding a special degree in pathology.
6. See your county's requirements.
7. Any three of the following: rigor mortis; skin discoloration; skin indentation; cooling
8. Any four of the following: clean the patient; place the patient in repose; straighten the unit; soften the lights; rearrange flowers; provide chairs
9. To prevent discoloration and indentation of the underlying hand if folded over the chest
10. a. IVs
    b. Nasogastric tubes
    c. Urinary catheters
    d. Oxygen equipment
11. An examination of the body after death
12. a. To determine cause of death
    b. To gather scientific knowledge
    c. To add to statistical data

714